# THE
# BIG
# FAMILY
# GUIDE
## TO ALL THE
# VITAMINS

# THE BIG FAMILY GUIDE TO ALL THE VITAMINS

## RUTH ADAMS

Keats Publishing, Inc. ✻ New Canaan, Connecticut

*The Big Family Guide to All the Vitamins* is not intended as medical advice. Its intent is solely informational and educational. Please consult a health professional should the need for one be indicated.

THE BIG FAMILY GUIDE TO ALL THE VITAMINS

Previously published as *The Complete Home Guide to All the Vitamins*
Eighteenth printing, October 1992

Library of Congress Cataloging-in-Publication Data
Adams, Ruth
    The big family guide to all the vitamins / by Ruth Adams.
        p.    cm.
    Includes bibliographical references and index.
    ISBN 0-87983-583-4 (trade pbk.) : $17.95
    1. Vitamins in human nutrition.    I. Title.
QP771.A33    1992
612.3'99—dc20                                            92-12869
                                                        CIP

Printed in the United States of America

Published by Keats Publishing, Inc.
27 Pine Street (Box 876)
New Canaan, Connecticut 06840-0876

# Contents

# CONTENTS

# CONTENTS

## VITAMIN E

## VITAMIN K

## AN UPDATE

# Publisher's Note

In its original edition, and in subsequent revisions, this book became established as perhaps the standard work on the role of vitamins in nutrition and health, selling out 17 printings and reaching—and educating—millions of readers.

In looking it over in preparation for this printing, it seemed to us that an overall revision was at this point unnecessary. The original text established clearly all the fundamental information on vitamins in general and their specific effects, and subsequent research has in the main confirmed than significantly added to or altered this information and the author's conclusions. We feel that a total revision would result in the removal of a number of references to early research studies which are historically important and which broaden the reader's understanding of the important work in this field. Revision of the main text has been confined to such essential new information as the new official Recommended Dietary Allowances, presented in Chapter 2, and to necessary changes in tense required by the passing of such important figures as Roger Williams, Carl Pfeiffer and Carlton Fredericks.

There have of course been important new developments, such as the wider "establishment" acceptance of the part vitamins play in promoting health and preventing disease, and research showing previously unsuspected benefits of vitamin C, niacin and other nutrients. These the author has explored in a new introductory chapter covering the exciting discoveries of the last five years and relating them to the main body of vitamin information.

Some of the books mentioned in the text are not as readily available in bookstores as they once were, but any large public library should be able to provide or obtain any that interest the reader—who can only benefit his or her health by learning more on this vital topic than even this most comprehensive and thorough work provides.

# Foreword

SOME MONTHS AGO I received a long-distance telephone call
from a man who wished to have me resolve a question.
This type of request is not uncommon in our office. What
made this particular incident unique was the fact that the
caller is a very prominent man, famous enough to appear
in the newspapers across the nation almost daily.

Clearly, as one might expect, anyone of such stature can
certainly afford the best medical counsel. Anyhow, the question he wished resolved was "Should I take vitamins?"

The real reason for the call was that he had already queried
his three attending physicians. His internist said, "Absolutely
no, if you do, you will get kidney stones!" His urologist
responded with, "It really doesn't matter, you will simply
excrete what you don't need." Finally, his ear-nose-throat
specialist said, "I insist that you take vitamins daily." Which
makes for a convenient array of answers, the only spectrum
of answers, absolutely yes, absolutely no, and it really doesn't
matter.

Had the famous patient-caller or any of his physicians
read this book, there would have been no need for the question
and, hence, no justification for the confusing answers.

E. Cheraskin, M.D., D.M.D.

# THE
# BIG
# FAMILY
# GUIDE
# TO ALL THE
# VITAMINS

# CHAPTER 1

# What Are Vitamins?

I CAN'T take vitamins. They give me heartburn."

"I never take vitamins. I've heard they make you fat."

"What vitamins will cure the disease I've got?"

"I'm allergic to vitamins, so I can't eat anything that contains Vitamin C."

"I eat a good, well-balanced diet. Why should I take vitamins?"

"I have no faith in vitamins. Something that comes in a tiny pill couldn't possibly do anything important for your health."

"Don't vitamins have calories? Won't they make me fat?"

Statements like these illustrate the confusion many of us are in when it comes to vitamins. We think of them as something like starches, fats, or proteins, and we imagine that we may need some of them, but not all of them. And, unfortunately, we tend to think of each vitamin as related to the prevention or cure of some specific disease.

Vitamins are not the same thing as starches, fats and proteins. We do not eat them in quantity and take them or not take them according to whether we feel hungry for that particular one on a certain day.

Vitamins are chemical substances which are necessary in extremely small amounts to bring about certain chemical changes or reactions in our bodies. They combine with other substances—minerals, proteins, enzymes, or, perhaps, all three—to change something chemically. Generally speaking,

9

vitamins cannot be made by the body but must be obtained from food.

Carbohydrates (starches and sugars) and fats are energy-providing foods. Proteins are building, repairing and protective foods. Vitamins help to process carbohydrates, fats and proteins so that they can perform their functions. In *Bridges Dietetics for the Clinician,* vitamins are defined as "substances which differ widely in chemical nature and physiologic function. They have the one common characteristic of being non-mineral substances required in relatively small amounts for the maintenance of normal structure and function of body tissues." Note that important word "required." It is impossible to sustain life without vitamins—without *all* the essential vitamins.

To put it more simply, carbohydrates, proteins and fats could not be used, broken down in digestion and later built into cells, turned into energy or stored in the body without a long chain of chemical reactions which must take place to transform cells of plants or food animals into human cells. Vitamins play an important part in this process, along with minerals, which are present in food and water, and hormones, which are manufactured by body glands. Vitamins occur naturally in food, and the charts throughout this book show the amounts of the vitamins in various types of foods.

A food rich in carbohydrate contains plenty of the vitamins and minerals necessary for processing that carbohydrate. If it did not, our ancestors would never have grown to maturity and had children. Protein food is accompanied naturally by the vitamins and minerals our bodies must have to deal healthfully with protein. In fatty foods, we find the vitamins, minerals and other substances we must have to deal with fats in food.

Most vitamins are manufactured by plants. We do not know exactly what functions they perform for plants. One vitamin which is almost non-existent in plants, however, is vitamin D. It is produced in human tissues by the action of sunlight on the skin. Some nutrition researchers believe that vitamin D should be classified as a hormone rather than a vitamin, since it is manufactured in the bodies of animals, rather than in plants.

This illustrates the great difference between a vitamin and a protein or a starch. Obviously, you could not obtain either of these from sunlight. They have bulk. You must obtain quite a large quantity of them, right there before you on a plate, in order to be well nourished. All vitamins exist and are needed only in extremely small amounts, generally speaking.

For instance, the recommended amount of protein needed by an adult male is 56 grams; for an adult woman, 46 grams. A serving of lean beef contains about 25 grams of protein. The recommended amount of B1 (thiamine) required in a day is one to one and a half milligrams. A milligram is one-thousandth of a gram. Some vitamins are needed in such small amounts that we measure them in micrograms. This is one-millionth of a gram. Vitamin B12 is one of these. If you have taken vitamin B12 in a pill, you have noticed that the pill is quite small but not microscopic. It contains a filler, in addition to the vitamin, to give it enough bulk so that it can be handled easily.

It is, for the most part, impossible to relate any one vitamin to any one disease, except for those disorders which we know are directly caused by a shortage of some vitamin. Scurvy is the disease that results when one lacks vitamin C. Beriberi is the disease that results when one lacks one of the B vitamins. Pellagra indicates lack of another B vitamin. Rickets is a crippling disease involving lack of vitamin D and/or calcium. In this case, both the vitamin and the mineral are important.

Today, we are apt to suffer most from what we call *subclinical deficiencies,* which means that we may be deficient in several vitamins or minerals—not enough to develop one of the classic deficiency diseases—but enough to result in chronic ill health, plus susceptibility to more serious conditions.

Said the authors of *Clinical Nutrition:* "Most physicians are familiar with the signs of advanced . . . deficiency disease

11

as they occur in classical starvation, protein deficiency, osteo-malacia, rickets, scurvy, pellagra and beriberi. Most malnutrition, however, is not of this advanced, easily recognized variety, but is manifested by signs less fully developed, less severe, or less acute than the classical textbook descriptions imply. Those lesser signs are frequently overlooked.''

If you lack one vitamin, you are probably deficient in a number of others as well. And you may not be getting enough protein or minerals either. So taking a pill that adds just one vitamin to your diet will probably not accomplish very much.

Do vitamins make you fat? Considering the complexity of the activity vitamins create and the small amounts of them in food, how could they possibly make you fat? Anyone who gets fat from eating too much starch or fat is involved with whole platefuls of such foods, meal after meal. A milligram or so of a vitamin weighs almost nothing. In addition, its function is not to provide energy or to store fat, so no vitamin could possibly cause anyone to gain weight.

It *is* true that people who are very thin and rundown, those who have not eaten enough for years, may gain weight when they are given enough nourishing food plus vitamins. The vitamins go to work immediately to process the food so that it is available to create energy or to build and replace cells.

On the contrary, there is considerable evidence that one reason for our nationwide problem of overweight is simply that we are not getting enough vitamins, minerals and other nutrients from our daily meals. So we suffer from pathological hunger. This means that we continue to crave and to gorge on empty-calorie foods, because we are actually hungry for the good, solid nutrients we need. Adding vitamins and minerals in good quantity may help to relieve this unnatural hunger and help us to reduce.

Can you be allergic to vitamins? Hardly. If you can't eat oranges, is there any reason to believe that it's the vitamin C in the orange that causes your difficulty? If you were really allergic to vitamin C and could not eat a mouthful of food that contains it, you would have died long ago of scurvy. You cannot live any length of time without vitamin C, and it is not stored to any extent in your body.

Of course, you might be allergic to the filler or binder in a vitamin tablet or capsule. If your doctor thinks this may be the case, try to ascertain from the manufacturer what kind of filler they use, or try another brand of vitamin.

Is it true that, if you get a well-rounded diet, you don't need vitamins? Possibly, depending on the person. Many of us, down through the millions of years while the human race has developed, have inherited a need for much larger amounts of vitamins than other people need, even among our own families. And what happens when the vitamins and minerals are removed from food by processing and we eat the depleted food? What happens when you eat food rich in starch from which most or all of the B vitamins have been taken? B vitamins are essential for processing the starch in foods.

White sugar is such a food. It contains no vitamins and almost no minerals. So, whenever you eat sugar, you may be creating a slight vitamin B deficiency in your body. The more sugar you eat, the more B vitamins you need. Almost all the B vitamins are removed from most cereals and grains used in baking. Only a few of the vitamins are restored synthetically by "enriching" the cereal or flour. And we do not as yet know much about the importance of those vitamins which are removed in the milling and are not put back in the finished product.

Surveys have shown that more than half the calories of the average American diet are made up of foods whose base is white sugar or refined cereals and flours. Isn't it possible, from this fact alone, that many of us desperately need to supplement our diets with the B vitamins?

The best source of vitamin E is also wholegrain cereals and breads. Most vitamin E is removed when the grain is refined, and nothing is done about restoring that which is lost. Can anyone say with justice that we should not take vitamin E or wheat germ products to help restore to our bodies this naturally occurring vitamin which is lost in processing? Dr. Evan Shute, founder of the Shute Clinic in London, Ontario, Canada, and one of the world's leading authorities on the vitamin, regularly treated heart patients with massive doses of vitmain E. He stated:

"One uses vitamin B1 to prevent neuritis because it has been found to cure neuritis.

"One uses vitamin B2 to prevent certain symptoms of riboflavin (vitamin B2) deficiency, because it has been shown to cure them.

"One uses niacin (vitamin B3) to prevent pellagra because it has been found so valuable in treating pellagra. . . .

"One uses vitamin K to prevent hemorrhagic disease of the newborn because it cures hemorrhagic disease of the newborn.

"Could vitamin E be the sole exception to the rule that vitamins tend to prevent what they relieve? . . . Why wait for your coronary (heart attack)? Why not prevent it?"

It seems more than just coincidental that heart attacks became the leading cause of death in the Western world about 30 to 40 years after refined cereals, sugar and flour became staples, making up about half of the average diet.

What about "having faith in vitamins?" Faith has to do with religion, not science. The necessity for vitamins is not a matter of faith. It's a matter of scientific fact that living things must have certain vitamins to survive. Don't think of vitamins as something magic in which you should or should not "have faith." Think of them as essential substances which exist in all natural foods and which perform certain functions in your body which cannot be performed by anything else.

How large a package they come in (like brewers yeast or wholegrain flour) or how small (like a 5-microgram tablet of vitamin B12) is not of the slightest importance. What is important is that you must have them. If you read labels carefully and take the suggested amounts, you cannot possibly get too much of any of them.

Vitamins are divided into two groups on the basis of their

solubility. The fat-soluble vitamins are A, D, E and K. The water-soluble vitamins are C and the B complex.

In the United States, the following vitamins are listed officially as vitamins, and recommendations for daily amounts are provided officially for most of them:

Vitamin A

The B complex of vitamins:

    B1 (Thiamine)
    B2 (Riboflavin)
    B3 (Niacin)
    B6 (Pyridoxine)
    Pantothenic acid
    Biotin
    Folic Acid or Folacin
    B12 Cobalamine
    Choline

(Two other vitamin-like substances associated with the B complex are: Inositol and Para-Amino-Benzoic Acid.)

Vitamin C (Ascorbic Acid)

Vitamin D (Calciferol)

Vitamin E (Alpha Tocopherol)

Vitamin K (Menadione)

Vitamin research is proceeding in many laboratories in many parts of the world. Perhaps more vitamins will eventually be discovered. The Russians, for instance, already recognize a substance in the B complex which they call vitamin B15 and they are using it in many interesting ways. But from the layman's point of view, the vitamins listed above are the only ones that need to concern you.

For the record, here are the minerals currently considered essential for human nutrition: calcium, zinc, phosphorus, iron, potassium, sodium, iodine and magnesium. In addition, certain trace minerals (that is, they occur in only traces in foods and soil) are vital to human needs, although the amounts have not yet been determined. These include copper, cobalt, manganese and others.

# CHAPTER 2

# Officially, How Much
# of Each Vitamin
# Do You Need?

THE OFFICIAL BUREAU which decides these things publishes a book on the recommended dietary allowances, by which is meant how much you and I need of the various vitamins and minerals. This book, titled, *Recommended Dietary Allowances,* is written by experts in the field of nutrition—university scientists and professors who have studied the subject for many years. The book is published by the National Academy of Sciences—National Research Council. It lists many scientific papers and books which were consulted by the committee in order to reach their conclusions.

The chart on page 24 (shortened a bit for simplicity) shows their recommendations. Most of us non-scientists need considerable explanation in order to know what such a chart is all about. First, why aren't all the vitamins and minerals listed? What about the rest of the B vitamins, potassium, vitamin K? What does the chart mean when it says "designed for the maintenance of good nutrition of practically all healthy people in the U.S.A.?" Does the chart mean that, if you get the recommended amount of every vitamin and mineral listed, you will be healthy no matter what else you do or do not eat?

Let's try to answer some of these questions, for if you plan to use the information about individual vitamins which

16

we give you later in this book, you will want to know how to use this chart.

Officially recommended allowances are made for only the nutrients listed in the chart. The experts agree that things like potassium, the other B vitamins and vitamin K are essential to life and health. We must get them in our food or we cannot survive. But even after years of research, scientists simply do not know how much the average healthy person needs of each of these nutrients and others like the trace minerals—which is a story all by itself.

Until 1968 the NAS-NRC experts did not consider vitamin E essential to good health and did not list a recommended allowance for it. Although they knew that we must get iodine in our food they had no suggested allowance for this element. Magnesium, too, was ignored in their recommendations, although they were aware that this mineral is essential.

In the case of vitamin E, any official recommendations must be made with one thing in mind: some people are at present replacing saturated fats with large amounts of unsaturated fats, in an effort to keep their blood cholesterol levels low. The more unsaturated fats anyone is taking, the more vitamin E he needs. The processing and refining of modern cereals and flours removes most of the vitamin E. So people who make sure they eat cereals and bread which are completely wholegrain and folks who eat lots of seeds, nuts, wheat germ and salad oils may be getting enough of this vitamin, while others who eat white bread and refined cereals and avoid other good sources of vitamin E may not be getting enough.

Vitamin K is another nutrient for which human requirements were hard to arrive at because some vitamin K may be manufactured by beneficial bacteria in the digestive tract. Different people have different kinds of bacterial activity in their digestive tracts, so there is no way of knowing how much vitamin K each individual is manufacturing for himself. However, an RDA of one milligram per kilogram of body weight was established for the first time in 1989.

Then, too, each person has a different pattern of absorbing

this important vitamin, which is essential for the proper clotting of the blood. Some people may eat food rich in vitamin K, but absorb little of it, while others may require very little, but may just happen to like foods in which there is lots of vitamin K and may be able to absorb it very well.

Iodine is a mineral essential for the proper functioning of the thyroid gland, whose hormones perform life-saving and life-preserving work in the body of each of us. Supposedly, people who use iodized salt and/or eat plenty of fish and seafood get enough iodine. But folks who live far inland and eat food grown locally do not get much iodine in their meals, unless they eat plenty of fish, for iodine is absent from inland soils. We are told that the average adult needs about 50 to 75 micrograms of iodine to scrape through. To insure a margin of safety, daily intake of 100–150 micrograms is suggested. What about people who don't use much salt of any kind, let alone iodized salt? Are they likely to be short on iodine?

Lack of vitamin C is known to cause the disease called scurvy. We have known this for many years. So much research has been done on vitamin C that experts feel pretty certain the amounts of vitamin C recommended in the official chart will prevent scurvy. However, there is a great deal of evidence that much larger amounts of this essential vitamin may be necessary for abundant good health. Biologist Linus Pauling suggested in his book *Vitamin C and the Common Cold* that most of us need vitamin C in massive doses to prevent colds the year round. He justified this theory by reminding us that human beings are almost the only animal which does not manufacture its own vitamin C. In the early days of man's history on earth he must have gotten immense amounts of this vitamin from the fresh, green fruits, berries and leaves which made up a large part of his diet then.

Following the publication of Dr. Pauling's book, other scientists confirmed his theory, many physicians and lay people wrote in medical and lay journals of their own experiences taking massive doses of vitamin C with nothing but excellent results so far as good health is concerned.

So the generally accepted precept "Get a little orange juice (or fake orange juice) at breakfast every morning and that will take care of your vitamin C needs" falls quite a bit short of what is currently being discussed in regard to optimum amounts of vitamin C.

Officially, we know that needs for vitamin C rise as stresses mount. What do we mean by stress? Illness, colds, chronic conditions of ill health, the effects of many drugs. Almost everything in our modern environment would classify as "stress" these days: noise, air pollution, water pollution, smoking, chemicals in food, worry over family affairs or even the perennial bad news on the evening news report.

Tests have shown that merely driving through heavy traffic on a busy throughway going to work is a form of stress which influences blood pressure, blood sugar, nerves, heart action and, possibly, the fate of vitamin C stores in the body. As a matter of fact, can you think of anybody you know who is not under some kind of "stress"? Hence should not everybody perhaps be getting lots more vitamin C than the recommended amount?

Iron is another nutrient essential for good health. It is not a vitamin, but a mineral. We bring it up here because it is on the chart of *Recommended Dietary Allowances*. Can we all feel comfortable about the amount of iron we get? Not at all. Officially, we are told there are no definite studies to determine to what extent iron deficiency anemia exists in the U.S. population. So no one knows whether there are large or small numbers of people who are not getting, in their food, the recommended amount of iron.

Many surveys have shown that there are serious iron shortages, probably in several age groups, especially teenagers, women and older folks. Recently so much concern has arisen over the fact that everyday food may not give enough iron for protection, that nutrition specialists are debating the addition of large amounts of iron to white bread.

The NAS-NRC book, *Recommended Dietary Allowances*, 1989 states many times that the RDA's are for the purpose of planning food for large groups of people, doing surveys of the nutritional state of the country, establishing regulations for health and welfare programs and school lunch programs, for nutritional labelling and so on. They are not to be taken as absolute levels for everybody in the country to decide that they will get just as much nutrient as the RDA recommends for their age group, no more and no less.

It is apparent, says the book, that special nutritional needs arise from metabolic disorders, chronic diseases, injuries, prematurity of infants, and "many other medical conditions require therapeutic treatment not covered by RDA for healthy persons. Infections, even mild ones, increase metabolic losses of nitrogen and of a number of vitamins and minerals. In addition, acute or chronic infections involving the gastrointestinal tract impair the absorption of nutrients . . . poor appetite may lead to curtailed food intake commonly resulting in depletion of body stores of nutrients and wasting of tissues. Severe or prolonged illness may precipitate malnutrition in individuals habitually receiving inadequate diets."

The book says, further, that almost nothing is known about the nutritional needs of older people, since little research has been done in this area. The book says that "Chronic diseases occur with increasing frequency as aging progresses, requiring special dietary modification for those affected. However, the role of long-term nutrient intake in pathogensis of these diseases such as osteoporosis, diabetes, hypertension and atherosclerosis (hardening of the arteries) remains uncertain. Aging also causes a reduction in function of most organs, but, in general, it is not known whether the rate of aging is influenced by dietary modification."

Literally, nobody knows what this means in terms of any individual. For nobody but you knows how old you are, how active you are, what and how much you eat, how healthy you are, what stresses you are under, what chronic diseases you may have and what you may have inherited in the way of special needs for one nutrient or another.

Does this mean you may need twice or three times more of some nutrient than someone else in your family needs? Of course. Or you may need less, or you may need twenty or thirty times more! This happens regularly with laboratory animals which have been bred to be as much alike as possible. Human beings vary much more than these animals in their individual biological needs.

So your husband or wife, sister or brother, mother or father may get along perfectly well with no more vitamins or minerals than they get at mealtime, but *you* may need far, far more of this or that vitamin or any other nutrient. What makes the difference? Your hereditary background which may make your natural need for one or more nutrients much higher than average. Or the circumstances of your past or present life which may dictate the necessity for larger amounts of some nutrients. Perhaps you do not assimilate or absorb your food well. Perhaps you are exposed to greater than average amounts of stress. Perhaps you have had accidents, burns or operations which have greatly increased your need for some nutrients.

Dr. Roger J. Williams, the late eminent biologist and vitamin researcher at the University of Texas, coined the term "supernutrition." Dr. Williams said that no living things have ever been studied who were living under absolutely optimal conditions of nutrition because we are not even sure what such conditions might be. If or when we finally have the knowledge to determine just which nutrients are needed and in what amounts, when we finally know just what the perfect diet is, we may be able to produce in everyone a state of "supernutrition" which might bring about such excellent health that we would live longer, happier, much more abundant and productive lives just because we were so perfectly nourished! It is indeed a perfection for which we should strive.

Is there any way for you to find out, at this moment,

just what your own nutritional state is? Can you take some
kind of test, or ask your doctor? In general, some physicians
may recognize some of the gross symptoms of malnutrition:
the bleeding gums and aching bones of scurvy, the skin
disorders and mental depression of pellagra, a vitamin B
deficiency disease, and so on. But, in general, most physicians
are unfamiliar with these symptoms and seldom think of
diagnosing any condition as a nutritional deficiency.

There are some very complicated and expensive tests used
in official surveys to determine just what the state of one's
nutrition is, in regard to B vitamins, vitamin A and so on.
But these are not available, generally, in physicians' offices.
So there is no way for you to know absolutely whether you
are short on this or that vitamin or mineral. And, in fact, it
is almost axiomatic to say that no one is ever short on just
one vitamin or mineral. The kind of diet that would produce
such a deficiency state would almost certainly be short on
lots of other nutrients as well.

What does the official chart mean when it says it is designed
for "practically all healthy people"? If you are perfectly
healthy, then you may be able to get along on these recommended amounts of protein, vitamins and minerals. This
means that you do not suffer from headaches, tooth decay,
indigestion, constipation, falling hair, baldness, overweight
or underweight, to say nothing of the far more serious disorders like diabetes, high blood pressure, heart trouble, colitis,
cancer, mental illness, cataract, and so on. On this basis
do you know anyone who is perfectly healthy?

National health statistics show that more than 50 million
Americans suffer from some form of serious chronic illness:
diabetes, epilepsy, multiple sclerosis, mental illness, circulatory and heart ailments and so on. Fifty percent of them
are under the age of 45. So just who *is* this completely
healthy individual for whom the recommended dietary allowances are designed?

If you are one of the many who cannot qualify as being
completely healthy, would it not be wise to provide yourself

with a form of health insurance, much as you might buy fire insurance, in the form of added nutrients? Isn't it possible that you may need considerably more of some or all of the nutrients listed?

Perhaps someone among your friends or family has derided you for taking food supplements. Chances are they quote some newspaper columnist who says, "The person who eats a good diet gets plenty of vitamins and minerals." The next time you get into such a discussion quote the official booklet on vitamin and mineral needs which states on almost every page that *individual* needs for things like vitamins and minerals cannot be estimated. The official estimates are very general. Deviations from the recommended nutrient allowances are significant only in terms of the *individual's* total health status.

Sure, eat the best possible diet you can afford. Be sure to include in this diet ample amounts of the four basic groups of foods which should be eaten every day: meats, fish, poultry, eggs, milk, cheese, yogurt and other dairy products; the seed foods like whole grain cereals, nuts, seeds, beans and legumes; fresh fruits and vegetables, especially those which are bright yellow or bright green. Eat as many foods as possible that have been organically grown, for in this way you can avoid ingesting many pesticide residues and some of the 10,000 or so chemicals which pollute our food supply, which are added either intentionally or somehow get into the food as remnants of pollution.

In addition to this good diet, just in case you're one of those people who have much greater than average nutritional needs or just in case you want to prevent some chronic illness or condition that has victimized other members of your family or circle of friends, why not use vitamin and mineral supplements as health insurance? They are inexpensive so what's to be lost?

The latest edition (1989) of the book *Recommended Dietary Allowances* is available from the Printing and Publishing Office, National Academy of Sciences, 2101 Constitution

FOOD AND NUTRITION BOARD, NATIONAL ADADEMY OF SCIENCES—NATIONAL RESEARCH COUNCIL
RECOMMENDED DIETARY ALLOWANCES,[a] Revised 1989

*Designed for the maintenance of good nutrition of practically all healthy people in the United States*

| Category | Age (years) or Condition | Weight[b] (kg) | Weight[b] (lb) | Height[b] (cm) | Height[b] (in) | Protein (g) | Fat-Soluble Vitamins Vitamin A (µg RE)[c] | Vitamin D (µg)[d] | Vitamin E (mg α-TE)[e] | Vitamin K (µg) | Water-Soluble Vitamins Vitamin C (mg) | Thiamin (mg) | Riboflavin (mg) | Niacin (mg NE)[f] | Vitamin B6 (mg) | Folate (µg) | Vitamin B12 (µg) | Minerals Calcium (mg) | Phosphorus (mg) | Magnesium (mg) | Iron (mg) | Zinc (mg) | Iodine (µg) | Selenium (µg) |
|---|---|---|---|---|---|---|---|---|---|---|---|---|---|---|---|---|---|---|---|---|---|---|---|---|
| Infants | 0.0–0.5 | 6 | 13 | 60 | 24 | 13 | 375 | 7.5 | 3 | 5 | 30 | 0.3 | 0.4 | 5 | 0.3 | 25 | 0.3 | 400 | 300 | 40 | 6 | 5 | 40 | 10 |
|  | 0.5–1.0 | 9 | 20 | 71 | 28 | 14 | 375 | 10 | 4 | 10 | 35 | 0.4 | 0.5 | 6 | 0.6 | 35 | 0.5 | 600 | 500 | 60 | 10 | 5 | 50 | 15 |
| Children | 1–3 | 13 | 29 | 90 | 35 | 16 | 400 | 10 | 6 | 15 | 40 | 0.7 | 0.8 | 9 | 1.0 | 50 | 0.7 | 800 | 800 | 80 | 10 | 10 | 70 | 20 |
|  | 4–6 | 20 | 44 | 112 | 44 | 24 | 500 | 10 | 7 | 20 | 45 | 0.9 | 1.1 | 12 | 1.1 | 75 | 1.0 | 800 | 800 | 120 | 10 | 10 | 90 | 20 |
|  | 7–10 | 28 | 62 | 132 | 52 | 28 | 700 | 10 | 7 | 30 | 45 | 1.0 | 1.2 | 13 | 1.4 | 100 | 1.4 | 800 | 800 | 170 | 10 | 10 | 120 | 30 |
| Males | 11–14 | 45 | 99 | 157 | 62 | 45 | 1,000 | 10 | 10 | 45 | 50 | 1.3 | 1.5 | 17 | 1.7 | 150 | 2.0 | 1,200 | 1,200 | 270 | 12 | 15 | 150 | 40 |
|  | 15–18 | 66 | 145 | 176 | 69 | 59 | 1,000 | 10 | 10 | 65 | 60 | 1.5 | 1.8 | 20 | 2.0 | 200 | 2.0 | 1,200 | 1,200 | 400 | 12 | 15 | 150 | 50 |
|  | 19–24 | 72 | 160 | 177 | 70 | 58 | 1,000 | 10 | 10 | 70 | 60 | 1.5 | 1.7 | 19 | 2.0 | 200 | 2.0 | 1,200 | 1,200 | 350 | 10 | 15 | 150 | 70 |
|  | 25–50 | 79 | 174 | 176 | 70 | 63 | 1,000 | 5 | 10 | 80 | 60 | 1.5 | 1.7 | 19 | 2.0 | 200 | 2.0 | 800 | 800 | 350 | 10 | 15 | 150 | 70 |
|  | 51+ | 77 | 170 | 173 | 68 | 63 | 1,000 | 5 | 10 | 80 | 60 | 1.2 | 1.4 | 15 | 2.0 | 200 | 2.0 | 800 | 800 | 350 | 10 | 15 | 150 | 70 |
| Females | 11–14 | 46 | 101 | 157 | 62 | 46 | 800 | 10 | 8 | 45 | 50 | 1.1 | 1.3 | 15 | 1.4 | 150 | 2.0 | 1,200 | 1,200 | 280 | 15 | 12 | 150 | 45 |
|  | 15–18 | 55 | 120 | 163 | 64 | 44 | 800 | 10 | 8 | 55 | 60 | 1.1 | 1.3 | 15 | 1.5 | 180 | 2.0 | 1,200 | 1,200 | 300 | 15 | 12 | 150 | 50 |
|  | 19–24 | 58 | 128 | 164 | 65 | 46 | 800 | 10 | 8 | 60 | 60 | 1.1 | 1.3 | 15 | 1.6 | 180 | 2.0 | 1,200 | 1,200 | 280 | 15 | 12 | 150 | 55 |
|  | 25–50 | 63 | 138 | 163 | 64 | 50 | 800 | 5 | 8 | 65 | 60 | 1.1 | 1.3 | 15 | 1.6 | 180 | 2.0 | 800 | 800 | 280 | 15 | 12 | 150 | 55 |
|  | 51+ | 65 | 143 | 160 | 63 | 50 | 800 | 5 | 8 | 65 | 60 | 1.0 | 1.2 | 13 | 1.6 | 180 | 2.0 | 800 | 800 | 280 | 10 | 12 | 150 | 55 |
| Pregnant |  |  |  |  |  | 60 | 800 | 10 | 10 | 65 | 70 | 1.5 | 1.6 | 17 | 2.2 | 400 | 2.2 | 1,200 | 1,200 | 320 | 30 | 15 | 175 | 65 |
| Lactating | 1st 6 months |  |  |  |  | 65 | 1,300 | 10 | 12 | 65 | 95 | 1.6 | 1.8 | 20 | 2.1 | 280 | 2.6 | 1,200 | 1,200 | 355 | 15 | 19 | 200 | 75 |
|  | 2nd 6 months |  |  |  |  | 62 | 1,200 | 10 | 11 | 65 | 90 | 1.6 | 1.7 | 20 | 2.1 | 260 | 2.6 | 1,200 | 1,200 | 340 | 15 | 16 | 200 | 75 |

[a]The allowances, expressed as average daily intakes over time, are intended to provide for individual variations among most normal persons as they live in the United States under usual environmental stresses. Diets should be based on a variety of common foods in order to provide other nutrients for which human requirements have been less well defined. See text for detailed discussion of allowances and of nutrients not tabulated.

[b]Weights and heights of Reference Adults are actual medians for the U.S. population of the designated age, as reported by NHANES II. The median weights and heights of those under 19 years of age were taken from Hamill et al. (1979) (see pages 16–17). The use of these figures does not imply that the height-to-weight ratios are ideal.

[c]Retinol equivalents. 1 retinol equivalent = 1 µg retinol or 6 µg β-carotene. See text for calculation of vitamin A activity of diets as retinol equivalents.

[d]As cholecalciferol. 10 µg cholecalciferol = 400 IU of vitamin D.

[e]α-Tocopherol equivalents. 1 mg d-α tocopherol = 1 α-TE. See text for variation in allowances and calculation of vitamin E activity of the diet as α-tocopherol equivalents.

[f]1 NE (niacin equivalent) is equal to 1 mg of niacin or 60 mg of dietary tryptophan.

Avenue, N.W. Washington, D.C. 20418. Keep in mind that the authors of the book recognize that each individual is different and that nutritional requirements may vary by wide margins, depending on the state of past and present health, inherited need for larger amounts of one nutrient or many, and the everyday stresses which may take much greater toll of one or another individual.

# CHAPTER 3

# Vitamin Thieves
# Are at Work
# All About Us

LET'S SAY YOUR diet contains plenty of all the known vitamins and you are quite sure you don't have any inherited special needs for larger than average amounts. Are you aware of the fact that many things you encounter in daily life may be inactivating or destroying those vitamins before they have a chance to do you any good?

Vitamins disappear rapidly from fresh foods that have been cut, chopped or otherwise exposed to air. Some vitamins are destroyed by heat, some by light, some by steam, some by soaking foods in water. Rancid fats destroy fat-soluble vitamins either in food or in the digestive tract. In addition to all this, many modern chemicals are extremely destructive of vitamins.

To take just one modern poison—a widely used, almost everpresent one in daily life, nicotine. No one knows for certain just how continuous, heavy exposure to cigarette smoke may operate to produce cancer, heart attacks, emphysema, Buerger's Disease and the many other conditions that appear to be closely related to heavy smoking. It seems quite possible that one reason for the damage may be that cigarette smoke destroys a very important vitamin.

As long ago as 1952 American researchers knew that nicotine added to a sample of whole blood in a test tube decreased the vitamin C content of that blood by 24 to 31 percent. As long ago as 1941 a German scientist demonstrated that vitamin C levels are much lower in the blood of heavy smokers than in the blood of those who do not smoke at all.

A Canadian physician, Dr. W. J. McCormick, wrote in the October 1954 issue of *Archives of Pediatrics* that he believes lack of vitamin C may be one factor that predisposes to cancer. Smoking may have three effects on health, said Dr. McCormick, all of them relating to susceptibility to cancer. Exposure to the tobacco tars accumulating in the lungs causes a vitamin C deficiency in the very area where the tissues have been broken down by this exposure. Vitamin C is essential for prompt and effective healing. But it is not available at the cell level in the lungs. Then, too, smoking may have destroyed the body's store of vitamin C, so not nearly enough of the vitamin to heal these tissues can be brought by the blood to the lungs.

Finally, people who smoke seem to need stimulating drinks like coffee, tea or soft drinks, rather than fruit juice which is rich in vitamin C. Dr. McCormick goes on to say that he has tested the vitamin C blood level of close to 6,000 patients and has never yet found a smoker with normal levels of vitamin C.

In the March 9, 1963 issue of *The Lancet,* a British medical publication, three scientists described their experiment with smokers and vitamin C. They say they have confirmed the fact that vitamin C is destroyed in a test tube when tobacco smoke comes into contact with it. Then they tested the blood levels of vitamin C in volunteers who smoked one cigarette every half hour and in volunteers who smoked 19 to 25 cigarettes within six hours. They could find no evidence of vitamin C being destroyed, they say. But when they tested the vitamin C level in the blood of long-term smokers and compared it to that of non-smokers, they found that the levels were considerably lower in the blood of those who had smoked for some time. They go on to say, "There was no evidence . . . that the difference in blood-vitamin levels was due

27

to a larger intake of vitamin C among the non-smokers.''

In other words, non-smokers were not getting more vitamin C in their food than the smokers. They were simply getting the benefit of the vitamin C they did eat. But the smokers—eating the same amount of vitamin C—were losing so much of it, due to smoking, that they consistently showed lower blood levels of the vitamin than the non-smokers.

We do not know as yet all the functions of vitamin C in the body. We do know that they include the following. Vitamin C is essential for us to use properly two kinds of amino acids or forms of protein. It also helps the body to use a B vitamin, folic acid. It is believed that vitamin C carries hydrogen, an important substance, to every cell. It enhances the absorption of iron from the intestine.

In addition, vitamin C is necessary for the formation of the substance between cells—the biological glue that literally holds our bodies together. It is essential for the swift and successful knitting of broken bones and healing of wounds. It maintains the walls of the capillaries, the smallest of the blood vessels. It is essential for healing burns where new intercellular cement must be created to replace what has been destroyed.

These are only some of the functions of this extremely important vitamin. No other substance, vitamin or mineral, can be substituted for vitamin C. It seems abundantly clear that, in any individual whose blood levels of vitamin C are consistently too low, year after year, all these functions will be impaired to some extent. Do you see now why smokers are likely to suffer from many ailments, some of them quite well known to doctors, some more mysterious, because we just don't know enough as yet to relate them to a lack of vitamin C in the blood?

Nor do we know what other nutrients may be inactivated or destroyed by the nicotine in cigarettes. There is now evidence that one eye condition, caused by smoking and drinking, is nutritional in origin. Amblyopia is a condition where vision is dim, with no organic reason for it. According to a writer in *Archives of Ophthalmology* for September 1963, there is no convincing evidence that this condition is the direct result of poisoning by nicotine or alcohol. Rather "it is concluded that the primary cause is probably nutritional."

According to a South African physician, writing in *The Lancet* for October 19, 1963, tobacco amblyopia is cured (note that word—cured) by vitamin B12, even though the individual goes on smoking and even though his blood levels do not indicate that he has any deficiency in this vitamin.

For people who cannot or will not give up smoking, large amounts of vitamin C taken every day will perhaps mitigate some of the damage being done. And the most helpful thing we learn from the story of vitamin C and smoking is that exposure to every-day poisons destroys some vitamins. The best way to protect yourself is to guard against such exposure if you can. This means avoid, as much as you can, everything in modern life that you know is or could be toxic: drugs, insecticides, weed killers, chemicals in food, household products like strong cleansers and paint removers, industrial solvents, dusts and sprays of all kinds. If there is any question about the safety of any product and you can possibly avoid using it—do so.

Since it is quite impossible, however, to avoid all such poisons, the best protection is an abundance of vitamins and minerals. Make sure you are getting more than you may need as added insurance against vitamin thieves, which you cannot avoid. Here are some other destroyers of vitamins. How many of these play an important part in your life or that of your family?

Antibiotics destroy B vitamins in the digestive tract.

Mineral oil destroys fat-soluble vitamins A, D, E and K.

Drugs containing mercury, procaine, gold or lead destroy vitamin C.

Bicarbonate of soda in food destroys vitamin B in the stomach.

Aspirin and barbiturates destroy vitamins.

Benzene, a solvent, destroys vitamins.

Lindane, an insecticide, destroys vitamins.

Other pesticides destroy other vitamins.

Raw fish destroys the B vitamin thiamine.

Raw egg white in excess destroys the B vitamin biotin.

Chlorine and other bleaches destroy vitamin E.

Antihistamines and sulfa drugs destroy vitamin C.

The following are antagonists to vitamin D—that is, they tend to destroy it: toxisterol, phytin in many fibrous vegetables and grains, phlorizin (from the bark and fruit of certain trees), cortisone and cortisol (drugs), thyrocalcitonin (a drug).

These are antagonists to vitamin E: any oxidants, cod liver oil, thyroxine (a drug).

These are antagonists to vitamin K: the drugs dicoumarol, sulfonamides, antibiotics, a certain drug form of vitamin E, aspirin preparations, warfarin, a drug given to prevent the formation of clots.

No one has investigated how many other vitamin "enemies" are present in any of the chemical pollutants to which we are exposed these days. If we were living in Eden, a pure, pristine, unpolluted paradise, we would not have to worry about vitamin enemies. But we're not. They are all around us and we have yet to discover how much harm they have done or can do in the future.

# CHAPTER 4

# Getting the Most
# Out of Your
# Vitamins

YOU BRING THE bottles home from the health food store and put them away. The label indicates the amount to take each day relevant to the present official Dietary Allowances. But how do you know when to take them? Should you take them all at the same time or spaced out through the day? Are some of them incompatible with others? Will one vitamin possibly cancel out the good effects of another? Is there danger of getting too much? If you take the amount indicated on the label can you be certain this is enough to answer your individual needs? What is the best way to store vitamins and for how long?

Studies seem to show that vitamin and mineral supplements are best absorbed and used if they are taken at breakfast. That means, with breakfast while you are eating, or shortly before or after breakfast. Apparently in the body's rested state in early morning, all body processes are purring along at their best and the vitamins and minerals get to the appointed spot and do their best work, most economically, when they are taken at breakfast.

If you don't eat breakfast, now is a good time to begin this very healthful habit. Your body has been on a 12- to 14-hour fast. Feed it! Feed it a good high protein breakfast that will stay with you until lunch time so you won't be tempted to sneak some sugary goody at coffee break. Vitamin and mineral supplements are food, not medicine. So they should be taken along with food, for every one of them has a number of important functions dealing directly with food. That is their purpose—to guide your food in the paths it should go, right through all the complicated body machinery into each cell and then into every activity that cell engages in. So always take your vitamins with food. Lunchtime is best, if you can't manage to take them at breakfast.

What about spacing them out during the day? In the case of the fat soluble vitamins—A, D and E—these are stored in your body, so there is no need to worry whether they will be present when they are needed most. If you are taking them regularly, they will be there, stored in fatty tissues or in your liver or wherever their storehouse is. With the water-soluble vitamins—C and all B vitamins—these are not stored to any great extent, so it is important that you get them every day. Body metabolism tends to excrete things on a four-hour basis. That is, it takes about four hours for any substance that has completed its tasks to be excreted in urine. So if you are taking large amounts of vitamin C or some of the B vitamins, it is best to divide the dosages to allow for this body activity. If you want to keep your cells flooded with vitamin C, it's best to space out the tablets every four hours or so.

Is there any chance that some vitamins and minerals are not compatible—that you should not take them together? No. Vitamins and minerals occur together in food where they certainly do not cancel one another out. Instead they work so closely together that scientists have discovered some of them can actually substitute for others, in emergencies. In cases of scurvy, for example. Laboratory animals which are getting enough of the B vitamins can somehow substitute them for vitamin C, so that they do not get scurvy as soon as those animals which are not getting so much vitamin B.

It is true, however, that certain forms of iron interfere with the body's store of vitamin E. This is medicinal iron— not the kind that is found in food supplements or in iron-rich foods like wheat germ. If you are taking iron pills prescribed by your doctor, chances are that this iron is in the form that interferes with vitamin E absorption. This does not mean that anything terrible will happen if you take the two pills at the same time, but you will probably be wasting some of the vitamin E. So, to be economical, take the iron pill in the morning and the vitamin E at night or vice versa, so that they will not be in your digestive tract at the same time.

Is there danger of getting too much of the vitamins? In the case of vitamin A and vitamin D, yes. A number of cases have been reported in medical literature, almost all of them involving mothers who have misinterpreted the label on a vitamin D bottle and given it as if it were cod liver oil. And there have been cases—mostly resulting from doctor's prescriptions—where people have taken too much vitamin A over long periods of time and have had quite serious side effects. These disappeared when the vitamin was discontinued, so there is no doubt that the vitamin caused the damage. But it was not permanent.

In any case, your vitamin intake should depend on your needs. If you are a devotee of vegetable juices and regularly quaff large glasses of carrot or spinach juice, you are getting enormous amounts of vitamin A in these juices. If you love liver, carrots, sweet potatoes, squash, watercress and other bright yellow or bright green foods, you are getting very large amounts of vitamin A in these foods. So you need less of this vitamin in supplements than does the person who avoids foods like these and lives mostly on meat, potatoes and desserts.

In general, 10,000 units of vitamin A taken in a supplement every day have never caused any trouble and many people feel their best while taking 20,000 units daily. Medical men have reported giving as much as 50,000 units daily to treat certain conditions harmlessly. On your own, it's best to stick with something around 10,000 units. If you need more vitamin A, get it in the highly nutritious foods mentioned above.

Vitamin C and the B vitamins are water soluble, hence

any excess is excreted harmlessly. A number of physicians and psychiatrists are now recommending massive doses of vitamin C to prevent colds, counteract cholesterol, fight infections and perform many other beneficial acts for the health seeker. Dr. Fred Klenner, who has been giving massive doses of vitamin C for longer than any other physician, says, "I have taken 10 grams to 20 grams (10,000 to 20,000 milligrams) of vitamin C daily for the past 10 years with nothing but beneficial results. With these doses at least three glasses of milk—regular, skimmed or buttermilk—should be taken every day. I have several hundred patients who have taken 10 grams or more of vitamin C daily for three to 15 years. Ninety percent of these never have colds; the other need additional ascorbic acid (vitamin C)."

Dr. Klenner sometimes gives as much as 150 grams intravenously in 24 hours to counteract such things as carbon monoxide or barbiturate poisoning. He gives enormous doses of the vitamin to combat all virus infections. In his fine book, *The Healing Factor, Vitamin C Against Disease,* Dr. Irwin Stone presents evidence that seems to show the versatility of large doses of vitamin C in preventing many common disorders—allergies, asthma, cancer, arthritis, strokes, ulcers and so on.

During the past few years researchers and physicians who doubt the effectiveness of vitamin C and vitamin E in preventing and treating many conditions of ill health have prophesied grim results—everything from kidney stones to prolonged fatigue. But somehow none of these predictions have materialized. Today hundreds of thousands of people are taking vitamin C in large doses and vitamin E in large doses with no results but beneficial ones. In the case of vitamin E, some high blood pressure patients may experience a temporary but uncomfortable rise in pressure if they begin abruptly with a large dose, so they should start with small amounts and increase them gradually.

How should you store your vitamin and mineral supplements and how long can you keep them? Vitamin and mineral supplements, like any other food, deteriorate with time, of course. If one leaves his bottle of vitamin C in a hot sunlit room, with lid off, for months at a time, he should expect to find some deterioration in quality. Like other perishable foods, vitamins should be treated gently and carefully. Light destroys some vitamins. Heat is destructive of others. Sealing the bottles they are packed in guarantees the freshness of the products you buy.

Once you have broken the seal, it is best to store your supplements in a cool spot—the refrigerator if possible. This prevents light from getting to those which are light sensitive and guarantees that differences in daily temperature will not affect the quality of your products.

How long can you keep them? Use your good judgment. Just as you would not expect a loaf of bread or an apple to keep forever, so you cannot expect your vitamin supplements to keep forever even under the most favorable conditions. Generally speaking, food supplements made today have been manufactured with every precaution to guarantee their freshness and quality. The careful way you store them will do much to retain that quality.

# CHAPTER 5

# Reading Labels on Vitamin and Mineral Supplements

Do YOU GET confused trying to figure out what all those tiny words and figures mean on the labels of food supplements? Some vitamins and minerals are spoken of in terms of milligrams or micrograms, some in terms of International Units. What's the difference or is there any?

Why do scientists use such confusing words and how is the average layman expected to find his way through this clutter of unfamiliar terms and meaningless figures? Why do some of the ingredients of a supplement have notes after them stating "the need for this vitamin in human nutrition has not been established"? Why are there combinations of things—like an iron pill which is called "ferrous gluconate" or a pantothenic acid pill called "calcium pantothenate"? Why don't the labels tell you exactly how much to take, instead of just saying "one tablet provides such and such a percentage of the daily requirement"?

These are some of the questions that arise, especially among people who are just beginning to supplement their diets with vitamins and minerals. The answers are not really as difficult to come by as you might think. Keep in mind that some of the vitamins are fat-soluble—that is, they dissolve in fats but not in water. And some of them are water soluble—they dissolve in water but not in fats. The fat-soluble vitamins are A, D, E and K. The water soluble ones are all the B vitamins and vitamin C. These are always listed in terms of milligrams or, in the case of some B vitamins, micrograms. Proteins, carbohydrates and fats are needed in relatively large quantities, so they are spoken of in terms of grams.

A milligram is one-thousandth of a gram. A microgram is one millionth of a gram. A gram is ⅟₂₈th of an ounce. Chemists must work in terms of grams, milligrams and micrograms. That's the way the laboratory apparatus is made, so we must put up with it and learn to read labels in these terms.

One reason why the fat-soluble vitamins are expressed in terms of International Units is that each of them consists of several compounds. Thus one International Unit of vitamin A (fat soluble) includes some retinol, some retinyl acetate and some carotene. So experts from the World Health Organization and official bodies of various countries have decided to apply the term International Unit to a measured amount of each of these three.

Vitamin D (fat soluble) exists in two forms: vitamin D2 (ergocalciferol) and vitamin D3 (cholecalciferol). Vitamin D3 is the natural vitamin which is formed in the deep layers of the skin when exposed to sunlight. Vitamin D2 is made by exposing a plant compound to ultraviolet light. This is the vitamin D which is used to enrich milk, so that, in most localities, a quart of milk contains 400 I.U. of vitamin D.

In the case of vitamin E, this is called by scientists alpha tocopherol. There are other related tocopherols also named with Greek letters: beta, gamma and delta. But we are concerned only with alpha tocopherol because it is the most active of the group. There are two forms of this—the natural and the synthetic. The natural form is d-alpha tocopherol. The synthetic is called dl-alpha tocopherol.

The confusion over whether to speak of vitamin E in terms of milligrams or International Units arises from the fact that the international standard for alpha tocopherol was set using the synthetic form (dl). One I.U. of dl-alpha tocopherol equals 1 milligram. But in the case of the "natural" vitamin E, 1 milligram equals 1.49 International Units.

The official USA book *Recommended Dietary Allowances* states that, since food analyses for vitamin E are chemical rather than biological, values should be reported in milligrams of vitamin E per serving of food. But, in terms of human beings, the biological nomenclature should be used—hence International Units for us. In general, labels of d-alpha tocopherol, which is the natural form, are labeled accordingly. A 100 I.U. capsule would be labeled: "Each capsule contains d-alpha tocopherol (or d-alpha tocopherol acetate) equivalent by bioassay to 100 International Units of vitamin E."

In other words, the vitamin E in such a capsule has been tested with living animals and found to be equivalent to the International Unit. So you can be sure, with such labeling, that you are getting precisely one I.U. of vitamin E—no more and no less. But when we print a list of foods and their vitamin E content, this will appear in milligrams.

Vitamin K is one of the craziest, mixed-up vitamins of all. We manufacture this vitamin in our intestines, complicating the establishment of a recommended dietary allowance. It exists in two forms—K1, in plants, chiefly green leafy vegetables, wheat germ and bran, and as K2 in animal cells: liver, kidney and egg yolk.

Vitamin K is not spoken of in International Units, but in dam units (named after Henrik Dam, discoverer of vitamin K) or ansbacher units. Twenty dam units are equal to 0.0008 milligrams of vitamin K, a fact which need not concern us at all since we do not usually take this vitamin in supplements and there is no reason for us to be concerned about it or try to learn its various names and ways of measuring it.

All the B vitamins are spoken of in terms of milligrams, except for folic acid and vitamin B12 which occur in such very small amounts that it is easier to speak of them in terms of micrograms (millionths of a gram). Vitamin C is spoken of always in terms of milligrams.

As we have seen, the fat soluble vitamins occur in various

forms. The vitamin is made up of different compounds, each of which has its own name. There are many members of the B complex of vitamins. Some of these are officially called vitamins; others are called "vitamin-like substances."

The official B vitamins are these: thiamine (vitamin B1), riboflavin (vitamin B2), niacin (also called nicotinic acid and niacinamide), folic acid, vitamin B6 (pyridoxine), vitamin B12, pantothenic acid, biotin, choline. Vitamin-like substances which are part of the B complex are inositol and para-amino-benzoic acid, (PABA).

Looking over the above information on vitamins, it appears to be a veritable hodge-podge of names and numbers. For goodness sake, why don't the scientists make it all names or all numbers? Why don't they refer to all vitamins either in units or in milligrams? Why are some of them called vitamins and others not called vitamins? Why are there official recommendations for some and not for others?

Scientific work with vitamins is in its infancy. It is going on in many laboratories all over the world, as it has for the past 50 years or so. When Dr. Roger J. Williams discovered pantothenic acid he gave it that name from a Greek word meaning "available everywhere." When he studied folic acid (which had no name then, but was just a chemical compound) he named it folic acid, because it occurs mostly in leafy green vegetables, or foliage.

Vitamin B12 is a generic name for "all cobalt-containing corrinoids" (this refers to the central structure of the vitamin). Between 1926 and 1955, many scientists were working with various substances in widely scattered laboratories to determine what the substance is in liver which cures pernicious anemia. In 1948 two researchers named it vitamin B12, since it was then thought that there might be vitamins already tentatively named vitamin B10, B11, etc. The chemical name for B12 is cobalamin or cyanocobalamin. (It's a lot easier to deal with the simple number 12, isn't it?)

"The need for this vitamin in human nutrition has not been established" means just what it says. Officially, we know that this is a vitamin. And, by definition, the word vitamin means something that is essential for life. But in the roundabout way of scientific bureaucracy, some committee or other decided that not enough laboratory work had been done to decide finally that this or that vitamin is absolutely necessary for good health. Para-amino-benzoic-acid is one such. Undoubtedly in the future much more research will turn up the many significant facts indicating that this substance is indeed essential to health. But for the present, manufacturers can legally only use the sentence above to indicate "yes, it may be a vitamin, but possibly it may not be."

The labels on food supplements cannot tell you exactly how much of any tablet or capsule to take, since this would be interpreted as prescribing medicine. "Take two aspirin and call me in the morning" is legal for your doctor to tell you over the phone. But only doctors can prescribe exact doses of medicine. Vitamins and minerals are not medicine. They are wholly beneficial, harmless (in reasonable amounts) elements of *food, not drugs.* And nobody but you can or should decide how much of any of these to take. You alone know what your health and diet circumstances are, as well as your way of life.

For example, if you regularly drink large amounts of freshly made raw fruit and vegetable juices, you probably have no need to take a vitamin A supplement. But someone who shuns all fruits and vegetables should certainly take a vitamin A supplement. How could anyone write a recommended dose on a label which would apply to both of you?

Why do you find words like "ferrous gluconate" and "calcium pantothenate" and "pyridoxine hydroxide" instead of just the words "iron" and "pantothenic acid" and "pyridoxine"? Just because, chemically speaking, things are usually combinations not single elements. Table salt is sodium chloride, not just sodium, because that's the way it appears in nature. The word "ferrous" refers to one form of iron. Ferrous gluconate is iron combined with glucose because this kind of iron has been found to be acceptable and easily assimilated by the body. Pantothenic acid combined with a bit of calcium is a convenient form in which to take this B vitamin. So don't be overly concerned about this chemical terminology.

Manufacturers of vitamin-mineral supplements must legally deal with all these facts and apparent inconsistencies when they label their products. They must also include on the label information on which vitamins, minerals and other food factors are recognized as "essential," and which have been given official recommended daily amounts. And they must include other information, somehow crowding it all onto a label which, in the case of a small bottle, may seem a near impossibility. In general, they do a good job.

# CHAPTER 6

# Might Not Massive Doses (Megadoses) of Vitamins Be Dangerous?

IF THE OFFICIALLY recommended amount of a vitamin is only several milligrams daily, isn't there a chance that doses far larger than that—megadoses as the doctors call them—might be dangerous? Couldn't very large amounts of vitamin C cause kidney stones? Niacin, the B vitamin, has an acid reaction in the stomach for some people. Could it cause ulcers? Of course, nobody should take immense doses of vitamin A and vitamin D over long periods of time, but what about taking all those other B vitamins in large doses along with the niacin?

It seems to us that the people who probably know more about this subject than anyone else are the physicians who regularly give their patients massive doses of vitamins along with whatever other treatment they give. Do these medical men also take the same amounts of vitamins every day? Do they give them to their families? What do they say about the possible dangers?

In March, 1972 a group of such physicians and scientists got together in New York under the auspices of the Huxley Institute for Biosocial Research to discuss problems of aging. Most of us must face these problems eventually. Most of us have such problems in our families already. Here are some of the statements made by various physicians present, chiefly in regard to the physical and mental problems of aging, senility among them.

Dr. Roger J. Williams of the University of Texas was one of the most distinguished researchers in the field of nutrition and vitamins. Speaking of old folks, Dr. Williams said in part, "A most important part of the environment of an aging person is the food that he or she eats. This provides an internal environment for the cells and tissues. This environment is never perfectly adjusted. That it is often poorly adjusted is due in part to the fact that our staple foods are often trashy and provide in scanty fashion the nutritional essentials which make possible the adequate maintenance and repair of body cells and tissues.

"My work with pantothenic acid (a B vitamin) and longevity was precipitated by the well known observation that worker bees that are fed ordinary food as they develop, develop into worker bees. But the very same larvae, if fed extraordinary food which we call Royal Jelly, develop into queens, fertile queens and live several years, even as long as 8 years. Workers do not live more than a few weeks . . . at one time royal jelly was the richest known source of pantothenic acid. . . . We tried an experiment on the longevity of mice. There were 40 animals in each group. We treated them exactly alike except for the fact that in one group of 40 we gave them extra pantothenic acid in their drinking water. The result was an almost 10 percent increase in the longevity of the mice that got this extra pantothenic acid. I would assume that for some of the mice this did not do any good, but some of them needed larger amounts of pantothenic acid and when they got it they lived longer."

Dr. Abram Hoffer is a distinguished psychiatrist in Canada, who was the first to use large doses of certain vitamins in treating mentally ill patients. He said: "Every time a physician has to treat a patient with a chemical, he has to decide which is more dangerous to that patient—the disease untreated or the chemical he is using for the treatment. This is always the decision we have to face and from this point of view 'optimum' nutrition is that which does the job without producing any harm. . . . You can start with certain levels and see what happens; and gradually increase the level until you get what you want without producing side effects.

"Are there any contra-indications for this regime of large vitamin doses? With niacin (vitamin B3) you may have acidity factors. Rarely there are skin lesions that are not very pleasant. You can have changes in color that you have to deal with. . . .

"Is niacinamide as good as niacin? (Niacinamide is the amide form—a different chemical form—of niacin). It depends on what you are using it for. If you are using it to prevent pellagra, they seem to be equivalent. If you are using it to lower blood cholesterol, the niacinamide will not do it, but niacin will. So in each case you have to decide what it is that you expect from the 'medication' and then you will be able to determine.

"Is there any danger of kidney stones from vitamin C? It has been suggested that large doses of vitamin C might prove to be harmful because it would increase the formation of kidney stones. I have gone over the medical literature very carefully . . . so far there is not a single report in the medical literature where this has been established and in fact many physicians have recommended that vitamin C be used to dissolve kidney stones. . . . I am sure there are at least 50 theoretical dangers but this one doesn't have any data yet to confirm it . . . I have given patients as much as one gram (1,000 milligrams) of vitamin C per hour, day and night, for certain conditions. I have never seen acidosis. It may be I don't know what to look for."

". . . There are two energy yielding chemicals commonly consumed for which self-selection often fails to work advantageously. One is sugar. The other is alcohol. Children who are raised on soft drinks and given a choice will choose more of the same in preference to nourishing food. Adults who commonly consume alcoholic beverages regularly and copiously for long periods of time not infrequently reach the point where they lose interest in nourishing food and have on the contrary a prevailing interest in consuming alco-

holic beverages. In each case, the appetite controlling mechanism in the brain goes awry. In children excess sugar consumption leads to general malnutrition. In adults, consuming
too much alcohol can lead not only to general malnutrition
but to severe damage to the brain. Brains of alcoholics are
so badly damaged that their cadavers are unfit for brain dissec-
tion by medical students. Alcoholism is a terrific health hazard
and elderly people are highly susceptible, particularly if they
have had extended drinking experience.

"The brain cells of individuals need a good environment
throughout their entire life history—from conception through
the prenatal months and into the postnatal years up to old
age. The environment of these brain cells is determined largely
by the quality of food made available during pregnancy and
consumed during youth, middle age and beyond. The environment of these brain cells is also determined in part by the
poisons and near poisons that we consume.

"It was shown many years ago, with animals, that if
you placed them on a vitamin B3 (niacin) deficiency program
and produced black tongue or pellagra, if you kept them
on it for a matter of a month or so, you could then bring
them back to relative health by giving them the usual vitamin
doses of niacin. If, however, you kept that same animal on
the same diet for up to six months, he no longer responded
to the usual vitamin dosages and now required what we in
human terms would call megadoses of niacin, merely to
bring him back to health and to maintain his health.

"It was also known by the early researchers in pellagra
that when you were dealing with chronic pellagra you might
have to give a daily maintenance dose of as much as 600
milligrams per day of niacin . . . I am suggesting that when
human beings are deprived over a period of many years of
the proper nutritional supplements, especially vitamins, that
in time they are converting themselves into an acquired dependency condition. I think that what senility is, in fact, is
merely a prolonged chronic form of malnutrition.

". . . You must provide the optimum quantity of nutrients in the right organ at the right time . . . in order to

stave off senility, not old age but senility—we have to take into account the following factors: an adequate diet, a good diet. Enough high quality protein; a proper balance of fats, a marked reduction in the consumption of refined sugars, especially of sucrose (table sugar), supplements, and here we must use those nutrients which seem to be most relevant: niacinamide which was used by Dr. William Kaufman in 1939—three to four grams a day of niacinamide on 600 cases of arthritis. The results were fantastic. He was able to reverse the arthritic changes which are so often associated with senility. Niacin is a vitamin that lowers cholesterol and fats, the subject of a large-scale $55 million experiment by the American government. The results are interesting and it seems they will now decrease the coronary death rate over a four-year period by about 65 percent.

"The next subject is ascorbic acid (vitamin C) . . . I can assure you that it is safe, and I myself have taken as much as 10 grams a day. We have given our patients as much as 90 grams a day. We have never yet seen any toxicity. If any person doubts that, I will challenge you to a duel. You eat a spoonful of salt and I will eat a spoonful of vitamin C and see who stops eating first. I think the average dose should be three grams a day. I take four. Pantothenic acid increases the longevity of animals . . . Vitamin E should be investigated for its ability to prevent free radical formation." (He is referring here to the ability of vitamin E to prevent rancidity from occurring in body cells.)

"What I am doing is taking at least 30 pills of vitamins a day: four grams of niacin, four grams of vitamin C, 800 units of vitamin E, 250 milligrams of thiamine (vitamin B1), 250 milligrams of pyridoxine (vitamin B6), A and D, calcium and a bit of iron and a mineral supplement. I feel fine."

# CHAPTER 7

# Vitamins Plus a Nourishing Diet Prevent Cataract in a Laboratory Experiment

PEOPLE JUST BEGINNING to learn about vitamins often ask, "What vitamin can I take that will cure this or that condition?" as if vitamins were drugs and you could pop one of them at meals for a week or so and cure high blood pressure, or diabetes or heart disease. Or cataract.

It doesn't happen that way. Vitamins are not drugs and you cannot cure some disease of long-standing by simply taking "a vitamin" and doing nothing at all about correcting that non-nourishing diet and unhealthful way of life that had a lot to do with creating the condition in the first place. Nor is it likely to do much good to take two vitamins or three, even if you throw in a few minerals. While one vitamin may make a difference in the way you feel, after the vitamin has had some time to "work," and you may even notice some additional good effects that you had not expected, chances are that you will do much better by taking a full schedule of vitamins combined with the best possible diet and a way of life that is conducive to good health.

The fallacy of demanding that one vitamin cure one disease is highlighted by an experiment once performed in the laboratory of Dr. Roger J. Williams. All his professional life Dr. Williams tried to educate the general public and his professional colleagues as well as government officials to the basic principle that vitamins and minerals are not drugs—that all of them work together as a team, that there is no such thing as one vitamin or one mineral curing a disease. They must all be involved.

Said Dr. Williams in an article in the *Proceedings of the National Academy of Sciences,* October, 1974, "No nutrient by itself should be expected to prevent or cure any disease; nutrients as such always work cooperatively in metabolism as a team . . . Unlike drugs, single nutrients always act constructively like parts of a complicated machine and are effective only when they participate as members of a team. This does not prevent nutrients from having drug-like actions when used in amounts higher than the physiological levels . . . When particular vitamins appear to cure specific diseases, it is because they round out the team, transforming a limping incomplete team into one that is complete enough to function with some degree of physiological adequacy . . . Testing nutrients for their effectiveness is thus entirely different from testing drugs. Unless a nutrient is tested under conditions which allow it to participate in teamwork, the results are likely to be seriously misleading."

Dr. Williams and a colleague set out to test this theory on laboratory rats. It is well known that rats lack an enzyme which is necessary to use properly a sugar which appears in milk—galactose. Since they lack this enzyme, they generally get cataracts when they are fed lots of milk or milk products. The Texas researchers set up an experiment using 18 groups of rats and 18 different diets. All the diets except one (the control diet) contained quite large amounts of galactose—up to 20 percent of the diet. The rest of the diet was arranged so that some of the rats got just the usual chow which adequately nourishes laboratory rats: some diets contained nothing but eggs in addition to the galactose. An all-egg diet has been found by Dr. Williams to constitute a complete and very healthful diet for rats. Some of the diets contained the usual laboratory chow plus vitamins in quite large amounts.

At the end of nine weeks cataracts had formed in the eyes of many of the rats which got the plain chow with no vitamins. Although they were getting the same large amount of galactose (the cataract former), those rats which got, in addition, the vitamin supplements had no cataracts at all. In every case the number of cataracts increased in direct proportion to the lack of nutrients in the diet. Those diets which contained most in the way of vitamins, in addition to the basic good diet, produced no cataracts. Those which contained no extra vitamins did produce cataracts. The diets in between—with fewer vitamins added—produced some cataracts, but not as many as the diets with no added vitamins. The control group of rats which got no cataract-producing galactose—also had no cataracts.

In a second experiment all the rats were fed a diet designed to produce cataracts. They were then fed a good diet plus all the vitamins to see if the cataracts would regress. The results of this experiment were not as clear-cut as those of the first experiment. Of 26 cataracts, 16 showed improvement from 40 to 80 percent. But, in general, the regressions were slow and incomplete, "though improvement in many cases was clearly manifested," said Dr. Williams. It seems that the lens of the eye (where cataracts form) has a slow rate of metabolism—that is, any improvement might be expected to be slow.

Dr. Williams pointed out that his experiments do not prove that one or another vitamin will prevent cataracts. Nor is it possible to decide which of the vitamins given to the test animals was responsible for preventing the cataracts. There is no way to know if leaving out one or more of the vitamins would have changed the results. There is also no way to know whether the vitamins given are in complete "balance"—that is, whether too much of one vitamin was given, perhaps, or too little of another.

The point is that, however complete the traditional nourishing laboratory diet for rats is, it can always be improved by the addition of vitamins—all the vitamins. It can be improved to such an extent that the mere addition of all these vitamins can prevent cataracts forming even when the rats are given very large amounts of a substance which is almost guaranteed to produce cataracts in rats!

How does this happen? What do the additional vitamins do to perform this near-miracle? We do not know, said Dr. Williams. It is possible that, with the extra nutrients, the animals build enzyme systems to substitute for the one they lack—the one that is necessary to handle galactose, the cataract-causing substance.

What about human beings? Cataract is a frequent accompaniment of diabetes. Can enough of all the vitamins provide enough extra nutritional building materials to overcome the tendency to diabetic cataracts? What about those cataracts that appear in older folks, called senile cataracts? It seems quite possible that here, too, providing the optimum nutrition—not just enough to nourish but lots more than that—may be effective in preventing these cataracts from forming in the first place.

Dr. Williams also believed that by treating the cataract with "supernutrition" as he called it, the moment it is discovered, rather than waiting until it has fully developed, we might be able to prevent it from progressing any farther. And if we afflict the eye with less of the toxic substance which causes the cataract, we may be able to prevent or stop its further growth. In the case of the rats, galactose is the toxic substance. Most human beings have no problems with galactose because they have the enzyme necessary to metabolize it with no difficulty. Those few people born without this enzyme may (probably will) be afflicted with the full range of symptoms which lack of this enzyme produces— failure to thrive in infancy, jaundice, involvement of liver and spleen, mental retardation and formation of cataracts.

It seems obvious that all the many cataracts now being treated or removed from the eyes of diabetics and older folks are not the result of inability to metabolize galactose. We do not know what causes most human cataracts. Some specialists think it may be the result of eating too much sugar, since cataract is common among us Westerners who consume such large amounts of sugar. No matter what it is that causes human cataracts, doesn't it seem possible that they might be prevented by following the design of the experiment described above?

Eat the most highly nourishing diet possible, like the laboratory chow which nourished the rats. Then add vitamins to achieve supernutrition. The best way to achieve the most nourishing diet for human beings is to eliminate sugar from your meals and snacks. Many modern people eat so much sugar and refined white flour products that half of the meals consist of these two foods. There is little that nourishes in either of these foods except for starch, sugar and otherwise empty calories. Laboratory rats die of malnutrition when they are fed diets like this.

Once you have eliminated the twin hazards of refined sugar and refined cereal and bread products, everything else that you eat is nourishing. There's no need to plan outlandish, difficult or expensive meals. Just be sure that you include the high protein foods: meat, fish, poultry, dairy products, all the seed foods like wholegrains, bran, wheat germ, seeds of all kinds, nuts, soybeans, peas, beans, peanuts, all the fruits and vegetables, especially those that have lots of bright yellow and/or green, like carrots, apricots, parsley, broccoli, spinach. Eating this kind of diet—as widely varied as possible—you will get the same highly nourishing food as the laboratory rats had.

Then, according to Dr. Williams's experiments, add to that excellent diet all the known vitamins, some of them in quite large amounts. The accompanying chart shows the amounts of vitamins Dr. Williams used for his animals. No vitamin C is included, since rats make their own vitamin C and do not need to get it in food. You, however, need it very decidedly and you should add comparatively large amounts of it to your supplement program.

To calculate the amounts for human diets, estimate the number of calories you eat every day. It's probably in the neighborhood of about 3,000 for an adult man and about 2,000 for an adult woman. These are the officially recommended number of calories for people who are of average weight and height. The nutrients given in the chart are for every 100 calories of food. If you are eating 3,000 calories multiply the numbers in the chart by 30 to get an estimate of how much you should be taking to achieve what was achieved in the rat experiment.

---

### Nutrients (Per 100 Calories) Furnished by Vitamin Mixture in Diets Which Prevented Cataracts

| | |
|---|---|
| Vitamin A | 1,333 I.U. |
| Vitamin D3 | 66.7 I.U. |
| Vitamin E | 40 milligrams |
| Thiamine | 0.83 milligrams |
| Riboflavin | 1.67 milligrams |
| Niacin | 10 milligrams |
| Pantothenic acid | 5.3 milligrams |
| Pyridoxine | 0.8 milligrams |
| Vitamin B12 | 3.3 micrograms |
| Folic acid | 3.3 milligrams |
| Biotin | 70 micrograms |
| Choline | 50 milligrams |
| Inositol | 33.3 milligrams |

**Plus some vitamin K and some fatty acid mixes.**

---

## VITAMINS PLUS DIET PREVENT CATARACT

It appears quite possible that the added vitamins may have such an excellent effect on your otherwise very nutritious diet that you will have achieved that "supernutrition" which Dr. Williams believed may be essential to prevent not just cataracts, but also other modern diseases like multiple sclerosis, muscular dystrophy, mental retardation, heart disease, dental disease, allergies, arthritis, premature senility, obesity, mental disease, alcoholism, and perhaps even cancer. It's worth a try, isn't it?

# CHAPTER 8

# The Special Vitamin Needs of Women on "The Pill"

*Medical World News* for August 24, 1973 reported on a National Institutes of Health study of medical records which showed that women on The Pill are nine and a half times more likely to suffer a stroke than women not taking The Pill. Another study in Boston showed that blood clots are much more frequent in women on The Pill, who were also found to be twice as susceptible to gall bladder disease as women not on The Pill.

We have known for a long time that blood-sugar-regulating apparatus is disordered by The Pill. This could lead to diabetes or low blood sugar. Medical journals recommend that any woman whose family has a history of fatty accumulations in blood which cause hardening of the arteries should not take The Pill because the drug increases levels of certain fats in the blood. Many women suffer depression and discoloration of the skin when they take The Pill.

The list of serious ailments which afflict many women taking contraceptives seems almost endless. But there is apparently little hope of discouraging the use of oral contraceptives. Indeed medical researchers now promise even more mysterious and potentially damaging substances as contraceptives of the future.

The least we can do, as health seekers, is to examine

what possible steps women can take to protect themselves against the more ominous threats they face from The Pill. Such information comes to us in *The Journal of Applied Nutrition* for Spring, 1974. An article by B. Pal, Ph. D., Research Associate of the Department of Medicine at the University of Rochester, discussed the metabolic and nutritional effects of oral contraceptives.

He told us that one hormone commonly used in The Pill causes high blood sugar problems and the other hormone used with it makes this situation worse. In women with an inherited tendency toward diabetes, overt diabetes may develop when the contraceptive is taken, and disappear when it is withdrawn. Quite often, high blood levels of fat are also present in diabetes. Since oral contraceptives create a false pregnancy, the body responds by increasing blood levels of the triglycerides, one kind of bothersome fatty substance. The effects on cholesterol levels are inconsistent. In some women these levels, too, go up. Since raised levels of fats are linked to hardening of the arteries and many circulatory disorders, it is obvious that such side effects as these are highly undesirable, especially in women so young.

In women taking The Pill, blood levels of the B vitamin pyridoxine are below normal. So serious and widespread is this situation that many physicians believe the B vitamin should always be taken in the same tablet as the contraceptive. If not, additional pyridoxine—at least 30 milligrams daily—should be taken. Four of the essential amino acids or forms of protein are also low in women on The Pill. Dr. Pal says these proteins are concerned with the production of pigments, so it's possible this deficiency may explain the discolored skin many women on contraceptives complain of.

Folic acid is another essential B vitamin which is deficient in pill takers. Quite often pregnant women are short on folic acid. So apparently pregnancy causes a drain on this vitamin, lack of which brings on a very serious anemia. Since The Pill induces false pregnancy, this B vitamin may be used up very rapidly while The Pill is being taken. Many scientists concerned in this research believe that folic acid supplements should be given to pregnant women and to women on The Pill. Another complication is that women may become pregnant after they discontinue The Pill and may be in a state of folic acid depletion during this pregnancy. Recent research has linked folic acid deficiency in pregnant women to spina bifida in their infants.

Researchers have reported a decrease of 30 percent in vitamin C in the blood of women on The Pill. Part of the reason may be that the copper content of the blood increases during this time and copper causes the destruction of vitamin C. Said Dr. Pal, "the requirement for vitamin C may be well above the normal level during the oral contraceptive use."

Vitamin A is another nutrient affected by The Pill. One of the hormones in this drug impairs the ability of the liver to store vitamin A. Now, vitamin A is fat soluble, meaning that it is *supposed* to be stored in the body, unlike the water soluble vitamins. If its storage in the liver is disrupted, this might mean that a woman who takes The Pill would have to get, every day, the full quota of vitamin A which she needs, rather than depending on stores of the vitamin in her body.

If one or two of the B vitamins are in short supply due to The Pill, it seems likely that all the rest of the B complex are lacking, as well. If vitamin A and fat metabolism are disorganized, this suggests that all is not well with the other fat soluble vitamins—D, E, and K. Is the body storage of these vitamins disrupted, too?

The only certain fact out of this review of scientific findings is that any woman taking oral contraceptives should go out of her way to eat the most highly nourishing diet possible and should certainly take food supplements in ample amounts to make up for the abnormal decrease in certain of these, due to the drug.

How much of each vitamin should she take? This depends on the individual. Some people require many times more than others just to stay healthy. Dr. Pal suggests 30 milligrams of pyridoxine (vitamin B6) daily. The official recommendation is a daily intake of 2 milligrams. So apparently the woman on The Pill needs 15 times this amount. She would have to get it from a high potency food supplement. On the same basis, should she be taking 15 times more of all the other B vitamins and vitamin C? We do not know, but certainly there is no harm in such a dose since these water soluble vitamins are not stored in the body and cannot accumulate. In the case of vitamin A, the woman on The Pill should make certain she gets, every day, a supplement containing at least the recommended daily amount of this vitamin which is 5,000 units.

The evidence on the way The Pill depletes vitamin stores has been piling up in medical journals year after year. As early as 1970 *The Lancet* published evidence that the depression of which many women on The Pill complain is caused by deficiency of vitamin B6, pyridoxine. Two Wisconsin physicians studied 58 patients who had been taking The Pill for an average of 14 months and who complained of at least three of these mental symptoms: emotional flareups and irritability, depression, fatigue, mild paranoia (they thought other people were persecuting them), difficulty with concentration and sleep disturbances.

Twenty-two of the patients had all five symptoms. Fifty had some of the symptoms before they started on The Pill, but the symptoms became worse on The Pill and new ones developed. The doctors gave them 50 milligrams of pyridoxine to take once daily when their premenstrual symptoms began. Eighteen reported complete cure of all symptoms. Twenty-six reported considerable improvement. Fourteen reported no change.

In those who noticed improvement with pyridoxine, the results were noticed within hours or by the next day at the latest. (This must have seemed like a miracle to women tormented with these troublesome symptoms.) The 14 patients who showed no improvement on 50 milligrams of pyridoxine daily were then given 100 milligrams—and still showed no improvement. No patients complained of any side effects.

One patient was so pleased with the results of the 50 milligrams of pyridoxine that she thought 100 milligrams would be even better. Every one of the 44 patients who improved on this vitamin therapy recommended pyridoxine to at least one friend or neighbor. One patient now has 12 friends taking the vitamin for mental symptoms.

Said these Wisconsin physicians, "These results support our clinical impression that pyridoxine is a valuable treatment for the five symptoms mentioned in patients taking oral contraceptives, and underlines the need for further research and controlled objective studies . . . the implications for treatment of premenstrual tension and pregnancy depression are obvious."

All 44 patients who improved were asked to discontinue pyridoxine to see if their symptoms returned. All refused to do so, because they were so pleased with the results. And even four patients who decided not to go on taking oral contraceptives because of their fear of side effects, went right on taking pyridoxine.

In November, 1970, another article appeared in *The Lancet* describing tests with 20 women using The Pill which showed that 16 of them had deficiency in vitamin B6. The authors, from New York and New Jersey, point out that pregnant women experience a similar pyridoxine deficiency for several months only, but the long-term use of The Pill can result in a "chronic and sustained derangement in a large segment of an essentially young, healthy population. In view of its ready correctibility by oral pyridoxine," they ask, "might it not be advisable to recommend a vitamin B6 supplement for users of The Pill?" Nobody answered their question, obviously, for few doctors seem to have noticed the pyridoxine deficiency produced by the pill they are giving.

In 1971 *The American Journal of Clinical Nutrition* printed an article by a group of New York physicians who studied 43 women all taking The Pill. They monitored the various changes brought about in the women as their supply of pyridoxine decreased. They point out that various processes involved in the way The Pill acts in regard to pyridoxine can produce defective regulation of blood sugar levels and supply of insulin and can cause concern.

They tell us that the recommended daily allowance of two milligrams of pyridoxine given to the women corrected the deficiency in only 10 percent of them. The rest required 25 milligrams. Because they were studying so few women and it was well known (or should be well known) that different people may have widely different needs for various vitamins, they concluded that all women taking The Pill should be given 30 milligrams of vitamin B6 (or pyridoxine) daily along with The Pill. A totally harmless dose of a totally beneficial vitamin. But still no notice was taken of this suggestion by any official medical group or government health group.

My extensive file on The Pill bulges with more and more medical articles relating newly discovered side effects of The Pill, all embellished with the quotation and disclaimer, "There is no such thing as absolute safety when it comes to contraception—you get nothing for nothing."

The Pill may be a cause of migraine headaches. The Pill may impair one's defense against infections. The Pill may bring vaginal discharges, urinary tract infections, susceptibility to chicken pox and other infections, eczema, loss of sex drive, mouth ulcers, high blood pressure, gall bladder troubles, serious alterations in results of laboratory tests which may throw off diagnoses of illness. Eighteen and a half million women were taking The Pill in 1969, undoubtedly many more than that by now. Periodically some researcher gives out a press release on research on the Male Pill but it's never any more than a press release.

And on March 5, 1975 the *New York Times* said that the development of safer methods of contraception is being seriously hampered because the multi-billion-dollar drug industry did not see any chance of making a pile of money out of a new pill before 1990—and we haven't seen one yet!

Barbara Seaman and Gideon Seaman, M.D. in their book *Women and the Crisis in Sex Hormones* quote two Australian researchers who said, "Many women taking oral contraceptives show biochemical evidence of a multifactor hypovitaminosis (vitamin deficiency) involving vitamin C, riboflavin, thiamine, vitamin B6, vitamin B12 and E." The Seamans continue, "Folic acid is seriously deficient in many pill users, as are B6, E and essential trace metals such as zinc and magnesium. The Seamans recommend as much as 400–800 micrograms of folic acid daily for pill users, plus 15–30 milligrams of zinc daily. Your public library may have copies of this book on the shelf.

# Vitamin A Is . . .

*Fat-soluble,* meaning it is stored in the body, so that it is not essential to provide vitamin A every single day.

*Responsible for* the health of the retina of the eye, the production of visual purple in the eye, which helps us to see at night, the maintenance of skin and linings of all body openings and organs, resistance to infections, bone development, maintenance of the myelin and membranes of our bodies, maintenance of color vision and peripheral (side) vision, maintenance of the adrenal gland and synthesis of certain hormones.

*Present* in most abundance in liver, kidney, carrots, spinach and all other dark green, leafy vegetables and yellow vegetables and fruits such as apricots, peaches, nectarines, yellow squash, sweet potatoes, butter, egg yolk.

*Not to be taken in excess.* Taking very large amounts of vitamin A over long periods of time can produce unpleasant and dangerous symptoms, which, in adults, disappear when the vitamin is withdrawn, but which may persist in infants and children.

*Destroyed* in the body by mineral oil laxatives, by several chemicals, estrogens and other drugs.

*Required* officially in amounts of 5,000 International Units by adults, somewhat less in children, depending on age.

*Available* in capsules of not more than 10,000 International Units.

*Safe* in amounts up to 20,000 units daily.

## Foods Highest in Vitamin A

| Foods | Units of Vitamin A |
|---|---|
| Carrots, raw, ½ cup | 11,000 |
| Sweet potatoes, 1 | 7,700 |
| Beet greens, ½ cup | 6,700 |
| Chard, ½ cup | 8,720 |
| Chicory, ½ cup | 10,000 |
| Dandelion greens, ½ cup | 15,170 |
| Endive, 10 stalks | 3,000 |
| Kale, cooked, ½ cup | 8,300 |
| Spinach, cooked, ½ cup | 11,780 |
| Turnip greens, cooked, ½ cup | 10,600 |
| Pumpkin, cooked, ½ cup | 3,400 |
| Cantaloupe, ½ small | 3,420 |
| Apricots, 6 halves | 2,790 |
| Apricots, dry, 8 halves | 3,700 |
| Peaches, fresh, 1 large | 880 |
| Prunes, dry, 12 | 1,890 |
| Tomato Juice, 4 oz. | 1,050 |
| Liver, beef, fried, 1 serving | 53,500 |
| Liver, calf | 32,200 |
| Liverwurst, ¼ pound | 5,750 |
| Eggs, 2 | 1,140 |

# CHAPTER 9

# Vitamin A Is Powerful Against Cancer

IN A 1968 SURVEY the United States Department of Agriculture discovered that 20 percent of the American population was eating a nutritionally poor diet. Projecting their figures onto the entire population of the country we may conclude that between 40 and 50 million people may lack in their diets the amount of vitamin A which experts believe we should have to be well nourished.

Cancer is today the most feared and most tragic disease we face. Lying in the pages of countless medical and scientific journals are accounts of experiments which showed without any question that vitamin A and/or carotene, which is the plant form of this vitamin, can prevent cancer and can prevent some of the growth of some cancers that have already formed. As long ago as 1966, Dr. Umberto Saffioti, then of the National Cancer Institute, reported at a Cancer Congress that vitamin A can prevent lung cancer in animals.

This astonishing news went almost unnoticed, although it was reported briefly in the pages of the *New York Times*. Since then many other scientists have reported the same results in laboratory experiments where animals were exposed to cancer-causing compounds and did not get the expected lung cancer. Animals on diets deficient in vitamin A or carotene did develop the expected lung cancers.

Other researchers have studied large populations of people and the diets they have eaten during their lives. They have found, without exception, that people who customarily eat diets that contain lots of vitamin A and carotene-rich foods have, in general, less cancer incidence than those who avoid such foods. Such studies have been conducted by experts in the field of epidemiology, which is what this kind of study is called.

The December 27, 1974 issue of *Science,* the prestigious publication of the American Association for the Advancement of Science, devoted a page to the unchallengeable fact that vitamin A prevents cancer in both laboratory animals and human beings. They were reporting on a symposium on vitamin A and cancer. Two scientists from the National Cancer Institute stated at the symposium that when they applied known cancer-causing substances to the breathing apparatus of animals, much more damage was done in those animals deficient in vitamin A.

Two scientists from the Massachusetts Institute of Technology reported that when laboratory animals are given cancer-causing substances in food there are fewer colon cancers among those which get plenty of vitamin A. Another scientist has found, he said, that animals not at all deficient in vitamin A can be protected against cancer of the breathing apparatus if they are given additional vitamin A. An Alabama scientist reported that when he applied vitamin A to prostate glands of animals he could prevent the cancers that would be expected from exposure to cancer-causing chemicals.

At Oak Ridge Laboratory (a government laboratory supported by your tax money) vitamin A was found to prevent lung cancers in animals exposed to a substance known to cause this kind of cancer. A cancer specialist at Hoffman-LaRoche laboratory transplanted cancers into his laboratory rats. Even after the cancers had started to grow in those locations they stopped growing when enough vitamin A was given. A Swiss expert reported at the same meeting that he had brought about a reduction in size of another cancer produced by still another chemical. He gave the animals vitamin A. This same scientist has also used vitamin A to prevent cancers in human beings. One of the participants at the symposium stated that at least one-third of all Americans are deficient in vitamin A. They do not get even that small amount of the vitamin that is officially stated to be essential for good health, let alone any excess to protect them from whatever cancer-causing chemicals they encounter in everyday life.

In 1976 Dr. Paul Newberne of Massachusetts Institute of Technology stated that if the epithelial cells do not have enough vitamin A to maintain their health, they are likely to succumb to cancer. The epithelial cells are those of the skin and the linings of all body openings and organs like the mouth, the lungs, the digestive tract and the excretory tract as well as glands. In addition to lung cancer, he pointed out, colon cancer is a risk for anyone who does not get enough vitamin A.

In 1977, Dr. Michael B. Sporn of the National Cancer Institute wrote in *Nutrition Reviews* that experiments on laboratory rats have shown that those who get enough vitamin A before exposure to known cancer-causing pollutants do not get the expected cancers. Dr. Sporn said that just such significant experiments have been carried out testing for cancer of the windpipe, the bronchial tubes that lead to the lungs, the uterine cervix, the stomach and the vagina.

He explained that cancer is, to put it simply, a disruption of the process of cell division and differentiation. In the individual who has cancer, certain cells do not reproduce themselves normally. They produce cancerous cells instead. In many kinds of cancer, they produce these cells rapidly and profusely, so that the body is overwhelmed with these sick cells that obstruct healthy organs and tissues, eventually causing death.

Dr. Sporn said, "Vitamin A and its synthetic analogs (retinoids) have been successfully used to prevent cancer of the skin, lung, bladder and breast in experimental animals. This is a pharmacological (drug) approach to prevention of cancer by enhancement of intrinsic epithelial defense mechanisms. Synthetic retinoids (the manufactured relatives of vitamin A) are definitely superior for this purpose."

In April, 1977 Dr. Sporn announced that the National

Cancer Institute (funded by your tax money) was beginning a test of more than 100 persons who face a high probability of developing bladder cancer. Scientists are giving these synthetic vitamin A preparations to volunteers who have already been treated for precancerous growths in the urinary bladder. He suggested that success in these tests would be very valuable for anyone likely to develop cancer—heavy smokers or people working in industries who are exposed to asbestos, uranium or other cancer-causing chemicals.

He added that no lay person should try to prevent cancer in himself by taking any vitamin A because he might do himself harm by getting an overdose of the vitamin. This is the usual scientific and medical point of view—that we lay people are childlike and totally unable to take care of ourselves. No, indeed, the researchers and physicians must tend to us and administer to us anything which goes into our mouths which is smaller than a potato—like a pill.

It's true that enormous doses of vitamin A (in millions of units taken over long periods of time) have brought toxic side effects to a few people. We cover these facts in another chapter of this book. But anyone capable of reading the label of a bottle of vitamin A capsules can easily see that 10,000 units taken daily will certainly pose no risk. The official recommendation is 5,000 units daily for adults.

In 1980 *The New England Journal of Medicine* published the story of a 43-year old man who had nodules or tumors growing on his skin from the age of seven. They had spread over the surface of his body until they covered large areas of his arms, legs, thighs, buttocks. Several fingers had been amputated when nodules appeared beneath the nails. The nodules were painful and so disabling that he was almost unable to walk or use his hands. They resembled skin cancers.

Over the past six years no treatment had given him any relief. Doctors at New York University Medical Center decided to try one of the relatives of vitamin A. They gave large doses of this synthetic "drug" to the man for 16 weeks. There were almost no unpleasant side effects and no permanent ones. Within three weeks of beginning the therapy, the patient noticed that some of the tumors were less tender and scaly. At the end of 16 weeks the drug was discontinued. The patient began to feel pain again in some of the tumors. He was put back on the vitamin A substitute again and no new tumors developed. Most of those that remained were removed with no difficulty and no recurrence. The doctors said, "Previously confined to a wheel chair, he has started to lead a normal life and reports that he now plays soccer with his family."

No diet history of the patient was given in the article, so we do not know whether this condition might have been caused by simple lack of vitamin A in his diet or whether he had some inherited or congenital condition which caused him to be unable to use the normally small amount of vitamin A he may have been getting at meals. Inability to adjust to glare at night is one early symptom of vitamin A deficiency. This man had, apparently, no such symptom. The thought of progressing from this annoying but harmless condition to something approaching the condition of this tumor-ridden man just from vitamin A deficiency is horrifying. Why not just encourage everyone everywhere to be certain to get enough vitamin A in meals and supplements and save the "drug" made from synthetic vitamin A for serious, untreatable conditions like this!

A study in 1984 showed that women with abnormalities of the female cervix were getting far less vitamin A in their diets than women who get plenty of this vitamin. The same was true of vitamin C. A lead article in *Science* discussed the possible ways in which carotene (the plant form of vitamin A) may give protection against cancer. The article showed that vitamin A is powerful in destroying compounds called "Free Radicals," substances in the blood which are known to cause cancer.

An article in *The New England Journal of Medicine* enthused about recent work in the area of vitamin A and carotene and prophesied that "there are indications that retinoids may in time prove of value in other areas of medicine such as rheumatic and connective tissue disorders as well." Over

1,500 compounds have already been synthesized as "drugs" by varying the basic molecule of vitamin A. Each of them may turn out to have beneficial effects in many disorders.

In the late 1970's researchers in many countries were working on vitamin A and carotene in relation to cancers of many kinds: breast cancer, colon cancer, lung cancer. In 1980 a Texas researcher used vitamin A and vitamin C to produce suppression of cancer of the lymph glands in animals. This disease is called Hodgkins Disease in human beings. A lead editorial in *The British Medical Journal,* October 11, 1980 discussed vitamin A as an extremely effective shield against many forms of cancer. The editorial reviewed as many as 200 different bits of research all showing essentially the same thing—enough vitamin A (and synthetic relatives of it) in the body appears to protect both animals and human beings from many different kinds of cancer.

A Norwegian study of more than 8,000 men showed less lung cancer among those who had more carotene in their diets. A Japanese study of more than a quarter of a million men showed that the risk of lung cancer was reduced by half in those who ate bright green and yellow vegetables and fruits daily as compared with those who ate them only occasionally. Two other studies showed that patients with lung cancer used fewer vitamin A supplements than those without lung cancer. Six studies showed a decreased intake of carotene in patients with bladder, lung, stomach and colo-rectal cancer. Another study showed that those with lower blood levels of vitamin A had a six-fold greater risk of getting cancer. Still another study found low blood levels of vitamin A compounds in patients with lung cancer and cancers of the mouth.

*The Lancet,* another British medical journal (October 18, 1980) had a lead article on a survey of 258 men, 86 of whom had developed cancer. The others who served as "controls" were healthy. The risk of cancer for the men with the lowest vitamin A levels in the body was more than twice as great as the risk for those with the highest levels of vitamin A. A letter to *The Lancet* on this article reported on autopsies carried out since 1948 by a group of London and Cambridge physicians. Forty years ago, they said, these studies showed low levels of vitamin A in those who died of hernia, cancer, valvular heart disease, prostate disease, chronic nephritis (kidney disease) and kidney and bladder infections. "If vitamin A is to prove valuable against cancer," they said, "it could well prove equally valuable against several other forms of common disease."

*Medical Tribune,* April 22, 1981 reported on experiments with vitamin A in animals exposed to cancer-causing compounds. The researchers found that there is an increased risk of bladder cancer in creatures who are deficient in vitamin A. The experiments also showed that human beings given the equivalent of a vitamin A compound that the animals got might expect to live six or seven years longer, even though they might eventually die of the cancer. Dr. Michael Sporn of the National Cancer Institute commented, "If an individual is grossly deficient in dietary vitamin A he is at risk for the development of bladder cancer . . . I continue to believe that a single multiple (vitamin) capsule is the best investment in health in America."

Drugs, surgery and radiation (the usual medical treatments for cancer) cannot change the way cells are reproducing. All they do is to destroy the sick cells in the hope of eliminating the cancer from the body. But always getting enough vitamin A will apparently prevent the entire disease process from getting started—at least in those parts of the body where epithelial cells are present. It goes without saying that the less exposure we all have to any compound that causes cancer, the better.

Experts studied 1,954 Chicago men, all employees of Western Electric, asked numerous questions about their diets and health and found that carotene, that bright-colored relative of vitamin A which exists in fruits, berries and vegetables, apparently helps to prevent lung cancer. Over the 19 years this study continued, the researchers found and reported in 1982 that *even in smokers* who ate lots of foods containing carotene there were far fewer lung cancers than in those men who shunned this kind of "rabbit food." Thirty-three of the men who were studied developed lung cancer, twenty-five of these men ate less than average amounts of foods rich in carotene. Fourteen of them were in the lowest percent for carotene intake.

*New Scientist* in 1984 described the cancers that form in the mouths of Filipinos who chew betel nuts. This is a form of addiction similar to smoking or chewing tobacco. Researchers studied cells from the lining of the mouths of residents who had never chewed the betel nut and compared these with scrapings from the mouth tissues of men who were habitual chewers of the betel nut. They found only 0.8 percent of precancerous cells in the mouths of nonusers and 4.3 percent in the mouths of the men who used the drug. Forty of the regular quid chewers were then given 50,000 units of vitamin A and 150,000 units of carotene twice weekly for three months. Excellent results were so astonishing that scientists double-checked them fearing they had made some miscalculation. Said *New Scientist,* "the figures seem to show a real effect and could go some way to preventing the hundreds of thousands of deaths every year from oral cancer in Asia."

By 1984 medical and scientific journals were describing vitamin A and carotene as protective against dysplasia (a precancerous condition) in the female cervix, also in the treatment of breast cancer. According to *Nutrition Reviews,* rats deficient in vitamin A have lowered levels of the male sex hormone testosterone. Severe deficiency in this nutrient can cause atrophy of the sex organs also small swollen testes and cessation of the formation of sperm. Couples troubled with sterility should certainly make every effort to include foods rich in vitamin A and carotene in meals and snacks.

So convinced are many members of the medical profession of the efficacy of vitamin A and carotene in protecting individuals from many kinds of disorders that "The Carotene Bunch" has been formed. This is a group of some 22,000 physicians who have volunteered to engage in a four-year study of the possibly beneficial effects of carotene, taken every day, with a 320-milligram aspirin tablet taken on alternate days. The researcher from Harvard University who is conducting the study told an international cancer symposium in 1985 that he hopes to discover the effectiveness of the carotene in preventing cancer and he wants to see if the small amount of aspirin makes any difference in "total all-cause mortality."

Half of the group are acting as "controls," taking either just carotene or just aspirin. The physician volunteers also send to Harvard every six months reports on other aspects of their lives: changes in diet, health status, smoking and alcohol intake. Dr. Kedar Prasad, director of the Center for Vitamins and Cancer Research at the University of Colorado, said of the study, "My belief is that we will learn over the next ten years how to markedly reduce the incidence of cancer by manipulating individual vitamins and dietary factors."

Anyone who prefers to change his or her daily diet to include plenty of vitamin A and carotene-rich foods can be certain that such change is bound to be beneficial where general good health is concerned and perhaps also in preventing cancer. For the hazards of taking too much of either of these nutrients see the chapter in this book which deals with this subject.

A British scientist, Sir Alexander Haddow, announced at a cancer symposium a number of years ago that as many as 80 percent of all human cancers may be due to environmental causes. If this is true, he said, "The implications for prevention are immense and exciting." He believes that scientists will be able to eliminate most cancers, even if they never find out what causes cancer.

What he is saying, in essence, is that, as soon as we have final irrevocable proof that air pollution, water pollution, toxic waste, chemicals in food, pesticides, drugs, cigarette smoke, radiation and the hundreds of thousands of other pollutants in our industrial societies cause cancer, then all we have to do is to eliminate these hazards and we won't have any more cancer. But what an impossible premise!

All men of good will admit today that these environmental hazards pose serious threats to health. But the job of eliminating them from the world we live in is impossibly immense. No government has made even a token start on such a job. Nor is there any assurance that, with the best will in the world and all the money that can be poured into the effort, any government will succeed in protecting us from the millions of environmental toxins to which our present technological society exposes us.

# CHAPTER 10

# Vitamin A for Fighting Infections and Improving Health In Old Age

In 1973 THE federal Food and Drug Administration decided, for no good reason, to limit the amount of certain vitamins and minerals that could be sold in one tablet or capsule. Since the official daily recommendation for vitamin A is 5,000 units, they decided that the general public should be protected from getting even a bit too much of this vitamin. So the F.D.A. proposed limiting all vitamin A supplements to no more than 5,000 units. It's perfectly obvious that anyone wanting to take more than this would only have to take two capsules or three in order to get more than 5,000 units, but apparently the F.D.A. pundits did not figure this out.

Speaking on this subject in the pages of *Medical Tribune* Dr. Frederick Klenner, a North Carolina general practitioner who specialized in vitamin treatment of all his patients, said, "These proposed safety regulations by the F.D.A. would indeed limit the freedom of the people, since each individual has the inalienable right to make his own decisions regarding his own person . . . There is very little chance of damage to humans from ingesting vitamin A. I have one patient with ichthyosis (a skin disease) who has taken 200,000 units of vitamin A daily for over ten years just to keep his skin within normal texture limits. No toxicity. I have taken 75,000 units of vitamin A up to 150,000 units daily for the past 25 years. No toxicity.

"I recommend to my patients who drive to take at least 50,000 units of vitamin A daily to improve their night vision. Many traffic deaths could be averted by taking not only vitamin A but also vitamin B1 (200 milligrams) and vitamin C (two grams) every hundred miles of driving."

Dr. Klenner's reference to the scaly skin condition, ichthyosis, demonstrates that individual requirements for vitamins may vary greatly. This patient obviously needs this much vitamin A just to keep his skin in the same comfortable, reasonably healthy condition the rest of us find normal. Night blindness is certainly a disorder that affects many of us. We will cover this subject fully in another chapter. Incidentally, so great an uproar was raised over the F.D.A.'s proposal to limit the content of vitamin supplements that they put the plan on the back burner. However, it still surfaces from time to time when the drug industry and the Medical Establishment decide that too many people are taking their health into their own hands.

A 1974 experiment in Thailand demonstrated some of the unexpected effects of a serious vitamin A deficiency. Laboratory rats, kept in a constant state of vitamin A deficiency, lost their appetites and had to be force-fed. They lost weight. Certain cells in the lining of their intestines deteriorated. Deposits of a foreign compound, porphyrin, in the space around their eyes, matted hair, changes in the lining of the windpipe and the salivary glands, crippled legs and peculiar movements afflicted these vitamin A deficient animals.

"Vitamin A Deficiencies Kill Children Worldwide" is a headline over an Associated Press Dispatch, October 21, 1984. It describes the work of Dr. Alfred Sommer of the Johns Hopkins School of Hygiene and Public Health who completed a study of thousands of children in Indonesia. He estimated that vitamin A deficiency causes an estimated 25 percent of all childhood deaths in developing countries, killing up to 10 million children each year. Scientists do not know exactly why lack of vitamin A should cause deaths from many diseases, as well as causing blindness.

It may be that the immune systems of these deficient children are weakened by not having enough of this fat soluble vitamin to fight off many serious diseases. Lack of vitamin A is known to cause drying of various tissues such as those of the eyes, the digestive tract and the urinary tract. This may allow microbes easy entrance, since this naturally moist protective shield is gone due to the vitamin deficiency. These children were not seriously deficient in vitamin A. But unfortunately it seems that even a slight deficiency in this nutrient can have grave consequences.

Crohn's Disease is an unpleasant and dangerous disorder of part of the excretory tract. It generally produces chronic diarrhea, cramps, pain, fever, lack of appetite and weight loss. *The British Medical Journal* reported in 1979 that 30 patients with Crohn's Disease were put on diets from which all refined carbohydrates were eliminated. The results were encouraging. *The Lancet* reported on one patient who found complete relief from Crohn's Disease within several days of adding vitamin A supplements to her diet.

In 1980 Dr. Eli Sifter of Albert Einstein College of Medicine in New York reported that mice deprived of vitamin A develop stomach ulcers. In his experiments he found also that such dangerous toxins as radiation and toxic chemicals can, to some extent, be protected against by increasing the body's stores of vitamin A. The doses of the vitamin that are necessary are "in the safe range," he says. In 1980 an editorial in *The Lancet* reminded its physician readers that lack of vitamin A can cause symptoms of distress in the respiratory system, the salivary glands, the pancreas and the prostate gland.

In 1982 a Central American researcher reported that low levels of vitamin A are linked to iron deficiency anemia in that part of the world. Surveys have shown that 20 to 30 percent of all rural children with anemia have blood levels of vitamin A far below normal. It seems there is plenty of iron in their diets, but it cannot be utilized without vitamin A. Giving vitamin A supplements to some of the children resulted in normal levels of the trace mineral iron in the blood of most of them. The recommendation is to take vitamin A supplements in addition if any iron deficiency does not respond to iron supplements.

In 1983 the publication *Science* reported on two physicians from Dartmouth-Hitchcock Medical Center who gave arthritic laboratory rats daily doses of a synthetic relative of vitamin A and found that it reduced the inflammation and reduced the production of a destructive enzyme which is involved in rheumatic disorders.

The immune system is that totality of body defenses which protects us from any outside enemy such as bacteria, viruses, foreign proteins, surgery, burns and so on. A further responsibility of vitamin A is to protect the immune system. In 1973, *Medical World News* reported on experiments by Dr. Benjamin Cohen of Massachusetts General Hospital who found that vitamin A stimulated his laboratory animals' "immune response"—that is, it gave them far more capability to withstand diseases and other potential health disasters.

He injected several groups of mice with virulent bacteria and gave some of the injected mice immense doses of vitamin A. Those animals which got no vitamin A died within 24 hours. The animals treated with vitamin A developed severe infection for the first three hours, but by the fifth hour Dr. Cohen could find no trace of any of the harmful bacteria in their blood. Dr. Cohen explained that people taking cortisone drugs are at risk of serious infections because this drug inactivates the immune system. He suggests that patients who must take this powerful drug should also be taking vitamin A which would help to protect them from infections.

Old age is a form of stress. Cancer takes a high toll in those age brackets. Cells are worn out. Resistance is low. Nutrition is very often inadequate. Meals may be skimpy and planned with little attention to vitamin needs. Many surveys have shown that the diets of older folks are often grossly lacking in vitamin A. For example, a study was done in 1971 at three homes for the aged. These happen to be in Switzerland but such establishments tend to be the same the world over. All of the 38 subjects studied were getting less than 85 percent of the recommended daily amount of vitamin A. Four of the guests were getting less than 1,200 units daily whereas the RDA is 5,000 units. In only one home were meals supplying the basic level of 5,000 units of vitamin A. Many of the guests were not eating all of the meals they were served, so they probably got very little of this important vitamin. The same was true of vitamin C which is also helpful in maintaining the immune system.

If you are caring for an older person, make sure the meals you serve are well-balanced in regard to all the vitamins and make sure the food is in a form the older folks can eat (puréed or chopped if there is difficulty in chewing). As added insurance, insist on a well-balanced complete vitamin and mineral capsule every day, containing ample vitamin A along with the other essential nutrients. If swallowing large tablets is difficult, such supplements are available in liquid form and may be given in milk, fruit juice or other beverages.

# CHAPTER 11

# Vitamin A May Prevent Acne and Other Skin Disorders

A UNIVERSITY OF PENNSYLVANIA dermatologist declared in 1974 that acne, the curse of teenagers, is not just very common, but actually afflicts 100 percent of American teenagers. Dr. Albert Kligman said that one should not speak of young people with or without acne. It's just a question of whether they have a mild or acute form, he said. They all have it.

Acne begins when the oily substance sebum is secreted into a skin cell. The sebum dries and becomes horny and infected. A small head of pus appears, crowned by a "blackhead." Doctors call these "comedones." Teenagers call them "pimples." If these are pressed out inexpertly the infection spreads to neighboring cells which begin to develop blackheads. The body tries to cover the whole mess with a layer of skin which causes the infection to fester, then drain, leaving a scar.

Dr. Kligman and his colleagues at the University don't speculate on what causes acne. They do use a synthetic vitamin A preparation to treat it. It is called retinoic acid, given in the form of a salve. It produces first redness, peeling and more pimples than before. After about ten weeks the peeling and redness disappear and so, in many cases, do the skin manifestations of acne.

Vitamin A appears to be an appropriate substance for use in any skin condition, for part of its job is to nourish the skin, as well as all the linings of things in the body.

The Pennsylvania doctors sometimes also give vitamin A by mouth in massive doses for a short time only, checking carefully on any indications of overdosage.

Two West German physicians have found that vitamin A acid (one form of the vitamin) is effective against acne. They treated 80 patients between the ages of 19 and 25 with this preparation in the form of a cream or jelly. Applied once a day for nine weeks, the vitamin A reduced the number of pimples by 90 percent.

Dr. Lendon Smith, popular pediatrician, says this of acne in his book *Feed Yourself Right,* "Dermatologists are taught that food has nothing to do with acne, but many of them and all the rest of the world know that 'you eat it today and wear it tomorrow.' Acne is aggravated by foods . . . blood sugar fluctuations will aggravate acne and will feed the germs that cause the infected pustules." He says he has used high doses of vitamin A on acne, hyperkeratosis, psoriasis and warts. Remember he is checking closely on those "high doses" to prevent any unpleasant side effects. He says also that the trace mineral zinc is useful in preventing and treating skin disorders, especially when it is used in conjunction with vitamin A. Vitamin E also helps to strengthen treatment with vitamin A.

In 1979 the National Cancer Institute reported on an experiment giving high doses of a synthetic relative of vitamin A to patients with extreme forms of acne resistant to all other methods of treatment. One of the N.C.I. physicians commented that experiments done in 1943 had shown the same good results. Dr. John Strauss of the University of Iowa has shown that the same vitamin A drug stops the flow of sebaceous material which is part of the cause of acne.

Dr. Carl C. Pfeiffer in his book *Zinc and Other Micro-Nutrients* describes experiments with zinc and vitamin A which were successful in controlling this skin ailment only when zinc was added to the vitamin A. He suggests 25,000 units of vitamin A daily for acne victims. *Medical World News* reported in 1974 on treatment of ichthyosis (a scaly skin condition) with massive doses of the vitamin A relative, retinoic acid. Two young children with this condition responded rapidly when treated with ointment containing the drug. A University of Miami dermatologist stated that treatment with the vitamin A salve is "probably the only useful treatment we now have for ichthyosis."

In 1973 *The New York State Journal of Medicine* reported successful use of synthetic vitamin A on psoriasis. The National Institutes of Health reported in 1976 that they had treated a number of serious skin disorders including Darier's Disease, Pityriasis Rubra Pilaris and Nevus Comedonicus with the vitamin A "drug" and got excellent results in all cases. Lichen planus is another skin disorder which responds fairly well to vitamin A treatment, according to Dr. Roger W. Pearson, a Chicago dermatologist.

*Nutrition Almanac* lists the following skin disorders that have showed improvement when treated with vitamin A preparations: abcesses, acne, athlete's foot, bed sores, boils, carbuncles, dermatitis, dry skin, eczema, impetigo, psoriasis, shingles, ulcers, warts. Rudolph Ballentine, M.D. in his book *Diet and Nutrition,* says "All the coverings and linings of the body are made up of tough, resilient sheath of several layers of cells called 'epithelium' . . . When the skin becomes unhealthy with, for example, the build-up of squamous cells that plug the pores, then there is an accumulation of oils and the resulting infection of these clogged pores is called 'acne.' Both unhealthy epithelium and an increased susceptibility to infection can be related to vitamin A deficiency and, not surprisingly, vitamin A has been found to improve acne.

"Teenagers . . . are a group whose diet is often deficient in vitamin A, but acne may not be due to a simple dietary deficiency of it. Zinc is necessary for the stored vitamin A in the liver to be released into the blood, and in the treatment of acne, zinc has been even more effective than vitamin A."

Dr. Carlton Fredericks wrote in his book *Eat Well, Get Well, Stay Well,* "Vitamin A in doses of 10,000 units daily has helped to control acne, but the medical nutritionist may wish to employ more . . . Vitamin A can be toxic, of course, but so can anything in overdoses—even water. So don't be astonished if your medical nutritionist takes you up to 100,000 units of vitamin A daily. He will monitor you for signs of toxicity, for they are reversible, when expertly managed." We discuss the potential toxicity of vitamin A in another chapter of this book.

# CHAPTER 12

# Vitamin A and the Health of Your Eyes

AN EYE DISEASE called xerophthalmia causes blindness in five to ten million children in the world every year. It has only one cause—deficiency in Vitamin A. A report from the Helen Keller Foundation in 1983 was written by Dr. Alfred Sommer, an ophthalmologist who is medical adviser to the Foundation. Research in Indonesia during ten years of study on this disease found that, year after year, it afflicts one percent of all the Indonesian people.

The name of the disease means "Dry Eye." It is rare in our country. It causes a greasy, dry cornea of the eye which gradually becomes denuded of its epithelium or skin. Tear glands and the whites of the eyes are also affected. Lack of tears causes extreme dryness in the eye. Each year in four Far Eastern countries an estimated five million pre-school children develop the disease. The worldwide total may be twice that number. Because of their poor nutritional status many of these children die. Of the ones who survive, 10 percent develop involvement of the eye cornea associated with permanent vision loss. Half of these children become blind.

The only effective preventive measure for these little ones is to give the children a high potency vitamin A capsule every few months at a cost of about two cents apiece. In Indonesia the Helen Keller Foundation has distributed fourteen and a half million capsules and has started training programs for health care workers there.

Although this blinding disease is supposed to be rare in our country, we must point out that every nutritional survey done in past years has demonstrated that large numbers of Americans, children and adults, do not get even the basic recommended amount of vitamin A. Since our physicians probably do not expect to find this rare disease in our country, it seems likely that many cases go undiagnosed.

The U.S. National Academy of Sciences National Research Council announced in their May, 1986 *News Report* that they are cooperating with the U.S. Agency for Development in studying the effects of vitamin A deficiency and the use of vitamin A supplements in Far Eastern countries. They have appointed a Sub Committee on Vitamin A Deficiency Prevention and Control which will engage in a three-year study of the problem.

Enough Americans suffer from a condition called "Dry Eye" that drug companies offer for sale several brands of synthetic "tears"—over-the-counter preparations that help to retain eye moisture. The medical literature on this subject does not mention vitamin A, but it seems possible that lack of vitamin A might be causing this condition just as it produces such symptoms among the malnourished, vitamin A deficient children of the Far East.

Why is vitamin A so extremely important for our eyes? The human retina contains a substance called "visual purple" which is essential for us to see. It can be manufactured in your eyes *only if enough vitamin A is present there*. Visual purple is used up helping you to see in bright light. It is reconstituted in your eyes after dark while you are asleep, but only if some vitamin A is present in your eyes.

A day at the beach in bright sunlight may use up so much of this compound that you may have trouble with glare driving home after dark. When you get home, you may have trouble finding the keyhole or even the path to the door because your eyes will temporarily have lost their ability to see in the dark.

Up until 100 years or so ago most human beings lived each day by rising at or about dawn and going to bed when night fell, winter and summer. Candles, open fires and oil lamps gave off very little light for seeing after dark. So there was always plenty of time after dark to regenerate the visual purple lost during the day.

Today we live exposed to extremely bright lights for perhaps 18 to 20 hours a day, if we stay up late watching television. We all extend the daylight with electric lights during winter. We pore over books, desk work and papers with brilliant reading lamps to light our way. We walk on streets brilliantly lighted day and night, where spotlights play and electric signs glitter.

Our young people go to "light shows" where they watch flashing lights of many colors in a dazzling array of electrical splendor which would challenge the best eyes in the world to survive this kind of punishment. Our actors, musicians, cameramen and speakers before audiences must expose their eyes to bright spotlights and footlights for long periods of time. What is all this doing to that precious substance in our eyes—visual purple—which is destroyed by light and can be renewed only in total darkness and then only if enough vitamin A is present?

The eye is one of the first organs to demonstrate vitamin A deficiency. Inability to see in the dark (after your eyes become accustomed to the darkness) is one of the first symptoms of deficiency in vitamin A. This nutrient also stimulates the secretion of fluid in the eye. Lack of fluid can result in a cornea which becomes dry and hard. It is then very vulnerable to infection from a scratch, for example.

It was reported in 1974 that protein is an important part of the diet too, since vitamin A is not stored very successfully in the liver unless there is enough protein in the diet. So a diet which contains enough vitamin A but not enough protein can also result in eye troubles which may lead to blindness. Keep in mind those surveys which have shown that many millions of Americans are not getting even the bare necessity of vitamin A and possibly many of these are also eating diets low in protein.

A popular magazine in 1965 told the story of one young man troubled with poor eyesight after dark. Driving at night he could barely see road signs, pedestrians or the edge of the road. At the movies he had to wait for 15 minutes before his eyes adjusted to the dark so he could find a seat. His diet was probably typical of many teenagers: coffee and a doughnut for breakfast, hamburgers and dessert for lunch, meat, potatoes, dessert and coffee for dinner. His daily vitamin A intake was about 1,000 units or only one-fifth of the recommended level.

He was given 25,000 units of vitamin A in fish liver oil and told to eat lots of foods rich in vitamin A: liver, whole milk, cheese, fresh fruits, spinach, raw carrots, squash, sweet potatoes and so on. Within ten days his night blindness had improved. Within two months it was normal. Many people on greatly restricted reducing diets are probably eating meals so low in vitamin A that they may be risking eventual serious eye problems.

*Federal World News* reported in 1971 that massive doses of vitamin A have been used in the treatment of a very serious eye disease, retinitis pigmentosa. This condition is hereditary, with slowly progressive blindness. Two patients with clouded vision from this condition were given 200,000 units of vitamin A by a team of doctors at the National Institute of Arthritis and Metabolic Diseases in Washington. Hours after they took the vitamin, their vision began to clear. Within a day they were seeing well. The protective effect of this one dose of vitamin A lasted for three months! One patient who started this treatment had relatively good vision seven years later. The other patient had since died of heart failure.

This eye condition which was hitherto considered incurable affects many children who have great difficulty absorbing the fat soluble vitamins. Vitamins A and E are fat soluble. We wonder whether the heart failure of one of the above patients may have been due to simple inability to absorb vitamin E. Dr. Peter Goursa, who treated the patients, feels that his success may indicate that vitamin A deficiency is the cause of most types of retinal degeneration.

One added note on vitamin A. Back in 1975 medical journals were reporting case of liver cancers in women on the oral contraceptive, The Pill. In *The Lancet* a British physician raised the question of whether this may be due to the fact that contraceptives decrease the amount of vitamin A in the liver. Dr. Isabel Gal stated that it is well known that hormones such as The Pill influence the way the body uses vitamin A. It is also known, she said, that cancer is a disorder of the process of cell division, and vitamin A participates in this process. She asks if a deficiency in this vitamin is caused by The Pill and if the woman's diet contains little vitamin A, is it not possible that just lack of this nutrient may be one cause of such tumors.

# CHAPTER 13

# How Much Vitamin A
# Is Too Much?

IN MANY ARTICLES on vitamins in the general media these
days you are reminded that vitamin A and vitamin D are
toxic in large amounts. You are told you must be very careful
about taking vitamin supplements containing these nutrients,
since you may poison yourself. Usually the impression is
given of hundreds of thousands of people sickening or dying
from vitamin A poisoning every year.

In 1970 a team of researchers at the U.S. Department of
Agriculture combed world medical and scientific literature
and uncovered all accounts of overdosages of vitamin A up
to that time. Fifteen cases of chronic adult hypervitaminosis
(too much vitamin A), 12 of which occurred in the United
States, had been reported. One of these people took 100,000
units every day for three and a half years before she reported
unpleasant symptoms. A physician tried to see how much
he could take without side effects. He took one million units
daily for about three weeks as an experiment. In other cases
people took too much vitamin A for as long as eight years
before experiencing any unpleasant side effects.

Very young children given doses of 300,000 to 400,000
units daily suffered great distress, some within days, others
not until the massive doses continued for two years. Five
cases in Sweden involved babies given from 7,500 to 10,000
units daily. Vitamin doses are set partly by weight, meaning

that the more you weigh the more you may need. So these were enormous doses for very small children.

Since vitamin A is fat soluble, it is stored in body tissues, chiefly the liver. Excessive amounts are not excreted rapidly as they are with the water soluble vitamins. So there is no need to take a vitamin A supplement every day, if you feel you should be getting more than you are getting in food. Your body probably has most of the vitamin A stored away that you took last week and the week before.

Recently, however, medical literature has produced a number of accounts of overdoses of vitamin A which have caused serious side effects. In 1981 a three-year old child was taking daily doses of 200,000 units of vitamin A because her parents wanted to protect her from winter colds. She was hospitalized with itching skin, dehydration, a severe tremor, and damage to kidneys and liver. Doctors assured her parents that she would recover from all the damage shortly after these high doses were discontinued as is usual in these cases.

In 1982 a 16-year old boy had been taking 50,000 units of vitamin A daily in an effort to cure his acne. He had headache, nausea, vomiting, stiff neck and dry skin. *The Journal of the American Medical Association,* reporting this case, pointed out also that a 79-year old man who had been taking 50,000 units of vitamin A for 17 years had suffered no signs or symptoms of too much vitamin A, although, at autopsy, his liver was found to have stored away an enormous amount of this vitamin. So individuals differ in their reaction to large doses.

An article in *Nutrition Reviews* (October, 1982) described several cases of massive overdoses of vitamin A over long periods of time. In one case the patient showed none of the usual symptoms except a liver disorder which was relieved when he was put on a diet with very little vitamin A. Another man, a vegetarian, took 100,000 units of vitamin A daily for ten years. He developed hepatitis, along with headache, dermatitis, confusion and a disorder of his body's use of calcium. Says *Reviews,* "These two cases may represent only the tip of the iceberg . . . we may be on the verge of an epidemic of vitamin A toxicity.'' The author believes that the publicity given to the potential of vitamin A and carotene in preventing cancer may be responsible for people taking too much of this vitamin.

The synthetic relatives of vitamin A such as retinoic acid (a prescription drug) which has been used in the treatments we have outlined in earlier chapters of this book, has also been shown to produce some severe side effects when it is given in extremely large doses. Said the *New York Times,* commenting on Accutane, one synthetic form of vitamin A used to treat severe cases of acne, "By all accounts Accutane is a miracle drug for people with severe cystic acne . . . Until recently, treatment involved long-term use of antibiotics and salves . . . Accutane has extraordinarily beneficial effects on skin tissue by combatting virtually all the mechanisms that create acne.''

But a number of reports have come in revealing birth defects in the children of young women who have been using this drug. When the ''drug'' (for that's what it is) was put on the market in 1982 there were clear warnings on the label and accompanying brochure that it should not be taken by pregnant women. In fact, the recommendation was that a pregnancy test should be given before the drug was administered.

In 1986 reports of retinal problems appeared in patients taking the drug for long periods of time. Since an estimated 700,000 acne patients are at present using the drug this suggests great caution in its use. Quite recently, a new ''tanning'' drug was introduced which contains another manufactured form of a vitamin A relative called Canthaxanthin. People who feel they must have ''a good tan'' every summer, but are rightfully afraid of too much exposure to the summer sun, have been taking this preparation. It has been used for several years in Europe and it produces a golden color on the skin which is apparently considered attractive. Although search of medical literature in 1984 turned up no information on unpleasant or dangerous side effects, we uncovered a note in *The Journal of the American Medical Association* in 1983 suggesting that women taking the suntan pill may develop menstrual problems. It was suggested that such problems may occur in women who are also eating diets that contain large amounts of carotene or vitamin A.

There seems to be good reason to avoid preparations in which the natural base of the compound (vitamin A or carotene) has been tinkered with in various ways to make it into a drug—something that does not exist as such in nature.

Two final comments on vitamin A. *The American Journal of Clinical Nutrition* reported in 1972 a study of autopsies on 372 people in four different states. The physicians found that liver stores of vitamin A "may be low in 12 to 37 percent of the population groups studied." To put it another way, more than a third of Americans may be at risk regarding their vitamin A status.

In 1976 E. Cheraskin, M.D., D.M.D. reported on a study conducted among a group of more than one thousand professional people—dentists and their wives—who had been cooperating with him in such studies for seveal years. A tabulation of vitamin A intake with general health and absence of symptoms of disease seemed to show that approximately 33,000 units of vitamin A daily from foods and/or from supplements are the "ideal" allowance. The author said, "It is recognized that the 'ideal' is non-existent as a theoretic end point since there is biochemical individuality and because the art of measuring leaves much to be desired. Nevertheless, the technique utilized here provides a mechanism and a goal not previously considered."

So the sensible thing to do, it seems, is to get as much vitamin A and carotene as you reasonably can in your diet. Don't eat liver every day. Don't drink quarts of carrot juice every day. But don't neglect your diet and think you can get all the vitamin A and carotene you need from supplements. If you prefer to take vitamin A supplements considerably larger than the RDA, don't take them every day. Twenty thousand units of vitamin A stored in your liver will keep you healthy. Read labels of baby food products carefully. Several of these contain levels that may be two and half times the RDA for babies which is 1,400 units. If you use these products, vary the vegetables you give from day to day, so the baby doesn't get too much vitamin A.

# Vitamin B Is . . .

A *complex* of water-soluble vitamins and vitamin-like substances including thiamine, riboflavin, niacin, pyridoxine, pantothenic acid, biotin, folic acid, vitamin B12, choline, inositol, para-amino-benzoic acid.

*Responsible* chiefly for the health and maintenance of nerves, eyes, digestion and skin, as well as the processing of carbohydrate, fat and protein, appetite, growth, production of hormones and digestive juices, prevention of anemia, maintenance of sex glands, sebaceous glands, bone marrow, and many more complex body functions.

*Present* in most abundance in liver, kidney, wholegrains, all seeds, nuts, dairy products, eggs, bran, wheat germ, brewers yeast, lentils, beans, peas, soybeans, leafy green vegetables.

*Safe* in very large amounts. Because the B vitamins are water soluble they are not stored to any extent in the body so whatever is not needed is rapidly excreted. However, a certain balance is advisable among the B vitamins, since they are closely related. So it is best to get plenty of all of them in food and supplements, rather than taking large amounts of just one or two.

*Destroyed* in food preparation by light, steam, long cooking, high temperatures, long storage and so forth. Destroyed by many antagonists in the form of drugs and chemicals, also by alkalinity in the stomach caused by taking antacids.

*Required* in very small amounts, according to the official Recommended Dietary Allowance which is on page 24 of this book.

*Available* in low or high potencies, in one-a-day supplements or individual supplements.

# CHAPTER 14

# Introducing the
# B Complex
# of Vitamins

VITAMIN A IS easy to understand. It comes in bright yellow and green foods. It's most abundant in fish liver oils. Vitamin C exists in fresh, crisp fruits and vegetables. It's important for many things in our bodies and many of us take it in large doses to saturate our tissues with it.

But what about the B vitamins? How does it happen we always speak of them as a "complex" and what does that mean? How many of them are there and are they all equally important or can we do without some of them? How are they discovered and why do scientists keep telling us that important supplements like brewers yeast and liver may contain more B vitamins than they have yet discovered?

Biochemists call them "the B Complex," because you do not find one of them in food or in a living tissue without the others being somewhere near at hand. They go together. They complement one another. They help one another out. If one of them is a little short, for some reason, another may be able to take up part of the work the first would have done, perhaps substituting for it in some complicated physiological function.

Vitamins do not suddenly appear in a laboratory labelled "vitamin B1" or "vitamin B2." The biochemist does not pick up a cup of brewers yeast, stir it around a little and decide that the big pieces of yeast must be vitamin B1 and the little pieces vitamin B2. Until about 50 years ago no one knew there were such things as vitamins, although scientists and physicians knew, in general, that there were some substances in certain foods which could prevent certain deficiency diseases. If these substances were destroyed by heat or soaking or exposure to light, the disease would not be prevented, no matter how much of the depleted food was eaten. This was about all the early nutrition scientists had to go on, and they made plenty of mistakes.

Until about 1926 scientists thought that vitamin B was a single element. Then several researchers showed that there were at least two kinds—one that could be destroyed by heat and another which was not destroyed by heat. Soon nutrition scientists in many parts of the world began to isolate different parts of these substances and, of course, called them by whatever name they happened to think appropriate. Vitamin B2 was called riboflavin in the USA and lactoflavine in Europe, because it is abundant in milk. For a long time it was also called Vitamin G.

What is now called pyridoxine has been labeled Factor Y, Factor I, Factor H, adermin and Factor B6. Other B vitamins were discovered and identified in the same way without, at first, much appreciation of the fact that they were all related, all part of one complex of vitamins. A B vitamin has been defined as "an organic substance which acts catalytically in all living cells and which is essential for the nutrition of higher animals."

By "catalytically" we mean that the B vitamins are involved all together in many of the very complex cellular functions inside the body. One B vitamin, biotin, is known to take part in at least 15 or 20 processes which involve many different enzymes. So it is not important for scientists to know only that lack of biotin brings about certain symptoms. They want to know, too, exactly what biotin does to the body to prevent these symptoms. Work is going forward in hundreds of laboratories all over the world, for scientists have only begun to untangle and understand these mysteries.

It may be many years before all the complexities are understood, or perhaps they never will be.

But we do know, basically, that the B vitamins are a complex, which means that they are closely related to one another, that they work together and they occur, generally speaking in the same groups of foods. Here are their names and some of their varying functions.

*Thiamine,* also called vitamin B1, prevents beriberi, a disease which was widespread and took many lives in the East when rice was first milled to eliminate the coating and germ of the rice in which thiamine is concentrated. Polished or refined rice was prettier and easier to cook. No one knew of the terrible health consequences which would follow. Thiamine is essential for proper nerve function. Its deficiency brings neuritis, paralysis, atrophy of muscles, edema or swelling, fatigue, loss of weight and appetite, depression, "pins and needles." Symptoms disappear almost magically when thiamine is given.

Deficiency in *Riboflavin,* also called vitamin B2, can bring a variety of symptoms: inflammation of mouth tissues, sores at the corners of the mouth, visual fatigue, a "sandy" feeling in the eyes, inability to endure bright lights. Seborrhea, a scaly skin disorder, is also a symptom of riboflavin deficiency. Many people today have such symptoms without knowing that they could easily prevent them by getting enough riboflavin. It's hard to get enough of this B vitamin from food if you slight the dairy foods—milk, yogurt and cheese, for it is most plentiful there. Liver, kidney and brewers yeast are other abundant sources.

*Niacin,* also called vitamin B3, is responsible for the health of skin, nerves and digestive tract—a big order for a substance needed only in milligrams. Pellagra is the deficiency disease when niacin is lacking. It produces three conditions: diarrhea, dermatitis and dementia—death if not treated. Today many psychiatrists and physicians are using niacin in massive doses to treat schizophrenia and other serious mental conditions.

*Pyridoxine* (Vitamin B6) has been found to be essential for many things that contribute to good health. Lack of pyridoxine causes anemia, skin disorders, nerve disorders including convulsions, mouth disorders and seborrhea. This is another B vitamin which has been found to be helpful in large doses in fighting mental illness and many other conditions. It is most plentiful in all seeds and wholegrains, wheat germ, bran, brewers yeast.

Lack of *Biotin* causes lassitude, lack of appetite, depression, muscle pains, scaling dermatitis, sometimes nausea, anemia, changes in heart rhythm. It occurs most plentifully in all those foods in which other B vitamins are abundant: nuts, wholegrain cereals, liver, eggs, brewers yeast.

*Choline* is not regarded as a B vitamin officially. In animals it protects against abnormalities in pregnancy and lactation. Lack of it brings anemia, heart and circulatory disease and muscle weakness. Many recent experiments have shown that it is important for the body to use fats properly.

*Pantothenic acid* was discovered by Dr. Roger J. Williams. It is involved in many enzyme systems in the body. Lack of it can bring apathy, depression, instability of heart action, digestive disease, abdominal pains, increased susceptibility to infection, impaired function of the adrenal glands which protect us against all kinds of stress, and certain nerve disorders including "pins and needles" and muscle weakness.

*Vitamin B12* prevents pernicious anemia, a kind of anemia that always proved fatal until it was treated with lots of liver which is the best source of vitamin B12. In this extremely serious disease nerves are involved and eventually the spinal cord. This vitamin is not present in fruits, vegetables and grains, so it must come from foods of animal origin only which is important for total vegetarians to remember.

*Folic acid* is closely related to vitamin B12. Lack of it also produces anemia which can be fatal. Some symptoms of deficiency are: intestinal disturbances, inflammation of mouth tissues and gums, gland disturbances, sprue and various blood disorders. It is plentiful in liver, green leafy vegetables, wheat germ and bran, brewers yeast, beans, lentils and other seed foods.

*Para-amino-benzoic acid (PABA)* is considered to be a vitamin by some scientists, though not recognized as such officially. It is an excellent protector against too much sun and is used in suntan lotions. It exists in the same foods in which all the B vitamins are found.

*Inositol,* not officially called a vitamin, is essential, along with choline, to make lecithin, that excellent emulsifier which may help to render cholesterol harmless.

Workers in other countries call several other substances B vitamins—Vitamin B15 and B17. These are substances which occur along with the other B vitamins. Ample demonstration that these are essential for life and health will undoubtedly result in their being classified as vitamins by our official classification experts.

The one lesson to be learned from studying the vitamins is the lesson our food technologists have never learned and apparently are incapable of learning. Nature likes things whole. Nothing worthwhile is achieved in nature with fragments. Removing all the B vitamins from our wholegrain cereals and flour then returning only bits of three of them is probably the worst possible thing we could do, for the imbalances thus created are complex. All the B vitamins work together.

One food may contain a bit more of this or that B vitamin, but, in general, they all exist most abundantly in these kinds of foods: liver and all organ meats, eggs, milk, cheese and yogurt, meat, fish, poultry, green leafy vegetables, wholegrains, seeds, nuts, legumes, wheat germ and bran and brewers yeast. A diet consisting of just these foods is a complete diet, if you add fruits and other vegetables for their vitamin A and C content. These foods are also the richest sources of protein which is what we are made of and which we must have in quantity for good health.

As soon as you begin to dilute such a diet with foods made from white refined flour, refined cereals and white sugar, you lose quantities of B vitamins as well as the precious minerals that accompany them. In nature the B vitamins are responsible for processing carbohydrates. By removing them from carbohydrate-rich foods like cereals and sugar, we invite nutritional disaster. One-half of all food eaten in our country consists of these depleted substances.

The B vitamin complex must be kept and eaten whole as it occurs in the excellent foods listed above. Make them the backbone of your diet. And when you buy a food supplement, make certain it contains all the B vitamins as well as yeast, liver, wheat germ or some other rich source, so that you will also be getting those B vitamins and related substances which have not as yet been discovered.

Here is a story which indicates how the B vitamins can be used by innovative and creative doctors to ease some of the problems of old folks. There are at present in our country about 20 million people over the age of 65. All of us will eventually attain this age, if we're lucky and cherish our health. Why not try to guarantee that life after 65 will be pleasant, rewarding and free from the mental and physical problems that torment so many of today's older folks?

Dr. Abram Hoffer, distinguished Canadian psychiatrist who successfully treats patients with massive doses of several vitamins, in addition to trace minerals and other therapy, tells how he brought his aging mother back to excellent mental and physical health by the simple expedient of suggesting that she take large doses of the B vitamin niacin, because she was suffering from arthritis, incipient blindness and failing memory.

He knew, he said—every doctor knows—that nothing can be done for such complaints of the aged. Senility and disability come and the only thing to do is to ignore it and keep the patient as happy as possible. The niacin could not hurt his mother, he knew, and she would feel her physician son had tried to help.

Six weeks later she wrote him a lively letter saying, "My vision is okay, my arthritis is gone and I feel marvelous!" Today, said Dr. Hoffer, "she is 86. Her mind is just as keen as it ever was and she spends her time writing her memoirs." She had been taking 3 grams a day of niacin— 3,000 milligrams.

An article in the *Journal of the American Geriatrics Society* some time ago reported on a British experiment in which 254 elderly patients were tested for their blood levels of the B vitamins and vitamin C. These folks suffered from Parkinson's disease, congestive heart failure, asthma, anemia, hardening of the arteries, bone fractures from falls, bronchitis, high blood pressure, kidney disorders, eye troubles, alcoholism and many other degenerative conditions which are commonplace among older people. Some of the patients were found to have pellagra and scurvy, disorders resulting from lack of B vitamins and vitamin C. All of them were confused.

They were given a concentrate liquid solution of the B vitamins and vitamin C. It contained 20 milligrams of vitamin B1 (thiamine), 2 milligrams of vitamin B2 (riboflavin), 80 milligrams of vitamin B3 (niacin), 2 milligrams of vitamin B6 (pyridoxine), and 40 milligrams of vitamin C. This liquid formula was given three times a day. In some cases twice this much was given three times a day, presumably with meals.

In almost every case the mental confusion disappeared completely and the patients were discharged as normal. One 66-year-old woman with hardening of the arteries and Parkinson's disease was discharged after only two weeks, her mental confusion cleared and the other conditions much improved. In an 88-year-old woman all mental alertness was restored in one month.

An 89-year-old woman suffering from anemia, dehydration and confusion went home mentally well. After two weeks an 81-year-old woman with bronchitis and mental confusion was able to go home in good shape much improved. A 75-year-old woman in "an acute confusional state" and congestive heart failure went home two weeks later. A 68-year-old alcoholic went home, mentally well, after two weeks of treatment.

Two aged women with pellagra were able to go home in two weeks. A 95-year-old woman in great pain if she was touched, and with bruise marks over her entire body, was given one gram of vitamin C (1,000 milligrams) every day for two weeks and went home in good health. A 70-year-old woman had been in a mental hospital for attempted suicide. She had bacterial endocarditis which was treated with antibiotics. She was confused and lethargic and had many bruises as well as painful legs. She was given one gram of vitamin C daily and in three weeks felt so well she wanted to go home.

During the time this triumph of preventive medicine was going on Dr. M. L. Mitra, who conducted the test asked six of the nursing personnel if they would act as "controls." To his great surprise he found that five of them were deficient in vitamins according to blood tests. They had no suspicion there was anything wrong with their health.

Many of the elderly patients had been put on drugs by their physicians. No allowance was made for the vitamin deficiencies that might result. Diuretics are those drugs given frequently for high blood pressure and other circulatory troubles. These drugs cause excessive urination. They naturally wash out of the body any of the water soluble vitamins which are in the digestive tract at the same time. They destroy minerals in the same way.

The doctors giving the drugs had made no allowance for such terrible losses, so understandably such patients were deficient in the B vitamins and vitamin C which are the water soluble ones. It seems likely that the only thing causing the supposedly irreversible confusion in the patients was vitamin deficiency. Until Dr. Mitra's experiment, no one recognized it. No one did anything about it.

We are not even sure that any of these patients, miraculously rescued from so many of the troubles of old age, were given any of the powerful vitamin preparation to take at home, or if they were given any instructions on how to shop for and prepare a reasonably nutritious diet for themselves, so that they would not succumb to mental confusion and other disabling conditions in the future.

Part of the reason for this, we suspect, is that no one appreciates the difficulties older people have in providing themselves with nourishing food. It's expensive, especially protein food, which is essential, far more expensive than cheaper refined carbohydrates. Older folks have great difficulty shopping for food. If they live some distance from a market they must take a bus or a cab or walk a long distance, carrying a heavy shopping bag on their return trip.

For those who live alone there is little incentive to prepare full course meals. It hardly seems worth the trouble. So they subsist on sandwiches or cereal, cakes or canned food which is easy to buy and easy to prepare. In a modern supermarket it is extremely difficult to buy small enough quantities for only one person. Meat is packaged for a family. Cheese comes in pound packages. Potatoes are bagged in five pound bags, and so on. In the average small apartment there is little room for storage, so frequent trips must be made to make small purchases every few days. In many stores where old folks buy prices are higher since management knows these people cannot go to the other end of town to seek out less expensive food.

If you are caring for the older person in your family or if you have reached the "golden years" yourself, you can work wonders with a nourishing diet, rich in high protein foods, with all the refined carbohydrates eliminated and the kind of vitamin supplements outlined in the story above. As Dr. Hoffer admitted, he did not think any treatment could bolster his aging mother's health and clear up the confusion in her mind. He gave her only one B vitamin and worked a near miracle. Undoubtedly by now he is giving her—and other elderly patients—massive doses of all the water soluble vitamins. That is, all the B vitamins and vitamin C. These are the vitamins in which older folks are most likely to be deficient.

But the fat-soluble ones are important, too—especially vitamin A and E. Vitamin A protects all the linings of things— the respiratory tract, the digestive tract, the reproductive tract and the skin. Recent research has showed it to be a powerful preventive of some kinds of cancer. Vitamin E has been shown by thousands of innovative physicians to be valuable for preventing the circulatory problems which beset us as we age. The mineral calcium is essential as we grow older to protect the health of bones. Dairy products are the best sources: milk, cheese, yogurt, buttermilk. Calcium supplements are available at the health food store, as are all the vitamin supplements mentioned above.

It is cruel and irresponsible to allow our old folks to degenerate into senility and a hundred related kinds of disability when we have the power to prevent many of them with nothing more than a good diet and an abundance of vitamins and minerals. Old age, with all the troubles it brings, is a form of stress. People under stress need more nutrients than those who are not under stress.

We do not know the name of the liquid supplement which Dr. Mitra gave his patients. And it is probably not available in this country. There is no reason why anyone must take just that special preparation. A vitamin is a vitamin, no matter in what form it appears. He probably gave the preparation in liquid form because this would be easier for the old folks to swallow.

You can, of course, find the same potency of vitamins in many preparations, either in tablet form or liquid. Any of these containing the same ingredients in approximately the same amounts would presumably work the same kind of near-magic.

# CHAPTER 15

# Thiamine Prevents Many Painful and Debilitating Disorders

NEAR THE END OF the last century a hideous disease ravaged some areas of the Far East. It attacked the nerves especially, with pain, irritability, depression, loss of memory, intolerance of noise, apathy, insomnia, hypochondria, lack of appetite, digestive complaints, eye disorders, heart ailments, breathlessness, paralysis, edema and many more symptoms serious enough to cause death. Between 1920 and 1929 an average of 17,000 deaths from this disease occurred in Japan alone.

Physicians were baffled. They called the disease beriberi meaning "weakness" in one of the Far East languages. After many years of medical sleuthing, physicians discovered that the disease was common where white rice was the staple food in the diet. Beriberi was caused by deficiency in the B vitamin thiamine which was removed from brown rice when it was milled into white rice. The cure for beriberi is an amount of thiamine which could be put on the point of a pin. But if this is not present in the diet, beriberi will occur. Thiamine is needed for the body to process carbohydrates—starch and sugar. When most of the diet is carbohydrate with no thiamine, this body function is disordered. By now, white rice and many high starch foods in the Far East and in our country are "enriched" with thiamine to prevent this disease.

Strangely enough, beriberi began to show up in 1977 in Japan among teenagers whose diets contained large amounts of soft drinks and other goodies rich in sugar, a carbohydrate. None of these foods contains any thiamine. The young people developed a variety of nervous disorders: loss of tendon power in legs, swollen legs and feet, dilated hearts, heart murmurs, "pins and needles" tingling in extremities. Giving them thiamine and directing them to much more sensible diets cured the disease. In birds and animals scientists can produce extremely serious nerve disorders by just withholding thiamine for a short time. In most cases the damage to nerves is irreparable.

*The American Journal of Clinical Nutrition* had an article in 1980 by two researchers from the Cleveland Clinic describing symptoms in a group of 20 teenagers which correspond closely to those of beriberi victims. Examination showed that all these children were deficient in thiamine. Symptoms were: abdominal or chest pains, sleep disturbances, restlessness, night terrors, personality changes, fatigue, excessive perspiration, lack of appetite and many more.

One 13-year-old boy had violent, unpredictable mood changes for seven years, stomach cramps severe enough to suggest appendicitis, intermittent diarrhea and depression. His father suffered from manic depressive illness. A seven-year-old girl had enlargement of the lymph glands, fever, vomiting, fatigue, stiff neck, restless sleep, loud snoring, constipation, nasal congestion, recurrent fever of unknown cause.

The diets of these children consisted almost entirely of "empty calorie" foods—sugar-laden drinks, pastries, candy, snacks such as potato chips and pretzels. Dr. Derrick Lonsdale, M.B., B.S. said the basic cause was malnutrition brought about by imbalance from the junk foods. He said, "The most dangerous aspect is . . . the carbonated beverages, powdered sweet drinks and fruit drinks . . . I think the record I've seen was 98 gallons of cola in two months . . . the diet is changing the balance of neurological transmission which is the hallmark of the function of the brain and central nervous system . . . the quality and quantity of nutrition can change your behavior.''

Said Raymond J. Shamberger, Ph.D., co-author of the article, ''Access to easily assimilable sweet beverages could represent a modern danger which is insufficiently emphasized in our society and may well be responsible for personality traits and symptomology that are regularly overlooked and considered to be 'the personality of a growing child or adolescent.' ''

An article in *The Journal of Orthomolecular Psychiatry* stated many symptoms of thiamine deficiency are found today among children and adolescents ''but are frequently considered to be the normal behavior of youth and excused as such . . . A vast industry has been built around the cult of sugar and 'soft' drinks are encouraged in excess in preference to 'hard' alcohol. Society condones the huge intake of sugar as a source of 'quick energy' and fails to recognize that it becomes a drug under these circumstances.''

In our country today many popular food products are based on white flour which has not been ''enriched'' with thiamine. Soft drinks, candy and many bakery products contain vast amounts of sugar which must have thiamine to be used normally by the body. But many of the foods contain no thiamine, so every mouthful of such foods increases the body's need for this essential nutrient.

There is an enzyme in raw fish which destroys thiamine. Captive mink fed on nothing but raw fish died of beriberi until owners discovered what was causing the disease. This does not mean that eating an occasional plate of oysters on-the-half shell will produce beriberi. But today many should be aware of too much sashimi (raw fish). Nitrates and sulfites in food are also destructive of thiamine. Nitrates are used as preservatives in many foods, chiefly delicatessen meats. Sulfites have recently been used to keep fresh vegetables crisp at salad bars and on supermarket shelves.

Diuretics (water pills) are also destructive of thiamine.

These are usually given to high blood pressure patients. Any heart patient taking these drugs should be certain to get enough thiamine in meals and supplements to replace that which is excreted. Digestive diseases which also destroy thiamine are colitis, diverticulosis, chronic diarrhea, celiac disease or any other condition that brings chronic diarrhea.

Live raw yeast (baker's yeast) was once given to sick people by doctors because they were told it contains B vitamins. It does, but yeast in which the plant cells are alive and growing needs moisture and warmth for these cells to grow as they do when bread is leavened. Once in the digestive tract they seize whatever nutrients they need to grow and the individual is robbed of these nutrients. When leavened bread is baked the yeast cells are inactivated. In brewers yeast, the live yeast cells have been inactivated and all the B vitamins are there for us to use for good health.

Alcoholics are notoriously deficient in thiamine. Ten to 15 million Americans have classic symptoms of alcoholism. Another ten million Americans are considered "on the verge of alcoholism." Over 30 percent of our suicides are alcoholics. Over 60 percent of county jailings are for alcohol-related crimes. Every ten years 250,000 car accidents are caused by drunken drivers.

Joseph D. Beasley, M.D., a specialist in this field, stated in *Medical Tribune,* January 9, 1986 that the alcohol-related disorder Wernicke-Korsakoff Syndrome, sometimes called "cerebral beriberi," is caused largely by lack of thiamine. And thiamine alone, given orally by mouth or intravenously, can dramatically reverse many of the symptoms and signs. He says that lack of vitamins, and especially of the B vitamins, "plays a primary role in the genesis of nerve symptoms produced by alcoholism."

In 1981 Dr. Carroll M. Leevy stated at a symposium on thiamine that 70 to 80 percent of alcoholics exhibit laboratory and/or clinical manifestations of thiamine deficiency. Deficiency begins early in the history of alcoholism, because alcohol causes excretion of thiamine. Later stages of alcoholism reduce thiamine levels even more, since other nutrients including protein and other B vitamins are also unavailable. In his center for treatment of alcoholics Dr. Leevy gives intravenous injections of thiamine for a week to ten days, and gives the vitamin orally from then on.

Dr. Beasley stated in *Medical Tribune* that a summary prepared by the National Institute of Alcohol Abuse and Alcoholism in 1979 listed the following nutrients that are absent or deficient in most alcoholics at any one time: decrease in zinc, calcium, thiamine, vitamin B12, folic acid, magnesium, potassium, *and an increase in cholesterol and triglycerides*—another kind of fat believed to be very detrimental. A 1978 study, reported in *Clinics in Endocrinology and Metabolism,* showed vitamin B6 deficiency in 75 percent of alcoholics, folic acid deficiency in 65 percent, thiamine deficiency in 60 percent, riboflavin deficiency in 52 percent and B12 deficiency in 15 percent of alcoholics.

Research on the great importance of loss of thiamine due to alcohol produced a movement in 1979 to put the vitamin into all liquor, wine and beer. An editorial in the *New York Times* pointed out that each dollar's worth of thiamine added to alcoholic beverages might save up to seven dollars in nursing home costs, to say nothing of the possibility of saving lives. Caring for victims of Wernicke-Korsakoff Syndrome cost the nation in 1978 some 70 million dollars. The 25-billion dollar alcoholic beverage industry protested that it would be almost impossible to put the vitamin into booze since this would appear to be recommending the beverage as a good source of nutrients which, of course, it is not. The Food and Drug Administration thought up a number of reasons why enriching booze with thiamine would not work out. The National Institute of Alcohol Abuse and Alcoholism suggested instead that alcoholics just take the helpful thiamine in pill form. Another specialist pointed out that alcoholics would probably not agree to take the pills or would just neglect to take them.

Several years ago a probation officer in Cuyahoga Falls,

Ohio, Barbara Reed, became interested in the health of the prisoners in her charge. In her book *Food, Teens and Behavior*, she says, "I discovered that a huge proportion of the people who were getting into trouble were junk food junkies. Many were alcoholics or heavy drinkers and were simultaneously living on booze and sugared snacks . . . If these men and women were living on processed foods and snacks how could their central nervous systems be functioning properly? Finally, if their brains and nerves were malfunctioning, how could one expect them to behave sanely in society?"

Because she was interested in nutrition, she experimented with any of the prisoners who would agree to go on her specified diet and take certain supplements. She says, "I was expected to keep my charges out of the courtroom and any legal way I could find to do that would be fine . . . I began using the diet and encouraging people . . . before long I was using the technique on everybody." Barbara put her charges on the diet to cure low blood sugar—a total ban on sugar, white flour products, chemical additives, caffeine and alcohol. She emphasized the consumption of fresh fruits, vegetables, wholegrains and such lean meats as chicken, veal and fish and plenty of water. She says that "an incredible number" of her charges managed to stay on the straight and narrow and out of the courtroom.

Barbara Reed soon became a celebrity, appeared on talk shows, testified before congressional and legislative committees, resulting, in the case of Los Angeles, in all junk and processed foods being removed from correctional facilities. She says, in her book, "A malnourished central nervous system will inevitably lead to serious physical and behavioral problems, problems which no amount of medication or psychiatry can touch." Her book tells stories of many of her charges, showing the changes in their personalities and lives when they followed her diet recommendations. The diet, of course, is rich in all the essential nutrients, especially B vitamins, so there is plenty of these to nourish brains and nerves and no chance for the B vitamins to be lost because of any "empty calorie" foods in the diet. "Keep the neocortex (of the brain) fed and the rest of the body will conform." Said Dr. Lendon Smith in the foreword to Barbara's book, "The brain and the body ARE connected."

An 1983 article in *New Scientist* told the story of Alexander Schauss, a psychologist who began his career as a probation officer. Schauss compared two groups of children with behavior disorders in a correctional institute, dividing them according to whether or not they had committed further offenses. Most of them had been eating very unbalanced diets. By correcting their diets in various ways and removing all junk foods, Dr. Schauss found that the children who ate the nutritious diet had far fewer behavior problems than those who continued to eat the former deficient diet they had been served. Dr. Schauss believes that thiamine deficiency is the one nutrient most often associated with deviant behavior in human beings.

Dr. Stephen Schowenthaler conducted similar trials at a children's detention home, producing the same results. Incidents of breaches of discipline decreased by 80 percent, judging by staff members' observation, although the staff members did not know which children were on the optimal diet.

There is no way to know how many people suffering from one or more symptom of thiamine deficiency have not been diagnosed or treated with thiamine. There is no way to know how many of us are born with "thiamine dependency," meaning that our inborn need for this vitamin is greater than the average person's or that some missing enzyme creates a deficiency in this nutrient. Deficiency can develop very rapidly in people who have lengthy bouts of diarrhea or vomiting, who have lost their appetites, or who are experimenting with some peculiar diet or fasting to lose weight. Ten years ago the *American Journal of Clinical Nutrition* reported a survey showing that more than one-fourth of all pregnant women in our country were deficient in thiamine.

In a massive volume, *Orthomolecular Psychiatry,* Dr. Alan Cott, a New York psychiatrist, described the megavitamin (massive dose) therapy he has used for many years for adult schizophrenics who have suffered one or more relapses requiring hospitalization and/or electroshock therapy. He and other physicians used intravenous injections of vitamins for patients already taking vitamins by mouth but not responding as rapidly as they should. In a sample group of 33 mental patients who had previously suffered relapses, 31 responded to the use of intramuscular injections and did not have to be hospitalized.

Dr. Cott used 200 milligrams of niacin (vitamin B3), 500 milligrams of vitamin C and a mixture of 100 milligrams each of thiamine and pyridoxine (B6) to every milliliter of intravenous fluid. He gave the injections three times weekly. Then, as patients began to improve doses were given twice weekly, and finally only once a week for several months. High doses of the same vitamins were also given by mouth. Some patients responded to the injections after less than two weeks, most by the end of three weeks. Remember that these were seriously ill patients, faced with hospitalization and electro-shock. Dr. Cott then used the same treatment on new patients, many of whom had been hospitalized because of the severity of their illness.

A British physician, Dr. John Gould, began to use megavitamin therapy in the 1930's for alcoholics with delirium tremens. He gave the vitamins in intravenous drip—1,500 milligrams of vitamin C, 1,000 milligrams of thiamine, 200 to 400 milligrams of niacin (B3), 20 milligrams of riboflavin (B2) and up to 35 milligrams of pantothenic acid. With this drip he successfully treated alcoholic psychosis, postoperative confusional psychoses, delirium due to drugs, barbiturate coma, psychoses following drug overdosage and drug withdrawal symptoms. Dr. Cott says that Dr. Gould often reported restoration to normality within 20 minutes to four hours. We cannot help but wonder why such harmless near miracles are not in use in every drug and alcohol treatment center in the world.

Dr. Abram Hoffer, the Canadian psychiatrist who has treated mental patients with megavitamins for more than 25 years, tells of two patients who were waiting to be admitted to a mental hospital. Unfortunately, their condition was deteriorating rapidly.

Dr. Hoffer treated them with megavitamin therapy and they responded so well that no hospitalization or electroshock therapy were necessary. Similar reports come in from other orthomolecular psychiatrists. The term orthomolecular, coined by Dr. Linus Pauling in 1968, means providing large doses of vitamins and other nutrients to certain body organs which may have special need at the time for much larger doses than doses that will prevent a simple deficiency disease.

Dr. Cott says, "The use of injected megavitamins in schizophrenic patients who show signs of relapse following the use of marijuana or other hallucinogenic drugs has been extremely valuable." He explains that "the daily requirement of vitamins is a significant proportion of the total body stores." The margin between plenty and not enough is very slim. "It has been shown," he says, "that recovery rates in vitamin deprivation experiments depend directly on the size of the replacement dose."

Why are not all psychiatrists using megavitamin therapy rather than drugs, all of which have serious side effects? Perhaps the reason has to do with the fact that drugs can be patented and immense amounts of money can be made selling them. Little money is made selling vitamins which cannot be patented.

*Executive Health,* September, 1976 reported on several children treated at the Cleveland Clinic. One eleven-year old boy had episodes of incoordination, sometimes following head injuries, infections or vaccinations. He was prescribed 600 milligrams daily of thiamine at the clinic. His general coordination improved greatly and episodes of incoordination declined.

One nine-year old girl from the age of one year, had been suffering from repetitive involuntary movements, seizures and physical and mental regression. No medication helped. She was treated with thiamine. Her coordination and ability to walk improved, as well as her school work. One child from infancy had shown serious abnormalities, failure to suck from the bottle, repeated vomiting and failure to thrive, signs of serious nerve disorders. At the age of three and a half massive doses of thiamine were prescribed— 600 milligrams a day. Five months later there was great improvement in development. She was alert, active and interested in her surroundings.

In *The International Journal of Biosocial Research,* volume 4. no. 2 an Ohio physician Derrick Lonsdale, M.D. related the story of a child with a number of complicated and serious disorders. When he was given gradually increasing doses of thiamine, until he reached 600 milligrams a day, his problems were over. By now a young man, he has found that any stress such as a cold may necessitate double or triple his daily dose of thiamine. Evidence that he had inherited a need for vastly larger amounts of this nutrient is confirmed by the fact that his brother suffers from the same condition, only to a lesser degree.

Dr. Lonsdale also treated an infant with mysterious symptoms including a series of heart attacks, anemia and many other defects. His urine was found to contain a substance known to block the body's normal use of thiamine. When he was given large doses of thiamine, his symptoms cleared within less than one week. "Of some interest," says Dr. Lonsdale, "his parents both excreted the same inhibitory substance and the mother has since then developed symptoms . . . diagnosed as multiple sclerosis."

The influence of thiamine on intelligence was clearly demonstrated by an experiment performed many years ago by a professor at Columbia University Teachers College, Dr. Ruth Harrell. She used two groups of closely matched children and gave one group a tablet of *only two milligrams* of thiamine daily, while the other group got a "dummy" tablet which contained nothing.

At the end of the experiment just this tiny bit of thiamine produced a superior mental response in the group which got the vitamin. They excelled in their studies. Say Dr. E.

Cheraskin and W. M. Ringsdorf, Jr. in their book *Diet and Disease*, "Thus it appears that mental achievement in children of presumably normal mentality consuming a presumably normal diet can be remarkably increased through the employment of daily supplements."

In 1980 an extremely serious anemia in a child was reported in *Nutrition Reviews* and nothing was effective in curing the disorder but thiamine, 100 milligrams given intravenously for nine days and thereafter by mouth for three weeks, and finally 25 milligrams of thiamine daily for the rest of her life. In 1973 *The Canadian Medical Journal* reported on work by Dr. H. T. R. Mount of Ottawa who treated multiple sclerosis with thiamine and liver extract which is a rich source of vitamin B12. With no other therapy his patients flourished, returning for more injections whenever their disorder began to reappear. Dr. Mount believes that these two nutrients can restore the myelin sheaths of nerves which are disordered in this disease.

A 1984 study by the National Institute of Mental Health found that *one in every five Americans* had some recognizable mental or emotional disorder. Only a small fraction of these people actually sought or received treatment for their mental problems. And only half of those went to specialists. "Such estimates raise questions about how to reshape the U.S. mental health care delivery system" said the psychiatrist who directed the study. It might be a good idea just to reshape the mental health care delivery system by delivering to the general public some information about the immense importance of certain brain nutrients for preventing mental illness.

If someone among your family or friends is faced with mental illness and wishes to use the megavitamin therapy which many physicians and psychiatrists are using today, get in touch with the Huxley Institute at 900 North Federal Highway, Suite 330, Boca Raton, Fla., 33423. They can send you literature on the subject, lists of books and perhaps the names of professionals in your area who are using this kind of harmless and apparently very effective therapy.

## *Thiamine (Vitamin B1) Content of Some Common Foods*

| Food | Milligrams |
|---|---|
| Almonds, 1 cup | 0.34 |
| Asparagus, 1 cup | 0.23 |
| Avocados, 1 cup | 0.16 |
| Beans, Lima, 1 cup | 0.22 |
| Beef heart, 3 oz. | 0.23 |
| Beef and vegetable stew, 1 cup | 0.12 |
| Brazil nuts, 1 cup | 1.21 |
| Bread: | |
| Cracked wheat, 1 lb. | 0.53 |
| Cracked wheat, 1 slice | 0.03 |
| French, enriched, 1 lb. | 1.26 |
| Italian, enriched, 1 lb. | 1.31 |
| Rye, 1 lb. | 0.81 |
| Rye, 1 slice | 0.04 |
| Pumpernickel, 1 lb. | 0.04 |
| White, enriched, 1 lb. | 1.05 |
| White, enriched, 1 slice | 0.06 |
| Whole wheat, 1 lb. | 1.17 |
| Whole wheat, 1 slice | 0.06 |
| Cashew nuts, 1 cup | 0.49 |
| Collards, 1 cup | 0.15 |
| Cowpeas (or Black-eyed peas), 1 cup | 0.41 |
| Dandelion greens, 1 cup | 0.23 |
| Dates, 1 cup | 0.16 |
| Flour, whole wheat, 1 cup | 0.66 |
| Grapefruit juice, frozen, 1 can | 0.29 |
| Grapefruit juice, dehydrated, 1 can | 0.41 |

Grape juice, 1 cup .......................... 0.11
Ham, smoked, 3 oz. ......................... 0.46
Ham, boiled, 2 oz. .......................... 0.57
Liver, beef, 2 oz. ........................... 0.15
Milk, dry, whole, 1 cup ..................... 0.30
Milk, dry, nonfat, 1 cup .................... 0.28
Oatmeal, 1 cup ............................. 0.22
Orange, 1 ................................. 0.11
Orange juice, frozen, 1 can ................. 0.63
Orange and grapefruit juice, frozen, 1 can ........ 0.47
Oysters, raw, 1 cup ........................ 0.30
Peanuts, roasted, 1 cup ..................... 0.47
Peas, green, 1 cup ......................... 0.40
Pecans, 1 cup ............................. 0.93
Pineapple, raw, 1 cup ...................... 0.12
Pineapple, canned, crushed, 1 cup ............. 0.20
Pineapple juice, 1 cup ...................... 0.13
Pork chops, 2 to 4 oz. ..................... 0.60
Pork roast, 1 slice ......................... 0.71
Raisins, 1 cup ............................ 0.13
Sausage, Bologna, 8 oz. .................... 0.36
Soup, bean, 1 cup ......................... 0.10
Soybeans, 1 serving ....................... 1.07
Soybean flour, 100 grams ................... 0.82
Spinach, 1 cup ............................ 0.14
Tangerine juice, 1 cup ..................... 0.14
Tangerine juice, frozen, 6 oz. can ............. 0.43
Walnuts, black or native, 1 cup ............... 0.28
Walnuts, English, 1 cup .................... 0.33
Watermelon, 1 wedge ...................... 0.20
Wheat germ, 1 cup ........................ 1.39
Yeast, brewer's, 100 grams ................. 9.69

# CHAPTER 16

# Riboflavin (Vitamin B2) Is Scarce in Food

OVER 70 YEARS AGO scientists were trying to find some solution to the problem of seborrhea, a skin condition involving greasy, scaly patches on the scalp, face, neck, underarms, genital areas. Trying different diets on their laboratory animals, they located one hitherto unknown nutrient—a yellow substance in milk—the B vitamin which they named riboflavin. Diets in which this vitamin was not present caused seborrhea in their laboratory animals.

Aside from this skin condition, some of the disorders produced when riboflavin (B2) is missing are: inflammation of the tongue causing pain and burning sensations, fissures at the corners of the mouth. The lips may look frayed or scaling, then develop slits or crevasses. Bloodshot eyes that may tire easily. Special sensitivity to light which makes an individual wear sunglasses even when the sun is not very bright. Itching and watery eyes also indicate deficiency in this vitamin.

Lack of riboflavin may produce nervous symptoms such as "pins and needles" sensations, difficulty in walking, muscular weakness and a condition called "burning feet" which developed in many prisoners of war when they suffered gross deficiencies in the B vitamins. A skin condition called acne rosacea may accompany lack of riboflavin. Deficiency may contribute to the formation of cataracts and one kind of anemia.

# RIBOFLAVIN IS SCARCE IN FOOD

In 1951 experiments at the prestigious Sloan-Kettering Institute showed that riboflavin can prevent liver cancer. Animals given desiccated liver (rich in riboflavin) were protected when exposed to chemicals known to cause liver cancer. Other animals not given liver developed the expected cancers. In 1973 physicians studied the riboflavin content of the blood of 22 alcoholics and found that half of them had none of this nutrient in their blood. Those who still had some of the vitamin suffered less than the others from characteristic symptoms of alcoholism. Several surveys conducted by the federal government have shown that deficiency in riboflavin is quite common in this country. Sore tongues and other unpleasant mouth symptoms are common among many pregnant women in the last six weeks before delivery.

An eye condition called amblyopia may be caused by toxins such as alcohol and nicotine. In fact, one form of this is called tobacco amblyopia. Exposure to carbon tetrachloride, lead, benzene, arsenic and quinine can produce amblyopia. So can simple lack of riboflavin.

In 1970 a woman was brought to a Singapore hospital complaining of pains in her feet. It burned "like fire" she said, both night and day for two weeks and was worse at night. The doctors tested her for all nutritional deficiencies they suspected and found none of the symptoms of riboflavin deficiency. They sprayed her feet with anesthetic which accomplished nothing. Nor did pain pills. Finally, they began to give her intravenous injections of riboflavin and "within three days the burning pain had subsided . . . and by the sixth day she was completely free from pain . . . ," the doctors reported in *The British Medical Journal*. The doctors discovered that this woman had an apparent inability to absorb all the nutrients in her food, although she had no symptoms of diarrhea, or other disorders that are usually present in such conditions.

*Nutrition and Physical Fitness* states that "Wide differences in requirements among individuals complicate the situation" when one tries to recognize riboflavin deficiency in an individual or a group of individuals. Roger

J. Williams explained this in terms of "biochemical individuality." Each of us is born with a different requirement for nutrients. One individual may need 20 or 30 times more of a given nutrient than another, even a close family member. Requirements are further complicated by lifestyle, by drugs taken, by stressful conditions such as pregnancy, illness, hard work, worry and so on. Since riboflavin is not all that easy to get in food, especially if one avoids dairy products, this is another life circumstance that might produce riboflavin deficiency even if an otherwise nutritious diet is being eaten.

In addition, it appears that a number of glandular conditions may affect the body's use of this vitamin. A number of commonly prescribed drugs may produce drastic deficiencies. Riboflavin is relatively inert and must be activated by various hormones. A hormone produced by the thyroid gland is essential in rendering riboflavin useful to the body. This suggests that either underactivity or overactivity of this important gland may determine the amount of riboflavin one's body has to work with.

A hormone, aldosterone, produced by the adrenal glands, is a very powerful regulator of the way the body uses sodium and potassium which are often unbalanced in the person who has high blood pressure. Dr. S. Rivlin, M.D. of Cornell University said in 1979 in *Nutrition Reviews* that some form of this vitamin might be used in treating the edema (water retention) that often accompanies this condition.

Thorazine is one of the most widely prescribed tranquilizers, used to control hyperactive children, severe psychotic disorders, alcohol withdrawal symptoms, anxiety and so on. It also destroys the body's riboflavin by causing it to be rapidly excreted. Wound healing, following surgery, raises requirements for riboflavin and many other nutrients. Certain oral contraceptives also cause loss of riboflavin. Anti-depressants deplete the body of riboflavin. Dr. Rivlin suggests that all pregnant women should be given supplements of this B vitamin since, in animals, it prevents the appearance of congenital defects caused by certain drugs. He also believes that all women on The Pill should be taking supplements of riboflavin.

One cannot help but wonder why we permit drug companies to play games with our nutritional health and then sidestep responsibility for the damage the drugs do. Why do doctors continue to recommend The Pill without mentioning the drastic defects in essential nutrients that may be produced? Evidence of the nutritional side effects has been available for many years.

A 1981 study of 210 teenagers in New York City found that 49 of the boys and girls were deficient in riboflavin. Those who used more than one glass of milk daily or took vitamin supplements were in the best condition where riboflavin is concerned. In a study of 484 high school students in New Jersey researchers found that only five percent were on diets that would be considered "good." Most diets were low in milk, fruits and vegetables. Said the researchers, "The adolescent is a high risk for nutritional inadequacy and it is likely that this inadequacy is not limited to riboflavin."

In 1983 Daphne A. Roe, M.D. reported from Cornell University that women who exercise rigorously but who maintain their weight by eating more need almost double the RDA for riboflavin while those who lose weight because of vigorous exercise need even more than double the RDA. Dr. Roe said, in a press release from Cornell, "Although we did not test men, we are assuming that findings would be pretty consistent." Just a couple of glasses of milk and some cheese every day should be adequate to supply the missing vitamin, she said.

Syracuse University athletes have a professional nutritionist and biochemist, Dr. Sarah Short, who watches over their diets and health. She has found that some of the athletes are eating up to 14,000 calories a day—as much as an ordinary man eats in a week. In spite of this, she found many nutritional deficiencies among them.

One wrestler was so deficient in vitamin A and the B

119

vitamin riboflavin that his lips were cracking and the inside of his nose had dried, his eyes teared and he was extremely sensitive to light. Fortunately, Dr. Short had read the literature on riboflavin and could recognize the symptoms. A number of years ago researchers in Kenya reported on baboons who were deficient in riboflavin. After only several months the animals developed swollen bleeding gums, scaly seborrhea dermatitis, bloody diarrhea, hemorrhages of the large and small bowel and drastic changes in blood components. Giving

## *Riboflavin (Vitamin B2) Content of Some Common Foods*

| Food | Milligrams |
| --- | --- |
| Almonds, 1 cup | 1.31 |
| Apricots, 1 cup | 0.24 |
| Asparagus, 1 cup | 0.30 |
| Avocados, 1 cup | 0.30 |
| Beef, hamburger pattie, 3 oz. | 0.18 |
| Beef, heart, 3 oz. | 1.05 |
| Beef, steak, 3 oz. | 0.16 |
| Beef, corned, 3 oz. | 0.20 |
| Bread: | |
| Cracked wheat, 1 slice | 0.02 |
| French, enriched, 1 lb. | 0.98 |
| Italian, enriched, 1 lb. | 0.93 |
| Rye, 1 slice | 0.02 |
| Pumpernickel, 1 lb. | 0.63 |
| White, enriched, 1 slice | 0.04 |
| Whole wheat, 1 slice | 0.05 |
| Broccoli, 1 cup | 0.22 |
| Buttermilk, 1 cup | 0.44 |
| Cashew nuts, 1 cup | 0.46 |
| Chicken, broiled, 3 oz. | 0.15 |
| Collards, 1 cup | 0.46 |
| Dandelion greens, 1 cup | 0.22 |
| Dates, 1 cup | 0.17 |

up to 500 milligrams of riboflavin for up to seven days either orally or intravenously cured all these symptoms in a short time.

Experiments dealing with the birth of imperfect offspring were conducted by Dr. Lorene Rogers, who found that animals not getting enough riboflavin bear defective offspring even though they are getting an otherwise highly nutritious diet, which, of course, many pregnant women are not getting. Testing various drugs on the animals, she also found that

| | |
|---|---|
| Egg, raw, 1 | 0.15 |
| Egg, scrambled (w/milk and fat) | 0.18 |
| Flour, whole wheat, 1 cup | 0.14 |
| Kale, 1 cup | 0.25 |
| Lamp chop, 4.8 oz. | 0.24 |
| Liver, beef, 2 oz. | 2.25 |
| Mackerel, 3 oz. | 0.23 |
| Milk, whole, 1 cup | 0.42 |
| Milk, dry, nonfat, 1 cup | 1.44 |
| Mushrooms, 1 cup | 0.60 |
| Mustard greens, 1 cup | 0.25 |
| Oysters, 1 cup | 0.39 |
| Peaches, 1 cup | 0.32 |
| Peas, green, 1 cup | 0.22 |
| Prunes, cooked, 1 cup | 0.18 |
| Pumpkin, 1 cup | 0.14 |
| Sausage, Bologna, 8 oz. | 0.49 |
| Shad, baked, 3 oz. | 0.22 |
| Soybeans, 1 serving | 0.31 |
| Soybean flour, 100 grams | 0.34 |
| Spinach, 1 cup | 0.36 |
| Squash, winter, baked, 1 cup | 0.31 |
| Strawberries, raw, 1 cup | 0.10 |
| Turnip greens, 1 cup | 0.59 |
| Watermelon, 1 wedge | 0.22 |
| Wheat germ, 1 cup | 0.54 |
| Yeast, brewer's, 100 grams | 5.45 |
| Yogurt, 1 cup | 0.43 |

Orinase (a drug given to diabetics to lower blood sugar) produced defective offspring in animals not getting enough riboflavin. She said, in part, "Our results suggest that all physicians administering drugs of any kind during pregnancy should make every effort to see that the patient's nutrition is as nearly optimal as possible."

In 1970 a Yale geneticist warned pediatricians that there is an increasing incidence of "inborn errors of metabolism" among today's newborn. These are congenital defects in some enzyme system that involves a vitamin, a mineral or a protein. He said that four new vitamin-dependent forms of genetic disease were reported in 1970, raising the number to about one dozen. Two of these are linked to pyridoxine (B6), another to vitamin B12. In this disorder the newborn child has need for 1,000 times the RDA of this vitamin to control this congenital disease.

This is what we mean by a "vitamin-dependent disorder." Because of an inherited defect, the baby is unable to transport the vitamin to the place where it will be used in the body, or else the body enzyme which deals with this vitamin is incapable of "binding it." Vitamin B1 (thiamine) and vitamin B2 (riboflavin) have been linked to anemias which may necessitate very large doses of these vitamins to keep the condition under control all during the individual's lifetime. Scientists do not know and may never know how many people are born with these handicaps.

Experiments conducted in the seventies showed a helpful relationship between pyridoxine (B6) and riboflavin. Studying red blood cells of various individuals, scientists found that part of the B6 in their cells was not converted into the usable form. When they gave the individual some riboflavin the pyridoxine situation became normal very soon and the volunteer stopped "wasting" pyridoxine. When the extra riboflavin was withdrawn the original situation once more prevailed and the volunteer "lost" pyridoxine. We stress often in these pages the fact that the B vitamins work as a "complex." They help one another out.

And they can sometimes substitute for another B vitamin,

as in this case. In another research, people known to be deficient in riboflavin were found to be deficient also in pyridoxine. So don't wonder whether you should take your pyridoxine supplement at one time and your riboflavin supplement at another time. All the B vitamins should be taken at the same time. They occur together in all foods in which they are plentiful. This is Nature's way to assure their helpfulness to one another.

Riboflavin is most abundant in liver, kidney, all dairy products, meat, poultry, fish, eggs, bran, wheat germ, lentils, beans, peanuts, nuts, peas, soybeans, leafy green vegetables and fruits. Gram for gram, brewers yeast contains far more riboflavin than any other food. Use it wherever possible in cereals, salads, soups, casseroles, blender drinks. Riboflavin is very sensitive to light, suggesting that milk should be stored in light-proof containers and exposed to as little light as possible when cooking. Cover any meats or vegetables while they cook.

Riboflavin has no known harmfulness when taken in large amounts, although there seems to be no necessity for taking massive doses, if you are eating a reasonably nutritious diet. Since any excess of this vitamin is excreted rather rapidly, you may notice a yellow color of the urine when large doses are taken. This is because this vitamin is yellow. Its appearance in urine indicates nothing harmful, just that your body didn't require quite that much to satisfy daily needs.

# CHAPTER 17

# The New and Exciting Potential
# of Niacin

"A SURPRISE LINK TO LONGEVITY: IT'S NIACIN." This was a headline in *Medical Tribune*, April 24, 1985. The article described the Coronary Drug Program Project, conducted between 1966 and 1975 by the National Heart, Lung and Blood Institute, a federal Institute funded by your tax money. In this project 8,341 men were studied. All had previously had a myocardial infarction (one kind of heart attack.)

For a period of nine years the researchers gave a daily dose of one or another of three drugs thought to have some helpful effects on circulatory disorders. The fourth group got a daily dose of the B vitamin niacin. No drugs. No other changes were made in the lives of the men, no special diets or exercise. A follow-up of the health histories of these men nine years later showed that fatalities among those taking the niacin decreased by eleven percent compared with the volunteers taking the drugs.

Dr. Paul L. Canner, Ph.D., chief statistician of the Maryland Medical Research Institute, said, "There were 70 fewer deaths in the niacin group," and those men with the highest cholesterol levels to begin with benefited more from the niacin treatment than those with lower levels. He also said, "the mortality benefit of the niacin group is present in each major category or cause of death—coronary, other cardiovascular, cancer and other causes." On the averge, the men who took niacin lived about two years longer than those taking drug therapy.

In February, 1986 *Medical Tribune* reported another triumph for niacin. "Cut Cholesterol for Five Dollars a Month?" asked this article. Physicians at the Beth Israel Hospital in Boston gave niacin in daily doses of two grams (2,000 milligrams) and found that "it offers more lipid (fat)-lowering benefits than traditional medication or diet alone and that it can be done at a cost of about five dollars a month, compared with the $217.00 cost of such drugs as cholestryamine." No special diets eliminating fats and protein! No special emphasis on exercise or any other aspect of life! By just taking the niacin every day for ten months the 72 patients who participated in this experiment lowered their total blood cholesterol and raised the level of the high-density lipoproteins which help to protect us against heart attacks and other circulatory diseases.

In 1983 a panel of the National Institutes of Health reported that certain "drugs" are known to reduce triglycerides in the blood by 30 percent. These are fats known to be destructive of arteries. One of these "drugs" is niacin, they said, and it works far better than any of the prescribed drugs in lowering low-density lipoproteins, those other promoters of hardening of the arteries and heart attacks.

Perhaps the attribute for which niacin is most famous is its ability to dilate blood vessels. It's well known that most of our circulatory problems are caused by clogged blood vessels which prevent the blood from flowing easily and safely as it should. The person who takes a large dose of niacin for the first time may be amazed at the almost instantaneous reaction. Mouth, throat and head begin to flush, tingle and itch. Face turns bright red. Some people find this reaction unpleasant and scary. Others, especially those taking the vitamin for a long time, don't mind it at all. Commenting on the use of niacin, professional people who conducted the study noted that the side effect of large doses of niacin ("The Flush") becomes less noticeable after the patient has been taking the vitamin for some time. Tricks to reduce the flush are to take the vitamin always with food, to avoid alcohol for at least an hour after taking it and take half an aspirin three times a day to decrease the flushing.

This B vitamin, niacin, plays an important role in cooperating with other vitamins to normalize the body's method of processing carbohydrates, protein and fats. It works closely with several trace minerals such as zinc and chromium. It helps to normalize body hormones, such as sex hormones and insulin.

Dr. Carl C. Pfeiffer said that the Research Director of the Miami Heart Institute has used niacin for heart patients in more than 1,000 cases. In one group of 600 patients, insurance companies had predicted 62 probable deaths over a ten-year period in these patients who had damaged hearts and circulatory systems. Instead, only six deaths occurred among those who took the large doses of niacin.

Dr. Pfeiffer also reported that niacin can decrease the effects of the hallucinogenic drugs such as LSD, help smokers reduce their use of cigarettes and increase the helpful effects of traquilizers so that lower doses of these drugs can be used. He recommended that anyone who wished to take niacin in large doses should start with smaller doses—50 milligrams, for example, and increase these doses very gradually. A medical textbook *Drugs in Current Use* published in 1978 speaks of niacin as a drug. It is used, said the author, "for improving circulation, acne, Ménière's Disease, migraine headaches and multiple sclerosis, also to lower blood cholesterol."

Interest in niacin began back in the early 1900's when a terrible disease called pellagra ravaged parts of the world including our own Southland where many thousands of people suffered from it and many died. In 1938 nearly half a million people in our country had pellagra and 3,500 died of it every year. *The cause was simple deficiency in niacin.* Symptoms were dementia, diarrhea and dermatitis. Diets consisting mostly of corn products with little or no food of animal origin, fruits or vegetables, produces pellagra.

# THE NEW AND EXCITING POTENTIAL OF NIACIN

Niacin is in charge of various enzyme systems dealing with the body's use of fat and carbohydrate. Many disorders of the skin and digestive tract may be related to deficiency in niacin. Many special conditions make heavy demands on this nutrient: pregnancy, lactation, dermatoses, high blood levels of cholesterol, high-calorie diets, sprue and glossitis (inflammation of the tongue).

Important enough to warrant first-page treatment in many newspapers was the announcement in 1966 by a researcher at the New Jersey Psychiatric Institute that a form of niacin was effective in treating 1,000 patients with schizophrenia (our most serious mental disorder). Dr. Humphry Osmond said that 75 percent of the patients treated were cured. "Cured" is quite a significant word not often used in regard to this terrible mental illness that afflicts most patients in our mental hospitals. Dr. Osmond mentioned one patient who had been ill for 29 years and was free of symptoms after only five days of treatment with niacin.

Dr. Abram Hoffer, a Canadian psychiatrist, has been reporting in medical journals for over 30 years on his almost miraculous results with many schizophrenic patients. The theory of Dr. Hoffer and Dr. Osmond is that schizophrenia is caused by a by-product of the adrenal gland, adrenochrome which builds up in the body and produces the hallucinations, the mania, the depression and other disturbances produced by this disorder.

Dr. Hoffer reported in *The Lancet,* a British medical journal, in 1962 "niacin has some, though not all, the qualities of an ideal treatment: it is safe, cheap and easy to administer and it uses a known pharmaceutical substance which can be taken for years on end if necessary . . . Why, then, have these benefits passed almost unheeded? One reason may be the extraordinary proliferation of the phenothiazine derivatives since 1954. These are tranquilizers. Unlike these, niacin is a simple, well-known vitamin which can be bought cheaply in bulk and cannot be patented, and there has been no campaign to persuade doctors of its usefulness." Dr.

Hoffer, formerly director of Psychiatric Research in the Department of Public Health in Saskatchewan, is now in private practice. He and Dr. Osmond published a book in 1974, *How to Live With Schizophrenia*. Dr. Hoffer and a colleague wrote a book *Orthomolecular Nutrition* in 1978.

On the shiny pages of *Psychology Today*, April 1974, appeared the story of a schizophrenic eleven-year old boy and the nutritional treatment which controlled his disease within several months. The author is Harvey M. Ross, M.D., a psychiatrist who uses mostly nutritional methods. The child (Mitch) had very serious symptoms. He talked to phantoms. He set fires. He stole. He attacked his sisters. Sometimes he stole candy bars and *sometimes he ate as many as 60 candy bars in one day*.

His parents had taken him to several psychiatrists whose treatment had done nothing for him. They counseled the parents against trying nutritional therapy—too dangerous, they said! Dr. Ross' tests discovered that Mitch had low blood sugar. He put the child on a diet high in protein with small meals and frequent between-meals snacks also high in protein. No sugar or sugary foods. After each meal Mitch took 500 milligrams of niacin, and the same dose of vitamin C, 100 milligrams of pyridoxine (B6) and pantothenic acid, 200 units of vitamin E and a multiple B tablet to provide the other B vitamins. Within a week his parents noticed a difference. After a month he had lost some of his overweight and was improving in his school work. He continued to improve and needed to see Dr. Ross only occasionally. Dr. Ross says that about 80 percent of schizophrenic patients have low blood sugar.

Dr. Ross' work is called ''orthomolecular'' psychiatry, meaning the administration to patients of massive doses of various nutrients which are needed in certain organs of the body in much larger doses than the ordinary person needs. This therapy has been shown to be helpful not only for schizophrenics but also alcoholics and drug addicts. The high protein diet plus massive doses of vitamins are now being used to treat autistic children, hyperactive children, minimal brain damage in children and learning disability. Dr. Ross has written a book, *Fighting Depression,* published by Keats Publishing Inc., New Canaan, Connecticut.

Sometime ago *Medical Tribune* published the story of a group of diabetics in Australia who volunteered to return to their aboriginal life in the "bush"—hunting and gathering, to see what happened to their diabetic condition. When they returned seven weeks later the diabetic condition had vanished and they were well. Blood pressure and triglyceride levels were also normal. Commenting on this story in the January 7, 1987 issue of *Medical Tribune,* John P. Cleary, M.D. said this story is "an excellent example of how a change in the diet is the real cause of diabetes. A diet of mostly meat [the diet the Australians ate in the forest] furnishes in excess of 100 milligrams of niacin per day and over a period of time a vegetarian or mixed diet can induce niacin deficiency in persons who normally take in 100 milligrams or more per day from meat. Complications of diabetes are the result of this same niacin deficiency state—which is not corrected by the current therapy for diabetes.

"The reason for chronic niacin deficiency in humans is that we were predators and hunters until 10,000 years ago when agriculture began to develop and change the diet for some humans. Others, like the Australian Aborigines have a more recent change, like our American Indian and Eskimos, who suffer more severely from this sudden change but really, all human have this potential problem. It now appears that NAD levels are part of the regulatory control mechanism—for the predator response. When NAD levels are low the animal begins to stalk and hunt prey, and when a kill is made and meat eaten, the brain NAD levels go back up and the animal is peaceful and rests. The addict exhibits this same frantic predatory behavior when in withdrawal and niacin corrects it.

"Medicine took a wrong turn in the 1930's and only now can we begin to understand that most of the diseases of unknown etiology [cause] now under study at the National

Institutes of Health are really caused by a vitamin deficiency. Offers to meet with a conference of various Institutes falls on deaf ears, postponing the day when people will be relieved of increasingly expensive medical treatment based on wrong ideas.'' The NAD to which Dr. Cleary refers is the form niacin takes in the body.

A Canadian reader wrote to *The Lancet* in 1980 suggesting that taking niacin might help smokers to quit smoking. She said, ''Although smoking has its social and psychological aspects, most people smoke to maintain a certain nicotine level in the bloodstream. In many cases, this need for nicotine becomes addictive. Morphine works by tricking the endorphin receptors—might not nicotine similarly dupe the niacin (vitamin B3) receptors of the central nervous system? Niacin is chemically very similar to nicotine, indeed the early name for niacin was nicotinic acid . . . If this hypothesis is valid, it might be possible to wean some smokers off their nicotine addiction by administering niacin.''

Dr. R. Glen Green, a Canadian psychiatrist who uses nutritional methods in treating mental patients, has found, he says, that about 10 percent of his patients have a ''subclinical'' case of pellagra. They complain of heartaches, difficulty in breathing, deep-seated chest pains, missing heart beats and many digestive complaints—taste changes, a lump in the throat, difficulty in swallowing, heartburn, gas, bloating, dyspepsia, cramps, nausea, constipation, diarrhea, pain in the side, loss of appetite. Dr. Green gets complete disappearance of all these symptoms when he gives such patients from 1½ to 6 grams a day of niacin or niacinamide, another form of this vitamin. *Executive Health* reported in 1983 that niacin stimulates the repair process in body cells which sustained damage to their DNA, the genetic material in the cell. The damage might have been caused by environmental poisons or drugs used in treating cancer.

A rare disease called Hartnup's Disease afflicts those who are born with inadequacies in certain amino acids or links of protein. This disorder causes strange nervous symptoms:

a peculiar gait, mental retardation, and a skin rash like that found in pellagra. *Nutrition Reviews* reported such a condition in July, 1984. A 12-year old boy in London had an unsteady gait, serious defects of sight and below normal intelligence. He was given 250 milligrams of niacinamide daily and in about two months most of the symptoms disappeared. He was symptom-free. Here is an obvious case of inborn need for this vitamin far above what the rest of us need.

Changes in perception of taste and smell occur in schizo-phrenia and also in people who do not have this disorder. *The Journal of the American Medical Association* reported on a Canadian physician who uses niacin in doses up to six grams a day for patients who complain that they cannot taste their food. Lack of a sense of smell can also be treated with niacin.

Dr. Abram Hoffer reported in 1984 on treating a psychotic patient who was also terminally ill with cancer. He was given three grams (3,000 milligrams) of niacin daily, plus the same amount of vitamin C daily—in divided doses, not all at once. Three days later, says Dr. Hoffer, he was mentally normal. After about a year his cancer was no longer visible in the chest x-ray. He survived for about two years and died of other causes. "Since then I have included niacin in my treatment program for patients with cancer, but I had no explanation of how it could work," he says. He also recommends niacin for people with allergies. He has found it helpful, he says, for epileptics for the vitamin can help anticonvulsant drugs to do their work better, so that less of the drug is needed.

Dr. John Cleary said in *Medical Tribune* March 7, 1984, "I found alcohol addiction could be cured by giving niacin in doses of 500 milligrams a day and I successfully detoxified a dozen chronic alcoholics in an outpatient setting using this treatment. I was certainly surprised when I tried to publish my findings in this country and in England to find that no one seemed to be the least bit interested in my breakthrough."

Several researchers have found that the amino acid tryptophane (a link of protein) helps to provide healthful sleep for insomniacs. It seems that this amino acid (which occurs in food) increases the amount of a nerve transmitter called serotonin in the brain which promotes sound sleep. Recent research has found that tryptophane breaks down into niacin in the body's processing. So it seems possible that just getting enough niacin might help the chronic insomniac to sleep.

Paraquat is a poisonous weedkiller which is used on a wide variety of crops in our country. *Science* in 1981 reported that paraquat has caused over 400 human deaths from accidental and suicidal ingestions. It has also caused lung cancer in drug users who smoke marijuana from Mexico. According to the *Science* authors from the U.S. Geological Survey rats poisoned with paraquat benefitted from daily niacin therapy. They did not develop lung injury until much later than did those animals which were not given the vitamin. The researchers called their niacin treatment "medically safe." This seems to indicate that getting enough of the nutrient may protect us from other environmental toxins as well.

Reading medical journals, we find accounts of old folks living in run-down tenements or nursing homes, or even in modern hospitals with many of the same symptoms we have described in detail above. Doctors appear to be unable to understand or treat them. Sore mouths and tongues and dermatitis are commonplace. Depression, confusion, insomnia, anxiety, irritability, tenseness—these are almost universal complaints among modern city dwellers. How many of these personal disasters are brought about by plain lack of B vitamins?

We don't know. But we do know that diets which are limited to any degree in any of the essential nutrients are likely to produce just such serious symptoms. Reducing diets or diets for allergic people which limit the amounts of meat, eggs, dairy products, wholegrains, fruits or vegetables are likely to bring on some of the symptoms of pellagra which probably no modern doctor would be able to diagnose.

Sugar is an "empty calorie" food. It contains no protein,

no vitamins, no minerals, no trace minerals and nothing else that provides good health. Every teaspoon of sugar we eat crowds out of our diets the nourishing food that can prevent vitamin deficiencies. Every "made" dessert loaded with sugar, every soft drink, every piece of candy dilutes the modern diet so that it is less able to maintain good health. For those who are born with especially high requirements for vitamins, or those whose jobs or way of life or health create a situation where there is a greater need for more vitamins, especially B vitamins, the answer is to correct your diet, first, so that every mouthful of food provides an abundance of nutrients and, as special insurance against any deficit, take vitamin and mineral supplements. They are inexpensive, harmless if taken in reasonable amounts and almost certain to benefit you in many ways you haven't even anticipated.

Many drug dictionaries list niacin as a preventive of high blood levels of cholesterol. *The 8-Week Cholesterol Cure* by Robert E. Kowalski, a medical researcher and writer, shows clearly that taking niacin daily along with a low fat diet and one other "magic" ingredient brought his blood cholesterol level down from catastrophic height to normal. The other magic ingredient is oat bran, shown by many studies to have a cholesterol-lowering effect, which he took every day, made into muffins or bread or simply added to casseroles and meatloaf. or spread over his breakfast cereal.

To begin with, Kowalski had a heart attack in 1978 at the age of thirty-five. It was so serious that his doctors recommended triple coronary artery bypass surgery. Six years later he needed another bypass surgery. Still his cholesterol levels stayed high, although he was by this time avoiding all those foods known to be high in cholesterol, such as fatty meats, eggs and fatty dairy products.

Then he found evidence of the helpfulness of a diet high in fiber, in his case chiefly oat bran, since this is the form of fiber that appears to have the best effect on lowering blood cholesterol levels. He found an article in the *Journal of the American Medical Association* 1983 saying that niacin, in doses of three to twelve 500-milligram tablets daily will lower blood levels of the "bad" kind of cholesterol and will raise to normal the helpful cholesterol levels.

"Amazing," said Mr. Kowalski, "Here was the medical community, the experts from the American Heart Association and the American Medical Association, actively advocating megadose vitamin therapy for a condition I was very personally interested in." So he began to search medical and scientific literature for everything he could find about this vitamin. He found that Dr. R. Atschul discovered in 1955 that niacin (three grams daily) effectivley lowers total cholesterol and triglycerides and that the Coronary Drug Project in 1975

## Niacin (Vitamin B3) Content of Some Common Foods

| Food | Milligrams |
|------|------------|
| Almonds, 1 cup | 5.0 |
| Apricots, dried, 1 cup | 4.9 |
| Avocados, 1 cup | 2.4 |
| Beef, 3 oz. portion | 3.1 |
| Beef, hamburger pattie, 3 oz. | 4.6 |
| Beef, steak, 3 oz. | 4.0 |
| Beef, corned, 3 oz. | 2.9 |
| Beef, heart, 3 oz. | 6.8 |
| Beef and vegetable stew, 1 cup | 3.4 |
| Bread: | |
|     Cracked wheat, 1 slice | 0.3 |
|     French, enriched, 1 lb. | 11.3 |
|     Italian, enriched, 1 lb. | 11.7 |
|     Rye, 1 slice | 0.3 |
|     Pumpernickel, 1 lb. | 5.4 |
|     White, enriched, 1 slice | 0.5 |
|     Whole wheat, 1 slice | 0.7 |

showed that niacin could be singled out as being responsible for a 29 percent reduction in nonfatal heart attacks.

In his book Kowalski says, ''The medical literature is filled with success stories in which cholesterol levels fall anywhere between ten and 25 percent for those taking niacin alone or with other approaches . . . when taken along with a sensible, modified-fat diet niacin produces even more dramatic results . . . depending on the individual, the combination of oat bran plus niacin could be sufficient to keep cholesterol levels well within or even below normal limits, even without changing the diet at all.''

He gives a suggested dosage schedule for beginning niacin therapy, in which you proceed gradually from one 100-milli-

| | |
|---|---:|
| Chicken, broiled, 3 oz. | 10.5 |
| Dates, 1 cup | 3.9 |
| Flour, whole wheat, 1 cup | 5.2 |
| Ham, smoked, 3 oz. | 3.5 |
| Lamb chop, 1 | 5.4 |
| Liver, beef, 2 oz. | 8.4 |
| Mackerel, 3 oz. | 6.5 |
| Mushrooms, 1 cup | 4.8 |
| Oysters, 1 cup | 6.6 |
| Peanuts, roasted, 1 cup | 24.6 |
| Peaches, dried, 1 cup | 8.4 |
| Peas, green, 1 cup | 3.7 |
| Pork chop, 1 | 3.6 |
| Salmon, 3 oz. | 6.8 |
| Sausage, Bologna, 8 oz. | 6.0 |
| Shad, 3 oz. | 7.3 |
| Soybeans, 1 serving | 2.3 |
| Soybean flour, 100 grams | 2.6 |
| Swordfish, 3 oz. | 9.3 |
| Tuna, 3 oz. | 10.9 |
| Veal cutlet, 3 oz. | 4.6 |
| Wheat germ, 1 cup | 3.1 |
| Yeast, brewer's, 100 grams | 36.2 |

gram table three times daily to two 500-milligram tablets three times daily. He suggests that if your cholesterol level is just a bit too high you may find that taking oat bran every day will be enough. For someone with a little higher level of cholesterol just one gram of niacin taken in divided doses during the day may be enough. Individuals differ.

They also differ in their response to niacin. Because it opens blood vessels rapidly, it may be accompanied by a flush and a tingling feeling usually on the face, arms, shoulders and back. This is limited to the skin and is harmless, although some people find it unpleasant. For these people he suggests time-release capsules of niacin which are available at most health food stores. However, experiments have shown, it seems, that taking large doses of niacin is not recommended for those with peptic ulcer, liver disease, diabetes or gout. He suggests, if you start with the niacin program, that you tell your doctor what you are doing. And he suggests showing his book to your doctor. He says Dr. Louis Cohen, a professor of medicine at the University of Chicago, has been treating raised levels of cholesterol with niacin for 20 years. He has had dozens of patients taking the vitamin for six years or more without any difficulties.

In other chapters author Kowalski discusses fiber and vitamin supplements, his own diet, his experiments with volunteers who followed the diet, how to shop for allowed foods and how to prepare them to avoid high cholesterol ingredients. He gives lists of foods with their fat and their cholesterol content and a great deal more that is helpful if you are concerned about high cholesterol levels.

He also publishes a *Diet-Heart Newsletter* at P.O. Box 2039, Venice, California 90291 and suggests that you write for a sample and subscription information. Send along a stamped, self-addressed LONG envelope.

# CHAPTER 18

# A B Vitamin Treats Arthritis

ALWAYS ON THE LOOKOUT for any new material pertaining to arthritis that might be helpful, we came upon a note referring to a book long out of print of which a few copies had been found which were for sale for $35, so rare and valuable they were. We sent for a copy and found it was well worth the price. Its author, William Kaufman, Ph.D., M.D., wrote the book for other physicians, so it is not easy reading for the layman. It deals with an astonishing story of many arthritis patients treated and greatly improved in most cases by a B vitamin given in large doses every few hours every day to saturate the tissues. Dr. Kaufman believed that arthritis is a disease of vitamin deficiency.

Here are case histories of several patients out of the hundreds Dr. Kaufman treated and reported on in this book back in the 1940's.

An accountant, sixty years old—arthritis. He was given 160 milligrams of a B vitamin to take every two hours for eight doses daily (1,200 milligrams in 24 hours). In 315 days of such therapy his arthritis improved from a rating of "severe" to "slight."

A 39-year-old woman came into Dr. Kaufman's office complaining of moderate arthritis, transient low back pain, right shoulder stiff, discomfort, persistent stiffness of joints. She had had a "nervous breakdown" several years earlier when her husband died. She had had "the usual" menopause symptoms. She was given 150 milligrams of a B vitamin to take every three hours for six daily doses. Within one month her joint troubles had greatly improved. On the advice of a friend, she decided to take less of the B vitamin. Her condition worsened again. When she went back to the original dose, it improved.

A 61-year-old engineer came to Dr. Kaufman's office with severe persistent headaches, from which he could get no relief. In the past two years they had become much worse. His joints grated, especially in the neck. He was stiff in the morning when first awake, also when the weather was bad. His shoulders had been painful with intermittent stiffness and pain in finger joints. He was given a certain B vitamin in doses of 160 milligrams at regular intervals to equal 975 milligrams per day. His headaches improved gradually. Within 190 days his arthritic condition improved from "severe" to "slight." He was also given large doses of vitamin C along with smaller doses of riboflavin and thiamine.

An attorney of 45 came into Dr. Kaufman's office with severe joint dysfunction, was given 1,800 milligrams of a certain B vitamin every 24 hours, along with other B vitamins and vitamin C. Within 178 days of therapy his condition was greatly improved.

The vitamin which was given in large doses in every case was niacinamide—the amide of the B vitamin niacin form of vitamin B3. The name of the book is *The Common Form of Joint Dysfunction: Its Incidence and Treatment.*

Dr. Kaufman, determined to conquer arthritis for at least some of his patients, developed elaborate devices for measuring what he called "joint dysfunction"—that is, anything which impaired the patient's ability to move about—any dysfunction in arms, legs, wrists, back and so on. By measuring the patient's grasp, reach and other extensions of joints, he was able to classify their ailment according to the numbers on the mechanism he had invented. As time went on, the same patient was asked to perform the same motions, so that improvement or lack of it could be measured and noted.

Dr. Kaufman was not content merely to ask the patient, "How are your joints today?" He could actually physically measure improvement or lack of it.

The stories in this book are almost unbelievable, especially in view of the fact that it was written more than 30 years ago when vitamins were almost never spoken of in terms of preventive medicine and when the idea of using vitamins in massive doses had not even been considered by most researchers or physicians. Dr. Kaufman was an innovator—years and years ahead of his time.

Also of interest is the fact that he made no other changes in his patients' lives except for the vitamins he gave them. There is no mention of revising their diets, asking them to exercise more or make any other changes in their way of life. So the record appears to be just a record of what one vitamin—niacinamide—along with several others in smaller doses, can do to improve the condition of patients with painful, stiff joints. It seems to us that far better or perhaps quicker results might have occurred had the patients been placed on diets in which all refined carbohydrates were restricted and emphasis was laid on high protein foods and whole, unprocessed foods. But Dr. Kaufman confined his treatment to vitamins alone.

He did not use just niacinamide. In most cases he also gave quite large doses of vitamin C, thiamine (vitamin B1), and pyridoxine (vitamin B6) and riboflavin (B2). He tailored the dosage of niacinamide according to the individual patient's needs. If there appeared to be little or no improvement, he increased the dosage. If improvement appeared to have stopped at a "plateau," he increased the dosage. He cautioned his patients to continue with the recommended dosage even if they became discouraged with slow progress. Improvement with this completely harmless therapy appears to take quite a long time, although in several cases described in the book almost miraculous improvement occurred in a matter of months in people who had suffered for years from arthritis.

He mentions several things which complicate treatment. These are things we might have neglected to notice ourselves. But a very detailed history sometimes turned up significant items in regard to the possible causes of the complaint.

Sometimes it was allergy. Some of his patients knew they were allergic to certain foods: wheat, chocolate, eggs, etc. When they carefully avoided these foods their improvement was assured. If they transgressed and ate even small amounts of the offending food, their condition always worsened.

Another drawback to continued improvement usually had to do with repetitive work done every day by the patient in an uncomfortable or awkward position. This is almost bound to create joint problems which will not yield to any treatment. Anyone working with tools or machinery, twisting a foot around the leg of a chair while sitting, holding the phone in an awkward position for long conversation, maintaining poor posture year after year, wearing uncomfortable shoes or high heels or socks that are too short. Dr. Kaufman describes a woman whose joint pains occurred only on certain days. It developed that these were the days when she ironed. She habitually held the iron in a tight grip and pressed hard on the ironing board, as well as pulling tightly on the object she was ironing. Correcting these improper methods of work greatly alleviated her joint pains.

Another complicating factor in arthritis, says Dr. Kaufman, is sodium retention. Many women complain of this several days before their menstrual period: bloating, weight gain, irritability, discomfort, insomnia caused by the body retaining sodium or salt. Some people appear to retain salt more readily than others. And of course some people eat far more salt than others. We have no need for salt. The modern American diet contains enough salt for good health without adding any in cooking or at the table. So specialists in kidney, heart and circulatory problems are recommending that you throw away your salt shaker.

Finally, Dr. Kaufman believes there is a kind of psychosomatic arthritis. People living under constant stress or under unbearable conditions which seemingly cannot be changed may develop joint symptoms which are not actually physical but are brought about by life circumstances, whether they are imagined or real.

Dr. Kaufman's conclusions are these: "During the first month of adequate therapy with niacinamide (alone or in combination with other vitamins) a patient with joint dysfunction (with or without rheumatic or hypertrophic arthritis) will have a rise in the Joint Range Index of at least 6–12 points, and thereafter will have a rise of at least ½ to 1 point per month of adequate niacinamide therapy, provided he eats the average American diet containing adequate calories and sufficient protein, and provided he does not mechanically injure his joints excessively. This improvement in joint mobility occurs regardless of the age or sex of the patient and regardless of whatever other health problems he may have. Subsequently, with continuously adequate niacinamide therapy, the Joint Range Index of 90–100 (no joint dysfunction) is reached and maintenance doses of niacinamide are required to keep the Index at this level." The only exception to this rule, he says, is the patient whose joints are ankylosed—that is, immovably fixed in one position. Such patients cannot ever achieve perfect range of movement, says Dr. Kaufman.

The patient must go on taking niacinamide. If he stops, the symptoms gradually recur. If, after he has achieved the best possible dosage *for him,* he reduces the dosage, he will regress to whatever degree of improvement such a dosage can produce for him individually. Dr. Kaufman says his patients derive other benefits from the vitamin treatment. Digestive complaints may disappear. They may tire less easily. Liver tenderness and enlargement may disappear. Muscle strength seems to improve.

"In the last stages of rheumatic arthritis there may be so much retrogressive tissue alteration in non-articular as well as articular tissue, that complete functional and structural recovery may not be possible, even with prolonged niacin-amide therapy," says Dr. Kaufman. He tells us, too, that he does not know how or why niacinamide acts to improve the condition of painful, stiff joints. He hopes that more research will be done on this. He does believe, however, that "the evolution of the common form of joint dysfunc-tion can be prevented by adequate niacinamide supplemen-tation of an adequate diet throughout the lifetime of an indi-vidual."

Other investigators in earlier years have turned up much valuable evidence that vitamin C is essential, in large amounts, to prevent and treat arthritis. Indeed, there seems to be great similarity between the joint symptoms of scurvy, the disease of vitamin C deficiency, and arthritis. In each case the collagen is disordered. This is the substance of which we are made, especially joints. Vitamin C is essential for the manufacture of collagen. In its absence, as in scurvy, collagen simply wastes away until the poor scurvy victim cannot walk or endure the pain of moving his joints. Is it not possible that modern arthritis may be caused in part at least by all the demands made on our vitamin C stores by all the poisons in our environment, along with the fact that many of us simply don't get enough vitamin C to meet our needs?

Practically all researchers on arthritis stress the need for an adequate diet with plenty of protein and elimination of sugar and all foods that contain it. Past researches have turned up the fact that arthritics tend to eat lots of sugar. Many are victims of low blood sugar which is corrected by a diet in which sugar is eliminated and protein is stressed. Early investigations turned up the fact that children who developed rheumatic heart conditions did not like or did not eat eggs when they were young. Perhaps the bounty of high quality protein plus the vitamins and minerals of eggs are far more important than we know in preventing the aches and disability of arthritis.

Three other books that devote pages to Dr. Kaufman's

niacinamide treatment for arthritis are: *Arthritis Without Aspirin* by George Berkley, Ph.D., *Arthritis: Don't Learn to Live With It* by Carlton Fredericks, Ph.D., and *Dr. Atkins' Nutrition Breakthrough* by Robert C. Atkins, M.D.

# CHAPTER 19

# There's a Lack of Pyridoxine in Our Meals

IN THE OCTOBER, 1975 ISSUE of the *Huxley Institute Newsletter*, Dr. Abram Hoffer, a Canadian psychiatrist who uses largely nutritional methods in treating mental patients, says, "Since there is no definite B6 deficiency disease as there is for vitamin C (scurvy) physicians have not been trained to look for evidence of pyridoxine deficiency. The daily B6 intake recommending up to two milligrams per day has no meaning, since it ignores wide-ranging differences between people. The need varies with the state of health—the more protein consumed the more B6 is required."

Dr. Hoffer believes that 75 percent of people who are severely ill with mental disorders need much larger amounts of B6. "As well as being mentally ill," he says, "these patients may have constipation and abdominal pains, unexplained fever and chills, morning nausea (especially if pregnant), low blood sugar, impotence or lack of menstruation and nerve symptoms such as amnesia, tremor, spasms and seizures. About one-third of all schizophrenic patients suffer from this need for very large amounts of the vitamin."

*Executive Health*, November, 1975 stated that mentally retarded children suffering from convulsions were controlled when B6 was given. Radiologists have found that B6 can prevent the nausea that accompanies x-ray treatment. Obstetricians use it to prevent morning sickness. One group of women and girls with acne took 50 milligrams of B6 daily for one

144

week before and during their periods and found that the acne was controlled.

Dr. Bernard Rimland of California, treating disturbed children, has given them from 2 to 3 grams of vitamin C daily, plus 150 to 400 milligrams of B6, 200 milligrams of pantothenic acid plus a high potency B complex supplement which includes the other B vitamins. Dr. Rimland said in *Science News*, April 18, 1981 that pyridoxine has been very helpful in treating autistic children. "There are now at least nine studies in world literature showing vitamin B6 to be helpful to autistic and autistic-type children. Four of these studies are classic, double-blind placebo-crossover design, and highly significant improvement has been demonstrated not only in the children's behavior but also in the urinary excretion of metabolites, and in the electrical activity of their brains. . . . There are no studies which contradict these positive results. In none of the studies have there been any significant side effects. Vitamin B6 is undoubtedly an extremely safe and inexpensive treatment as well as a rational one. Normal, as well as autistic children, require B6 daily. No one requires Thorazine (a popular tranquilizer) . . .

"The real reason there has been such wide neglect of the therapeutic potential of vitamin B6 in autism may be found in the longstanding, deeply ingrained hostility of the medical profession toward the concept that something as simple and innocuous as a vitamin can have profound effects upon human health and well being."

In 1981 *Medical Tribune* reported on the Brain Bio Center in New Jersey where psychiatrists treat mental disorders, mostly schizophrenia, using chiefly nutritional therapies. They report improvement in 90 percent of the 12,000 patients who had been treated there at that time. Carl Pfeiffer, Ph.D., M.D., founded and directs the Center. About half its patients are referred by psychiatrists for severe psychoses. Some prescriptions at the Center are for 200 to 1500 milligrams of B6, along with thiamine, folic acid, inositol, pantothenic acid, vitamin C and several trace minerals. Dr. Pfeiffer bases his dosages of vitamin B6 on whether the patient can remember his dreams when he wakens. If not, the dose is increased. Dr. Pfeiffer has written a number of books, including *Mental and Elemental Nutrients,* which is listed in our bibliography.

A publication of Hoffman-LaRoche, producer of vitamins and drugs, describes a number of cases of individuals born with a "dependency" on vitamin B6. They describe a 13-day old infant who suffered from constant and intractable convulsions from three hours after her birth. Giving the baby B6 stopped the convulsions, yet they recurred when the child was not taking enough B6. This is an instance of "dependency" on this vitamin. It means that the individual must take considerably larger amounts of the vitamin throughout life than the rest of us need if we do not have this condition.

The publication states that early recognition of this condition and the administration of B6 can save the newborn from serious troubles and possibly mental retardation in later life. In some cases there is a familial pattern—brothers and sisters of the patient with this dependency also are afflicted with convulsions unless they are taking B6 throughout life. It seems possible that this extreme need for very large doses of this vitamin in a few individuals may be important for all of us to remember. Perhaps many of us may have needs for B6 that are not this urgent or life-threatening. But we may have inherited needs for much more B6 than the average person.

In 1985 Dr. Karl Folkers of the University of Texas received the American Chemical Society's highest award— the Priestley Medal. In his acceptance speech he described his use of B6 in treating a very common disorder of the wrist, Carpal Tunnel Syndrome, which causes numbness and stiffness of the hands. Working with Dr. John Ellis, a Texas general practitioner, he gave the vitamin to victims of this condition and brought about relief in most of them. During this study, he said, he came to the conclusion that nearly 95 percent of Americans are deficient in this B vitamin.

He said that vitamins have been abused and the public suffers because of it. One might ask, "What is the effect

of going through many years of life with a vitamin B6 deficiency" or "Is it all right to be a little deficient in B6?" If
you replace the word "deficient" with the word "sick"
then the question becomes "Is it all right to be a little sick
many years of your life?"

Fortunately Dr. Folkers' work with Dr. Ellis has aroused
great interest. A number of letters came in to *Chemical and
Engineering News* when an article on Folkers was printed.
Several letters told of taking B6 for years and curing painful
wrists. The *New York Times* described the work of a physician,
Dr. Allan Bernstein, chief of neurology at Kaiser Hospital
in California, who experimented with B6 in 40 patients and
found that taking 50 milligrams of B6 three times a day
resulted in "dramatic improvement" in 80 percent of the
cases of Carpal Tunnel Syndrome.

Numbness, tingling, pain and stiffness in fingers and hands
are early symptoms of vitamin B6 deficiency—"signs of
winter rheumatism which has made people ill for 2,000
years," says Dr. John Ellis. He has treated many thousands
of patients with vitamin B6 (pyridoxine). In his county in
Texas for ten consecutive years local drug stores sold annually
two million vitamin B6 tablets and during that time no medical
man reported any adverse side effects from taking the vitamin
in much larger doses than the RDA.

Dr. Ellis listed the following conditions that are linked to
longterm deficiency in vitamin B6: Carpal Tunnel Syndrome,
tenosynovitis, tendonitis, DeQuervain's disease, diabetes
mellitus, diabetic neuropathy, periarticular synovitis; shoul-
der-hand syndrome; premenstrual edema; menopausal arthritis; edema of pregnancy, use of birth control pills, arterial
subendothelial proliferation and arteriosclerosis (hardening
of the arteries).

Dr. Ellis said that animals on vitamin B6-deficient diets
do not produce insulin normally. This is the body hormone
which regulates blood sugar levels. Diabetic patients are more
prone to have numbness, tingling and loss of sensation in
their hands. They may also develop the painful wrist condition
called Carpal Tunnel Syndrome. He has successfully treated

these conditions with pyridoxine in doses of 50 to 100 milligrams daily for 12 weeks. He thinks diabetics should consider taking pyridoxine supplements every day for all their lives.

From 1975 to 1982 Dr. Ellis, working with Dr. Folkers, demonstrated a correlation between degree of deficiency in B6 and crippling in shoulders, arms and hands. When B6 was given daily for 12 weeks the symptoms disappeared. Dr. Ellis suggested that white bread be enriched with one milligram of B6 to every slice of bread and one milligram to every cup of milk. "We have to begin somewhere," he says, "to prevent crippling vitamin B6 deficiency in the United States."

Dr. Ellis for some 25 years in his practice of obstetrics and gynecology has found that women who take between 100 and 300 milligrams of B6 daily during pregnancy have far fewer childbirth complications than those who are deficient in B6. Edema or swelling of the hands and feet can be prevented if enough B6 is taken during pregnancy. This is especially important for the pregnant woman who is diabetic. If the mother has eaten wisely during her pregnancy, has avoided smoking and alcohol and is getting enough of all the essential nutrients, the baby will come into the world equipped with the enzymes that are necessary for normal function. More than 100 of these enzymes depend on vitamin B6 for their healthful functioning.

Pregnant women need about 5.5 to 7.6 milligrams a day of pyridoxine, according to Dr. Karen Schuster of the University of Florida. She studied 196 mothers-to-be who were given various doses of B6 ranging from none to 20 grams a day. One minute after the babies were born the heart rate, breathing, reflexes, color and muscle tone of the babies were evaluated. Babies of mothers who had a total B6 intake of 7.6 milligrams daily had higher scores in all these aspects of health than those mothers who had an intake of 5.5 milligrams or less. Studies with animals have demonstrated the same thing. Vitamin B6 is especially important in the development of the nervous system of the unborn child.

In 1980 a Purdue nutritionist, Dr. Avanelle Kirksery,

Ph.D., reported in *Medical Tribune* that women who have been on The Pill for long periods may supply their infants with breast milk that is deficient in B6. She said, "Long-term use (of the Pill) can result in a reduction of this vitamin in the blood and possibly in the tissues of the mother. Then, if we don't have adequate supplementation with the vitamin during pregnancy and during lactation, it can affect the vitamin level in her milk." Lack of pyridoxine in one brand of formula in the 1950's resulted in very serious symptoms in babies who got the formula. The convulsive seizures which affected them caused a number of the babies to die. In 1982 another commercial formula was found by FDA to lack B6. This product has been removed from sale.

An article in *Nutrition Reviews,* March 1967, described B6 dependency showing that drugs commonly prescribed for epileptic convulsions are not effective in alleviating the ones caused by B6 deficiency. But giving the vitamin intravenously will stop the convulsions within minutes. In 1974, Dr. David Coursin reported in *Family Practice News* that B6 is of great value in treating schizophrenics, Down's Syndrome, myoclonic seizures and mental retardation.

Adelle Davis in her book *Let's Get Well* gave well-documented accounts of using magnesium and pyridoxine for muscle and nerve disorders of many kinds. She also related many documented stories of epileptic attacks alleviated with B6 alone. She pointed out that many years ago Dr. Tom Spies, the distinguished physician who stopped the pellagra epidemic in our Southland gave vitamin B6 to epileptics with excellent results. She told of 30 epileptic children given 340 milligrams of magnesium daily who could discontinue all drugs usually given for this disorder. Only one child of the 30 did not respond, possibly because this child was deficient in B6. Doesn't it seem only common sense for anyone who has this serious and destructive disorder to take B6 and magnesium supplements along with whatever medical prescriptions are already being taken?

In 1979 two neurologists at Massachusetts Institute of Technology wrote an article *Beyond Cholesterol* which they later developed into a book of the same name, in which they challenged the widely held theory that cholesterol in meals is the basic cause (or maybe the only cause) of our epidemic of heart and other circulatory diseases. They based their theory on an early study of a number of children who were mentally deficient because of very high levels of a compound called homocysteine in their blood. These very young children were all suffering from advanced hardening of the arteries and blood clots.

In 1969, Kilmer S. McCully of Harvard Medical School announced that pyridoxine is essential for the body to process normally this harmful compound. If the vitamin is not present in large enough amounts homocysteine may cause hardening of the arteries in adults, as well. A number of animal and human experiments here and abroad showed that homocysteine does indeed bring about clogged arteries when there is not enough vitamin B6 in the diet. Surveys have shown that heart attack victims have much less B6 in their blood than healthy people. They are also much more likely to have high levels of homocysteine in their blood.

A question addressed to one of the syndicated columnists recently asked if it is true that B6 can help prevent blood clots that may cause strokes. The physician columnist replied that the original article theorizing that this might be true appeared in *The Lancet*. He went on to say that if this is true under real lifetime conditions, then there may be some rationale for considering vitamin B6 as effective in preventing heart disease. Then he added, as all such columnists usually do, that we must investigate this matter thoroughly, and meanwhile all of us should be eating well balanced diets! There's a conservative answer to a most provocative question!

Over 40 years ago, J. F. Rinehart and L. D. Greenberg fed monkeys a diet deficient in B6 and produced hardening of the arteries of these animals—the very condition which is most likely to result in heart attacks and strokes. Their research appeared in *The American Journal of Pathology*, 1949, volume 25, pages 481–96. It was apparently ignored by the medical establishment.

# THERE'S A LACK OF PYRIDOXINE IN OUR MEALS

In *The Lancet* for October 10, 1981 three Canadian physicians commented on new discoveries that B6 is powerful against the unnatural blood clotting process that produces strokes. It seems that the vitamin stops the formation of fibrin (a protein substance in blood that encourages clotting) and also stops aggregation or clustering of those blood cells called platelets which form the clot. The physicians believed these new discoveries should make the role of B6 as a possible anti-stroke agent worthy of careful consideration. In the years since then we have found little evidence that the medical establishment has made any effort to confirm this extremely important discovery.

One hospitalization in every 1,000 in our country is for kidney stone removal. A 1974 article in the *International Journal for Vitamin and Nutrition Research* described experiments with rats fed a diet complete in all essential nutrients except magnesium, phosphorus and B6. The animals were stunted and their kidneys retained calcium and phosphorus indicating that kidney stones would result. A January, 1976 article in *Nutrition Reviews* described an experiment with human volunteers in the "stone belt"—that part of our country where the incidence of kidney stone is highest.

The researchers studied 265 volunteers separated into two groups, one of which was given supplements of pyridoxine and magnesium. In the group which got the supplements the average number of stones per year was reduced to almost zero and all stone formation was limited to only 17 of these people. The rest had no symptoms of stone, although they had a long history of forming kidney stones over the past years. The experts who conducted the study say they do not know why or how this treatment works. It's possible, they think, that the person who persistently forms kidney stones is just not getting enough of these two nutrients in the diet.

Do you see any reason why any chronic kidney stone victim should go on suffering from this painful disorder when the answer probably lies in a few pills of a harmless mineral and an equally harmless vitamin? The reason probably lies in the number of supermarket foods almost totally depleted of these two nutrients and the astronomical profits the food industry makes from these foods. Magnesium and B6 appear together most abundantly in the same foods. We give lists of these foods elsewhere in this book.

Environmental things that cause bladder cancer are all about us. At least 14 chemical compounds have been identified as potential causes of bladder cancer. We face at present some seven million new manmade chemical compounds. Essentially all of these have not been tested for toxicity and many of them are already in our environment. Six thousand more are manufactured and turned loose upon us every week. Incidence of bladder cancer in smokers is twice that of non-smokers. Dr. Balfour Mount, a Canadian physician, says that one of the reasons is probably that smoking depletes the body of vitamin C which is protective against cancer.

Dr. Mount also recommends B6 as protective against bladder cancer since it tends to restore the cancer victim's tryptophane metabolism to normal. About half the patients who get bladder cancer excrete elevated amounts of the breakdown products of this amino acid which are believed to be cancer-causing. Since B6 is harmless and appears to be essential for cooperating with tryptophane in body functions, Dr. Mount believes that 200 milligrams of B6 taken every day might "rectify the whole metabolic picture where some cancer-causing chemicals are concerned."

Malignant melanoma is a very dangerous skin cancer which tends to spread rapidly to other parts of the body, invading them with new cancer cells. *Medical World News* reported in 1985 on an experiment in which two patients with this form of cancer were treated with the pyridoxal form of B6 in a salve which was applied to the skin four times a day. After 14 days the application produced more than 50% regression of the lesions and destruction of the tumor. Untreated tumors on the same patients showed no improvement. Dr. Larry Nathanson, who conducted the experiment, said that lack of toxicity of this salve should allow its use against other cancerous skin growths.

Gyrate atrophy of the corona of the eye is defined as "progressive atrophy of the choroid and pigment of epithelium of the retina." Night blindness and scotomas (blind spots) are common. The disorder is frequently familial. Finnish and American researchers have tried B6 which is involved with an enzyme which converts a protein into a form that is harmless to the eye. An Oregon scientist who has tried this vitamin stated in *The Journal of the American Medical Association,* "If gyrate atrophy can be treated in some persons, it will become only the fourth of approximately 50 choroidal and retinal diseases of this class to be treatable."

*Merck's Manual,* a medical textbook, says that pyridoxine, 50 to 100 milligrams intramuscularly or orally, has been valuable in some cases of nausea. Adelle Davis in *Let's Get Well* stated that the vitamin has been used not only in pregnancy's morning sickness, but also in treating nausea from car, sea, air, and radiation sickness.

Cramps—both menstrual cramps and those nighttime cramps in legs and feet that bother so many people have been treated successfully with B6 and magnesium. Once again, the two work together, just as all the B vitamins work together. Speaking of the edema of pregnancy, Dr. John Ellis says, "Many doctors have come to accept it as being normal during pregnancy and patients have grown resigned to suffering through it. It is not normal at all. It is not normal at any time. The patient feels bad. There is nothing healthy about being swollen with fluid." He treats it with B6.

Of course, many other conditions also cause edema or fluid accumulation. It seems likely, does it not, that plenty of B6 might work just as well under these circumstances. In any case, there is no reason not to try it—in reasonable amounts, along with whatever medical treatment is being given. The diuretics (water pills) which are usually prescribed for this condition very often cause grievous loss of many essential minerals and vitamins. B6 and magnesium are among these.

Alan R. Gaby, M.D. of Baltimore believes that B6 deficiency is a modern epidemic. He mentions hyperactivity in children as one condition that responds to B6, as well as premenstrual syndrome. Children suffering from asthma are often deficient in this vitamin. Giving the children a B6 supplement brings fewer asthma attacks. Kidney stones are twice as common today as they were 20 years ago, he says. Vitamin B6 supplements, along with the trace mineral magnesium, can reduce the recurrence rate of kidney stones by more than 90 percent.

"Research has also shown," he says, "that B6 helps relieve M.S.G. intolerance (Chinese Restaurant Syndrome) and some cases of depression. Furthermore, there is evidence that B6 may help prevent cardiovascular disease and bladder cancer." Dr. Gaby points out that many toxic substances in our environment make demands on our store of B6. Hydrazines and hydrazides are sprayed on our food as pesticides and for other reasons. Yellow Dye #5 (tartrazine) is broken down into hydrazine in the body. PCB's and many industrial contaminants find their way into our food. These are potent enemies of B6.

Some prescription drugs also cause loss of B6: birth control pills and some drugs for high blood pressure, heart disease and depression. More than 400 drugs contain the yellow dye mentioned above. "Thus," he says, "modern man is being bombarded from all directions with chemicals that increase the need for vitamin B6. It is no wonder that this vitamin has recently become so helpful for such a wide range of ailments."

Dr. Gaby thinks that probably all of us should be taking a B6 supplement daily. True, there have been reports of unpleasant side effects from individuals taking 2,000 milligrams of B6 daily. There is no need to take that much. The Pill causes deficiencies not just in B6 but also folic acid, vitamin C, magnesium and other essential nutrients. If you can, avoid all foods and drugs that contain the yellow dye. Eat foods as little processed as possible.

Isoniazid is a drug given to tuberculosis patients which may have very serious side effects. If an overdose is given the side effects may be grand mal seizures (epilepsy), coma or acidosis. Three Boston physicians gave large doses of pyridoxine to five patients who had been given overdoses of the drug. They gave the same amount of B6 which had been given as an overdose of the drug. Within two hours of the beginning of the seizures, all five patients given B6 were free of seizures, with no other side effects of the overdose. *Drug Induced Nutritional Deficiencies* by Daphne Roe detailed experiments conducted as long ago as 1954 showing that overdoses of this powerful drug produce nerve defects brought about by destruction of B6.

Studies in England have shown that women on The Pill need far more of this vitamin than the rest of us. Other studies have shown that other drugs destroy pyridoxine in the body: certain drugs for hypertension, the drug penicillamine, used to treat many disorders, and a drug given to Parkinson's patients also destroys vitamin B6.

B6 deficiency isn't just a potential danger to young folks. At Virginia Polytechnic and State University a study of the diets of 17 elderly men and 20 elderly women showed that almost half the women and one-fifth of the men were getting less than half the recommended RDA for B6. Ninety percent of the women and half the men were found to be getting less than 70 percent of the RDA.

Since Chinese cooking became fashionable in our country, monosodium glutamate (MSG) has become a favorite flavoring ingredient of most dishes served in Chinese restaurants. Often it is used in very large amounts. And often some people get disturbing side effects from such dishes. There may be sensations of warmth, stiffness, weakness of arms and legs, tingling, pressure, headache, light-headedness, heartburn or digestive discomfort.

Cases have been reported where the victims had to be hospitalized so severe were their symptoms. *Nutrition Reviews*, January, 1982 theorizes that the people who are thus affected are deficient in B6. Of a group of students taking a capsule containing MSG without knowing what it contained, 12 developed the nerve symptoms described above.

Given 50 milligrams of B6 every day for 12 weeks, eight of the nine students getting the B6 had no symptoms. Three students taking a "nothing" capsule developed their original symptoms. One student needed more than 100 milligrams daily of B6 to prevent the symptoms caused by MSG.

Which foods are devoid of pyridoxine? Only those foods which make up half the diets of many Americans—the refined

## *Pyridoxine Content of Some Common Foods*

**(We list milligrams per serving of about three ounces. Remember that foods like brewers yeast are used in much smaller amounts than this. Even so, their pyridoxine content is remarkable.)**

| Food | Milligrams |
| --- | --- |
| Almonds | .100 |
| Avocados | .420 |
| Beans, dried | .560 |
| Brazilnuts | .170 |
| Breads, cracked wheat | .092 |
| Pumpernickel | .160 |
| Wholewheat | .180 |
| Broccoli | .195 |
| Brussels sprouts | .170 |
| Bulgur | .225 |
| Cheese, cheddar | .080 |
| cottage | .040 |
| Swiss | .043 |
| Chestnuts | .330 |
| Chickpeas | .540 |
| Chicken | .683 |
| Codfish | .225 |
| Corn on the cob | .161 |
| Corn grits | .147 |
| Crab | .300 |
| Eggs | .110 |

carbohydrates (white flour and white sugar) since essentially all vitamins have been removed from these two foods in the processing. Probably one important reason why so many Americans are deficient in B6 is that, even if you are eating a reasonably good diet, lots of B6 is lost in the preparation of food. Back in 1979 Dr. W. H. Sebrell of the Institute of Nutrition Sciences, Columbia University, stated that, "Some investigators believe that a surprisingly high percentage of

| | |
|---|---|
| Filberts | .545 |
| Flounder | .170 |
| Halibut | .430 |
| Kale | .300 |
| Kidneys | .430 |
| Lamb | .275 |
| Lentils | .600 |
| Liver | .840 |
| Mackerel | .660 |
| Milk | .040 |
| Oatmeal | .140 |
| Peanuts | .400 |
| Popcorn | .204 |
| Pork | .350 |
| Prunes | .240 |
| Rice, brown | .550 |
| Salmon | .700 |
| Sausage, liverwurst | .190 |
| Shrimp | .100 |
| Soybean flours | .570 |
| defatted | .724 |
| Sunflower seed | 1.250 |
| Tuna | .425 |
| Turnip Greens | .263 |
| Walnuts | .730 |
| Wheat bran | .820 |
| Wheat germ | 1.150 |
| Yeast, brewers | 2,500 |

Americans are not getting enough of this vital nutrient in their meals."

Typical home and restaurant meals analyzed in laboratory tests at Massachusetts Institute of Technology were found to contain much less B6 than expected, indicating significant losses of the vitamin during the processing and preparation of foods. Roman J. Kutsky, Ph.D., in *Handbook of Vitamins, Minerals and Hormones* states that up to 30 to 45 percent of this vitamin is lost in cooking, also lost in anyone with diseases of the digestive tract, anyone taking diuretics or anyone undergoing radiation treatment. This suggests using as many vegetables and fruits raw as possible and as fresh as possible. It also suggests that, in the modern process of irradiating foods to prolong their shelf life, much of the B6 may be lost.

Can you get too much pyridoxine? As we have shown above, many physicians are using B6 in quite large amounts and achieving almost miraculous results in many cases. However, in 1983 *The New England Journal of Medicine* reported on seven patients who had been taking between 2,000 and 6,000 milligrams of B6 each day for periods between two months and 40 months. They developed nervous symptoms, chiefly inability to coordinate movements. There was no evidence of damage to the central nervous system, and the individuals improved after they stopped taking these very large doses.

At once newspapers and magazines across the country featured headlines warning the public of instant disaster if they take even one tiny bit over the RDA of any vitamin. Since then, various government bureaus have been calling for restriction on the amount of vitamins that may be put into any one tablet or capsule. Government bureaus are urging physicians to report any cases of overdosage of vitamins to them so that, presumably, they can continue to warn against their use.

It seems perfectly obvious that the individuals reported in *The New England Journal* were taking too much B6. However, as Dr. Linus Pauling pointed out in a letter to the *Journal,* "there is no more reason to use the reported toxicity of pyridoxine at very high intakes as the basis for recommending against its use at a lower orthomolecular range than there would be to use the lethal single dose of aspirin . . . and the deaths of hundreds of people per year by aspirin poisoning as the basis for recommending against the present practice of physicians of prescribing three to seven and a half grams of aspirin per day to patients with arthritis." *The Newsletter of the Linus Pauling Institute of Science and Medicine,* Fall, 1983 concluded, "The report of neurological damage of patients taking 2,000 to 6,000 milligrams a day for several months indicates that there is an upper limit to the recommended orthomolecular dosage, perhaps around 1,000 milligrams per day. There is no justification, however, for the authors of this investigation to have recommended against any megavitamin therapy with vitamin B6."

# CHAPTER 20

# Biotin Deficiency Has Serious Consequences

EARLY IN THE 1980's a mystery was solved in regard to a number of puzzling disorders in a newborn baby. The doctors had no idea what might be wrong with this child. His blood sugar was low, blood levels of lactic acid and ammonia were high. These symptoms were so unusual that attending physicians had no idea what could be wrong. They had known of one other baby with somewhat similar symptoms and they decided to try the therapy that had been used then.

They gave the baby high doses of the B vitamin biotin. The treatment worked. In a very short time the baby recovered and developed normally, although he still needed, throughout life, supplements of this vitamin. Apparently, the difficulty was lack of an enzyme needed to process biotin normally. Since this was not present, the child needed very large doses of biotin to live a normal life.

Another case was reported in *The New England Journal of Medicine*. This baby developed normally until the age of three months, when she began to have convulsions and developed an eczema-like rash. She lost her hair, including eyebrows and eyelashes. Testing her blood, doctors found that she suffered from a congenital need for large amounts of biotin. When they gave her 10 milligrams of the vitamin daily, she improved greatly within 12 hours. After four months on biotin she was a perfectly normal baby.

An adult who suffered from Crohn's Disease (regional

enteritis) for 17 years was fed intravenously in a hospital because he had lost so much weight. He soon developed skin troubles around his eyes, nose and mouth, also lethargy and depression. He complained of "pins and needles" sensations in his feet. He lost most of his hair. What remained became gray. Biotin was added to the intravenous fluid and within three months his skin returned to normal, his mental and nervous symptoms improved. It had taken three years for this biotin deficiency to develop due to lack of this nutrient in his intravenous fluid. Over the years he had been given many antibiotics which had destroyed his intestinal bacteria so that they could no longer manufacture any of this essential nutrient in his intestines. The same may be true of many people who take antibiotics for long periods of time.

Almost any kind of peculiar diet might cause lack of biotin and some of the strange symptoms reported above. *The American Journal of Clinical Nutrition* told of a woman whose doctor placed her on a diet supplemented by six raw eggs a day and two quarts of skim milk. She had cirrhosis of the liver. The diet was supposed to increase her intake of high quality protein.

The patient soon developed lack of appetite, nausea, vomiting, inflammation of the tongue, pallor, depression, lassitude, pain, scaly dermatitis (seborrhea) and loss of tissue from her lips. She was given 200 micrograms of biotin daily and within five days all her symptoms cleared or greatly improved. What could have produced the deficiency? The answer is that raw egg white contains a protein called avidin which destroys biotin.

Animals given essentially nothing to eat but raw eggs develop serious symptoms from lack of biotin. This does not mean that an occasional raw egg will bring disaster. But it is not wise to use raw eggs every day (mixed in a blender drink, for example). Cooking the eggs lightly destroys the harmful protein and makes the eggs quite safe.

A Swiss physician theorized in a 1977 *International Journal for Vitamin and Nutrition Research* that lack of biotin might be a contributing cause of Sudden Infant Death Syndrome or "crib death." This tragic occurrence in our country kills about 10,000 babies every year. It occurs most frequently in the second to the fourth month of age, as is also the case of infant seborrhea dermatitis. *Medical World News* in 1984 discussed the possibility of giving pregnant women megadoses of biotin to prevent the effects of the genetic disease which creates the biotin deficiency.

In 1986 Virginia physicians decided to test every newborn baby for biotin deficiency, just as they test for several other genetic conditions which can produce serious complications later in life. For the past two years, three of every 176,000 babies born in Virginia tested positive for this disorder. Dr. Barry Wolf, professor of human genetics and pediatrics of the Medical College of Virginia, estimates that a deficiency in biotinidase (the enzyme necessary for normal use of biotin) occurs in one of every 50,000 to 60,000 babies born.

If the symptoms of such a child are not recognized by the attending physician the child may suffer convulsions, skin rash, loss of hair, difficulty in walking, hearing loss, developmental delay or mental retardation, coma or death. Such conditions may appear anytime from two to three weeks of age up to a few years of age. "Biotinidase deficiency should be added to the group of metabolic diseases for which screening is done in the neonatal period," said Dr. Wolf. Other countries, as well, are conducting tests for determining if a baby's mysterious disorders may be caused by simple lack of enough of this nutrient.

Aside from children with inherited inability to deal normally with biotin, why should the rest of us be very careful to get enough of this vitamin? It is considered a "minor" sort of vitamin and we don't generally hear very much about it. But there is no such thing as a "minor" vitamin as the case histories above demonstrate clearly. Skin, hair, nerves, digestion, sex glands, muscles, all depend partially on the presence of this nutrient in ample amounts. It seems to be impossible to get too much of the vitamin, although very little is needed for good health. True, this vitamin can possibly be manufactured in the healthy digestive tract. But anyone who has taken large amounts of antibiotics by mouth probably does not have such a healthy digestive tract. In addition, persistent diarrhea for any reason, pregnancy, athletic exertions, old age, post-surgery, alcoholism or certain medications may cause anyone's need for biotin to be greatly increased.

A genetic need for much larger doses than "normal" is shown in the case histories cited above. No one knows how the genetic need for many other nutrients may affect our health and the health of newborns. Some day scientists may be able to discover all such inherited defects and provide the remedy in supplements which can be taken throughout life. Until that time, it seems only sensible to eat the most nutritious diet possible and take supplements to make up for any deficits in our diets and any special inborn needs we may have.

How much biotin does the average healthy person need? In 1980 the official book, *Recommended Dietary Allowances,* suggested that, "it is believed that conventional mixed American diets containing approximately 100–300 micrograms of biotin will meet the needs of practically all healthy adults." Would you believe that the 1989 edition of these guidelines *reduced* the RDA to 30–100 micrograms per day! Note that the recommendations for this B vitamin are given in micrograms, rather than milligrams, which suggests that our need for it is quite small—but very important. Keep in mind that, if we are healthy (no skin, hair, nerve, digestive problems) we may need as much as 300 micrograms of biotin daily. Dietary sources may provide amounts like this: 100–400 micrograms in one serving of liver; 10–100 micrograms in one serving of eggs, chicken, wheat, rice, corn, oats, barley, cowpeas, chickpeas, lentils, soybeans, cauliflower, fish, nuts and seeds; 1–100 micrograms in fruits and most vegetables, beef, lamb, veal, pork, tuna, halibut and oysters. How does your family's diet stack up in relation to biotin?

Today, bizarre diets are popular, especially for reducing. Many of them are so badly planned that deficiency in many nutrients is quite possible, biotin among them. An all-fruit diet, for example, might contain almost no biotin, depending on which fruits you eat. A diet of just meat and potatoes with plenty of gravy may contain almost no biotin. A breakfast of coffee and Danish contains none. A snack of potato chips and a soft drink contains none. Just because biotin is probably not listed on the label of contents on packaged foods in the supermarket, don't underestimate its importance for good health.

## *Biotin Content of Some Common Foods*

**(We give the microgram content of a serving, which is a bit more than 3 ounces.)**

|  | *Micrograms* |
|---|---|
| Bananas | 4 |
| Beans, dried limas | 10 |
| Beef | 4 |
| Cauliflower | 17 |
| Corn | 6 |
| Eggs, whole (2) | 25 |
| Filberts | 16 |
| Halibut | 8 |
| Hazel nuts | 14 |
| Liver, beef | 100 |
| Milk (1 cup) | 5 |
| Mushrooms | 16 |
| Oysters | 9 |
| Peanuts | 39 |
| Pork | 7 |
| Salmon | 5 |
| Strawberries | 4 |
| Wheat, whole | 5 |
| Yeast, brewer's (3 tablespoons) | 75 |

# CHAPTER 21

# Vitamin B12 Prevents
# Pernicious Anemia

In December, 1986 two researchers at the University of Alabama reported that treatment with vitamin B12 and folic acid reduces the incidence of pre-cancerous cells in the lungs of long-time smokers. Charles E. Butterworth, M.D., Chairman of the Department of Nutrition Sciences at the University, stated that this vitamin therapy may enable doctors to prevent cancerous growths from developing into lung cancer. By the time a tumor shows up on x-ray, it may be too late to reverse it, he said. But giving the two nutrients earlier can perhaps prevent the growth of cancerous cells.

Dr. Butterworth and Dr. Carlos Krumdieck conducted a four-month study testing sputum samples from 88 men who had a history of smoking up to 30 cigarettes a day for the past 20 years. Half the smokers were given a daily dose of 10 milligrams of folic acid and half a milligram of vitamin B12 while the other half were given a placebo (a "nothing" pill). At the end of the test the group given the vitamins showed fewer pre-cancerous cells than the group which got no vitamins. Dr. Butterworth believes that cigarette smoke inactivates certain vitamins causing localized vitamin deficiency when the smoke hits the surface of the lungs.

The experiment is just another in the long history of vitamin B12 which goes back to 1926 when two researchers cured pernicious anemia by giving the patients liver—the best food source of B12. By 1948 the vitamin was identified and designated as a vitamin. Its uses in the human body include these: it maintains growth, nucleic acid synthesis, also synthesis of protein and fat. It maintains the cells of the skin and the linings of body organs, as well as the nervous system, including the myelin sheaths of the nerves which are disordered in a number of diseases. It also creates red blood cells which are essential for preventing anemia and white blood cells which protect us from germs of various kinds. Deficiency in B12 results in retarded growth, pernicious anemia (which causes death if untreated), and three other kinds of anemia, inflammation of mouth tissues, spinal cord degeneration, sprue—a disease of the digestive tract which causes inability to digest food. Since the early days when the only way to cure or prevent all these disorders was to give liver in large amounts, our researchers now know that giving the actual vitamin B12 either by mouth or intravenously can produce near miracles of cure in disorders associated with the above list of deficiency diseases.

As long ago as 1965 European doctors were reporting great success in treating various mental illnesses with vitamin B12. By testing for B12 deficiency in all patients who did not respond to any therapy for mental illness, European psychiatrists discovered that large numbers of these patients had nothing wrong with them but deficiency in B12. One researcher reported that over one-third of nearly 1500 patients examined had psychiatric symptoms such as irritability, mental apathy, memory defects, mental slowness, fluctuations of mood and other symptoms which appeared before there was any indication of pernicious anemia. Nevertheless, the cause of the symptoms was simply lack of vitamin B12.

One woman brought to a British hospital with numbness and tingling in arms and legs suddenly became psychotic and confused with delusions and hallucinations. The doctors injected vitamin B12 and within 48 hours all mental and emotional symptoms disappeared. One physician declared in 1971 that, "It may be desirable to measure blood B12 levels routinely in all new mentally disturbed patients."

Lhermitte's Sign is a bizarre symptom that involves a

sensation as of an electric shock which appears to shoot into arms and legs from the spine when the neck is stretched or turned. In 1981 *The Journal of the American Medical Association* published an article on this condition, stating that it is caused by a simple deficiency in vitamin B12. Tests on one woman with these symptoms showed very low levels of B12. She was given injections of 500 micrograms of B12 every two weeks. Blood levels rapidly returned to normal. All symptoms disappeared in five months.

In a second case a 44-year old man complained of fatigue, numbness of extremities and intermittent electric shock feelings when he moved his neck. Blood levels of B12 were very low. Treatment with the vitamin for four months brought him back to good health. In a series of 44 such patients referred to neurologists in England, injections of B12 cured the condition.

Roger J. Williams said once, "If I were afflicted with a disease of obscure origin that is virtually untreatable, or if I were a physician in charge of such a case, I would certainly wish first to see if 'supernutrition' might help." Note that the physicians treating the above patients used massive doses of B12.

In 1981 the case of a 77-year old man with the same symptoms was discussed in the *Journal* of the A.M.A. The doctor who treated him successfully with nothing but injections of B12 stated that deficiency of this vitamin is common among elderly people, that almost one-third of them have it, and they should always be tested for deficiency in B12 before other therapy is suggested.

Diabetics suffer from many nerve disorders including tingling in hands and feet, aching pain, disturbed vibration sense and, in men, gradual impotency. Three London physicians writing in *The Lancet* in 1983 theorize that vitamin B12 deficiency may be the cause. They produced similar symptoms in diabetic laboratory animals and cured them with B12. They said, "A possible metabolism of cobalamin (vitamin B12) co-enzymes may be an important factor in the development of acute diabetic neuropathy (nerve disorders) and clearly deserves further investigation."

Is it possible that some people cannot absorb vitamin B12 normally? Yes. A certain substance called "intrinsic factor" must be in the stomach in order for B12 to be absorbed normally. In such conditions, very large doses of the vitamin may result in some B12 being absorbed. Laboratory animals on diets deficient in iron lose their ability to absorb B12. People suffering from any condition that does not permit them to absorb their food normally will almost invariably be deficient in B12. This means people with chronic diarrhea, dysentery, sprue and those who have had part of the digestive tract removed.

Overgrowth of unfriendly bacteria (chiefly E. Coli bacteria) in the colon may result in little absorption of B12, suggesting that yogurt, which supplies the friendly bacteria (Lactobacillus acidophilus) should be part of everyone's diet. Alcoholism also prevents the absorption of B12. Strict vetegarianism results in diets in which this nutrient is almost completely lacking.

The importance of supplements of B12 for vegetarians was highlighted by the story of a fruit bat which flourished in the wild on a completely vegetarian diet but cannot survive on a similar diet in a zoo. Scientists studying the problem came to the conclusion that the bat living in the wild had eaten a lot of insects along with his fruit, and insects, like all living creatures, contain vitamin B12. So giving the fruit bat vitamin B12 made it possible for him to live in the zoo.

In 1978 *Nutrition Reviews* told of a man brought to a doctor with complaints of loss of weight, lack of balance, dizziness, swollen ankles, peculiar gait, numbness in hands and feet and impairment of the sense of touch. He had been a vegetarian for many years and blood levels of B12 were very low. The doctor gave him injections of 1,000 micrograms of B12 every day for three weeks, then for six months he got monthly injections. He was sent home, well, and told to take 100 micrograms of B12 every day from then on.

# VITAMIN B12 PREVENTS PERNICIOUS ANEMIA

In 1978 a six-month old baby was brought to a California hospital near death. He was in a coma, suffering from severe anemia. His arms and legs were covered with blotches of black and blue marks. Pale and limp, he was unresponsive even to painful stimuli. His eyes rolled about unseeingly. He could not control the movements of his head. His hands could not grasp. He had a diaper rash—a fungal disorder.

The doctors gave the baby a blood transfusion and an injection of folic acid, then they started intramuscular injections of B12. The doctors state in the *New England Journal of Medicine* that "the response to vitamin B12 therapy was dramatic." Four days after the initial dose he was alert, smiling, responding to visual stimuli and maintaining his body temperature. The fungus infection disappeared. He went home in two weeks apparently completely well.

He had been breast-fed exclusively since birth by his mother who had been a vegan for the past eight years. She ate no food of animal origin and took no supplements. The baby soon developed B12 deficiency again. The doctors gave him 100 micrograms of B12 each week and he soon returned to normal health. A year later his mother developed very low blood levels of B12 and she began to take supplements.

"These observations indicate that the requirement for vitamin B12 is greater in the infant than in the adult," say the doctors, "The presence of severe symptoms in this infant and their onset at the age of four months suggest that he began uterine life with marginal body stores. Experience with this infant indicates the importance of supplementation with vitamin B12 in the breast-fed infants of vegetarian mothers. Severe deficiency may develop in the absence of any signs or symptoms in the mother . . ." An editorial in the same journal said, in part, "the potential for irreversible neurologic (nerve) damage is already present at birth, and breast feeding with milk low in . . . vitamin B12 merely aggravates an existing problem."

A Canadian physician, D. L. Kotkas, M.D., has been using B12 and folic acid in treating his patients for many years. In 1978, speaking before a meeting of the Canadian

Schizophrenia Foundation, he said he asks for blood counts of folic acid in all his patients. Between 25 and 50 percent have low levels, he said, and these patients tend to be less healthy all around than those who have higher levels. Giving them a combination of B12 and folic acid brings "dramatic improvement" in all cases in the field of depressive illness and a little less improvement in a wide variety of other mental conditions.

Most interesting of all, he said, is that most of these patients have normal levels of B12. When he gives them folic acid the levels of B12 in their blood drop, almost as if the B12 had been substituting for the folic acid, and now that there was enough folic acid, there was no need for raised levels of B12. He believes, he said, that this important relationship between the two vitamins is one reason why some physicians have reported disappointing results in treating mental illness.

He said that deficiencies of both vitamins should be treated before there are symptoms of the extremely serious anemia which is caused by such deficiency. He uses both vitamins in mental illness in the aged, and in so-called "neurotic depression," also in women with conditions related to the reproductive cycle—depression after childbirth, for example. He uses the two vitamins, also, for underactivity of the thyroid gland and low blood sugar. Also for conditions when the body is absorbing large amounts of foreign chemicals like alcohol, drugs or treatment given for epilepsy. In iron deficiency anemia, also, these two vitamins should be given, he says.

Because of the difficulty many people have in absorbing B12, he usually gives it in injections. He often gives immense doses—about 10,000 micrograms a day if necessary, along with folic acid in doses of 10 to 20 milligrams a day. We deal with folic acid in another chapter of this book.

An estimated two to three percent of Americans suffer from psoriasis, the scaly skin disease which may attack anyone from 10 to 50 years of age. A 1960 issue of *Medical World*

*News* reported that two Russian physicians were getting excellent results with vitamin B12 combined with folic acid and vitamin C. They treated 72 patients with injections of the above vitamins twice daily for about 20 days. After three weeks of no treatment, they gave the injections again for another 20 days. Only 14 of the patients reported no improvement. An American physician writing to the *News* stated that he has been using B12 along with a proteolytic enzyme in resistant cases of psoriasis with "marvelous results."

An article in *The Lancet* described the bone marrow and blood condition induced in a number of surgical patients who were given nitrous oxide (laughing gas) during surgery. The physicians tested a number of surgical patients, giving them this anesthetic with or without vitamin B12. The results suggest "an abnormality of vitamin B12 metabolism in the patients as severe as untreated pernicious anemia."

*Medical Tribune* reported in 1978 that nitrous oxide can cause serious nerve abnormalities. Five dentists were studied who had deliberately inhaled the gas regularly for periods of up to six years. Results were numbness in fingers and toes, muscle weakness and lack of coordination, plus difficulty in walking and, in some cases, impotence and loss of bladder control. Nitrous oxide "sniffers" also report the peculiar electric shock sensation from the neck down to the feet. Doctors believe that something about the drug creates a condition in which vitamin B12 cannot be used by the body. If, at any time, you are faced with taking nitrous oxide for surgery, better fortify yourself with plenty of vitamin B12 before the operation. *Merck Manual* reported that improvement in the painful herpes disease of shingles has been found after daily injections of 1,000 micrograms of vitamin B12.

Dr. Roger J. Williams in his book *Nutrition Against Disease* said "Vitamin B12 is definitely a link in the nutritional chain that protects against mental disease. In pernicious anemia caused by deficiency of this vitamin, the mental symptoms are by no means uniform; they can range from such mild symptoms as having difficulty remembering to stuporous depression, severe agitation, hallucinations or even manic or paranoid behavior.''

In general, the reason for using injections of this vitamin is usually the chance that the digestive juice called ''intrinsic factor'' may be missing which means that the vitamin cannot be normally absorbed. Elderly people may suffer from this lack of absorption. If parts of the stomach have been removed, chances are that the vitamin will not be absorbed. Intestinal diseases that cause chronic diarrhea may also make absorption of this vitamin difficult or impossible.

A number of years ago a nutrition scientist published an article in the *Journal of the American Medical Association* saying that anyone taking vitamin C at mealtime is likely to be short on vitamin B12, since, he said, the vitamin C

## Vitamin B12 Content of Some Common Foods

**(We give the number of micrograms in 100 grams, the average serving)**

|  | Micrograms |
|---|---|
| Beef, kidney | 18–55 |
| Beef, liver | 31–120 |
| Beef, round | 3.4–4.5 |
| Bread, whole wheat | 0.2–0.4 |
| Cheese, American | 0.6 |
| Cheese, Swiss | 0.9 |
| Egg, 1 whole | 0.3 |
| Fish, haddock | 0.6 |
| Fish, sole | 1.3 |
| Ham | 0.9–1.6 |
| Milk, whole | 0.3–0.5 |
| Milk, powdered | 1–2.6 |
| Soybean meal | 0.2 |

has a destructive effect on B12. Although a number of physicians disagreed immediately with this theory, confirming their statements with evidence from their own patients, it was not until 1976 that an article in *The American Journal of Clinical Nutrition* published a detailed refutation of these facts. The four authors of the article tested the vitamin B12 content of a meal high in the vitamin, and a meal with not nearly so much of the B vitamin. They added vitamin C up to half a gram (500 milligrams). They could detect no destruction of vitamin B12 in either meal.

They pointed out that B12 is very stable in foods, since it is bound closely to a protein in the food, so closely that "a prolonged chemical attack" could be withstood and the vitamin B12 would not be separated from the food. They believe the incorrect results published earlier were brought about by inadequate methods of extracting the B vitamin from the food being tested. However, this erroneous claim is sometimes still repeated in articles on vitamins. Don't be misled. If you are taking an all-in-one supplement it will contain both vitamins, as it should. If you take massive doses of either or both of the vitamins, you can be certain that one will not "cancel out" the other.

# CHAPTER 22

# Folic Acid Is Absolutely Essential for Us All

C. E. BUTTERWORTH, JR., M.D., of the University of Alabama said in the December 1980 issue of *Contemporary Nutrition* "When chicks and monkeys are grown on a folic-acid deficient diet the female genital tract fails to develop normally in response to estrogen stimulation." In 1973, he said researchers discovered certain abnormal cells in the female cervix which responded to folic acid supplements, so they were evidently caused by deficiency in this nutrient.

He said also that the risk of developing endometrial cancer is four or five times greater in women taking estrogen for long periods. In 1976 a clinical trial tested the theory that cervical disorders are associated with deficiency in folic acid and oral supplements of this vitamin can correct the defect. A test involving 47 young women with mild or moderate disorders of the cervix showed improvement when they were given folic acid supplements, while another group with the same problems given no folic acid did not improve. In four women the trouble progressed to cancer, while none of the women given folic acid had this experience.

*The Lancet* (June 11, 1977) reported on folic acid deficiency as a cause of disorders of the lining of the small intestine in children, especially on those drinking goat milk which is deficient in this nutrient. Giving the babies folic acid supplements brought the condition back to normal. *Nutrition Reviews* (July, 1979) reported on experiments that seemed to show that zinc deficiency may result in lack of ability to absorb folic acid. Possibly many modern Americans are deficient in zinc, since this trace mineral is removed entirely when sugar cane is refined into white sugar and when flour is refined into white flour. It is not replaced by "enrichment." So one reason for deficiency of folic acid may not be just lack of it in your diet, but lack of enough zinc in your diet to help you to absorb the folic acid.

*Nutrition Reviews* for August, 1979 told of a patient who drank heavily and ate little meat, fresh vegetables or fruit. She was suffering from severe anemia brought about by deficiency in folic acid. When the condition was corrected and she responded to the folic acid supplements, she went back to drinking and the anemia returned even in the presence of plenty of this B vitamin. The authors suggested a two-fold approach to the rehabilitation of alcoholic patients. "Eat well and stop drinking."

Dr. Victor Herbert, M.D. tested the essential nature of folic acid by going on a diet in which all folic acid was removed, although all other nutrients were present. After 16 weeks on the diet he became sleepless, forgetful and irritable. He lost weight. By the 19th week his bone marrow showed unmistakable changes in the cells indicating anemia from lack of folic acid. Within 48 hours of taking a folic acid supplement his bone marrow tests returned to normal and other problems disappeared.

Dr. Herbert and a colleague tested alcoholic patients by giving them a few drinks in the hospital. First, they cured the anemia of the alcoholics, then gave them daily alcoholic drinks. Within ten days the symptoms of folic acid deficiency appeared again. Folic acid supplements did no good as long as the patients continued to drink. These researchers believe that one reason alcoholics improve in hospitals is that alcohol is unavailable and folic acid is available in the hospital diet.

Arthritics have been found to be deficient in folic acid. Also patients with many kinds of skin disorders. But pregnant women are most likely to develop this deficiency, possibly the chief cause of the many childbirth disasters—spontaneous abortions, miscarriages and hemorrhaging in pregnancy. One London physician believes that about 60 percent of all pregnant women are unable to meet the demands for folic acid in pregnancy. In 1969 the *Journal of the American Medical Association* printed a number of articles on the widespread deficiency of this vitamin in women on The Pill although the blood of some of these women showed no deficiency. It appeared to be localized in the tissues of the cervical area.

Today two children out of every thousand born come into the world with a serious spinal deformity called *spina bifida*, or neural tube defect. There is a defect in the closure of the vertebral column through which protrude membranes that normally cover the spinal cord. The problem of treating such patients has been successful only with surgery for many years.

Recent research and experiments in England have shown without any question that the defect is caused by nutritional deficiency and one of the deficient nutrients is folic acid. In a trial with pregnant women who had already borne children with spina bifida these women were given supplements of folic acid. Their next child was normal. Women who got no folic acid continued to produce children with spina bifida. A second trial reported in *The Lancet* showed that, of 254 pregnant women with a history of having these defective children, rates of recurrence among those given folic acid supplements were only 0.5 while women who did not get the vitamin had 4.2 percent incidence of these defective births. Deficiency in folic acid occurs in about one third to one half of all pregnant women throughout the world, according to an early study by the World Health Organization. During pregnancy the need for folic acid may double or triple.

Children who are breastfed usually are not deficient in folic acid while children fed on cow's milk formula may be. *Nutrition Reviews*, March 1982, described a "binder" in human milk which helps us to absorb this vitamin. Human milk is rich in this binder. Cow's milk which has been pasteurized does not seem to contain it. This suggests still another reason why breast feeding is the best idea for all babies.

Patients with Crohn's Disease may suffer from deficiency in folic acid, simply because it is not normally absorbed in individuals with this condition. Because anemia caused by lack of this vitamin may be confused with that of deficiency in vitamin B12, it is recommended that the two always be given together or that, in the case of anemia, tests be made to determine the patient's condition in regard to both nutrients.

*Executive Health* reported in 1976 that deficiency in folic acid has often been found in patients with congestive heart failure when fluids accumulate in the body. Diuretics (water pills) given to eliminate the excess fluid may cause loss of folic acid at the same time. Folic acid deficiency is also found in many children with rheumatic heart disease. A 1966 experiment with patients who had hardening of the arteries produced improvement in vision and circulatory problems when five to 7.5 milligrams of folic acid were given daily.

Celiac disease (or sprue) which involves inability to tolerate certain proteins in grains, can cause serious loss of folic acid. Various drugs can induce deficiency in folic acid. One is methotrexate used in treatment of cancer. Patients treated for malaria often develop deficiency in folic acid because of the drugs given. Anticonvulsant drugs given for epilepsy also deplete the body of this nutrient. Giving vitamin B12 and folic acid together has been found to be effective in epileptics.

Seven of nine patients in a mental hospital who were getting the drug phenytoin (Dilantin) were suffering from severe gum disorders apparently brought about by long-time treatment with this drug. Doctors gave the patients five milligrams of folic acid once a week. This brought their blood levels of folic acid up to normal and repaired the damaged gums.

*Nutrition Reviews* reported in 1982 on efforts to "enrich" many common foods with folic acid, both here and in other parts of the world, so common is the occurrence of deficiency.

177

Apparently no steps have been taken in this direction either here or abroad. The same issue of *Reviews* describes a "schizophrenic" teenager whose trouble was finally diagnosed as a congenital absence of several enzymes which are necessary for absorbing and using this vitamin. Sent to a hospital, she was withdrawn, had hallucinations, feelings of persecution and night terrors. She had to be fed, bathed and dressed. Given folic acid and pyridoxine she improved greatly, re-

## *Folic Acid Content of Some Common Foods*

**(We list micrograms per serving of 100 grams)**

|  | Micrograms |
|---|---|
| Almonds | 46 |
| Apricots, fresh | 3.6 |
| Apricots, dried | 4.7 |
| Asparagus | 89–140 |
| Avocados | 4–57 |
| Barley | 50 |
| Beans, Lima, fresh | 10–56 |
| Beans, Lima, dry | 100 |
| Beans, Navy, dry | 130 |
| Beef, round steak | 7–17 |
| Beef, liver | 290 |
| Beef, kidney | 58 |
| Blackberries | 6–18 |
| Bread, rye | 20 |
| Bread, wheat | 27 |
| Bread, white | 15 |
| Broccoli | 34 |
| Brussels sprouts | 27 |
| Buttermilk | 11 |
| Cabbage | 6–42 |
| Cauliflower | 29 |
| Cheese, cheddar | 15 |
| Cheese, cottage | 21–46 |

lapsed when she left the hospital, then returned with the same history of disorders. Given B6 and folic acid again she returned to near normal and, on 10 milligrams of folic acid daily she became normal for several years.

Richard A. Branda of the University of Minnesota said in 1982 that patients with certain anemias also have chromosome abnormalities. When folic acid is given to them these breaks improve. Grant R. Sutherland of Adelaide Children's

| | |
|---|---|
| Coconut | 28 |
| Corn, sweet | 9–70 |
| Dates | 25 |
| Egg, 1 whole | 5.1 |
| Egg, yolk | 13 |
| Endive | 27–63 |
| Flour, enriched white | 8.1 |
| Flour, rye | 18 |
| Flour, whole wheat | 38 |
| Ham, smoked | 7.8 |
| Kale | 50.9 |
| Lentils, dry | 99 |
| Lettuce | 4–54 |
| Liver, beef | 290 |
| Liver, chicken | 380 |
| Liver, lamb | 280 |
| Liver, pork | 220 |
| Mushrooms | 14–29 |
| Oats | 23–66 |
| Peanuts | 57 |
| Peas | 5–35 |
| Potatoes | 2–130 |
| Rice, brown | 22 |
| Spinach | 49–110 |
| Tangerines | 7.4 |
| Turnip greens | 83 |
| Watercress | 48 |
| Wheat | 27–51 |
| Zucchini | 11 |

Hospital in Australia said there are at least 15 fragile sites along human chromosomes, most of which can be protected by folic acid supplements when the cells are grown in a test tube. It seems likely that the same would occur in the human cell inside the human body. Another Minnesota scientist, Professor George J. Yunis, M.D., found that folic acid seems to bolster chromosomes against cancer.

A French researcher, Dr. Jerome Lejeune has given folic acid to children with Down's Syndrome. He has found, he says, a gap at the end of the X chromosome when there is not enough folic acid present. His experiments with children have shown great improvement in the number of healthy chromosomes when folic acid is given. According to *Executive Health,* other conditions that respond well to supplements of folic acid are porphyria, infertility, psoriasis, acne rosacea and eczema.

Finally, let's review the possible side effects of folic acid deficiency. They may include many kinds of nervous symptoms, problems with sex life and especially pregnancy and childbirth, defective children, health troubles in infants given formula rather than breast milk, psychological problems, broken chromosomes which may result in almost any kind of health problem, eye and circulatory problems, greater risk of cancer in the female reproductive tract, a variety of disorders in those taking drugs which destroy folic acid, a special kind of anemia which cannot be cured by giving vitamin B12, iron or any other therapy.

Older folks are more likely to lack folic acid than young folks. In addition, the fluid that accumulates in the body of a patient with congestive heart failure or other circulatory problems may respond to folic acid supplements. The Pill destroys folic acid in the body, so that women on The Pill who decide to become pregnant may have a devastating folic acid deficiency when the pregnancy begins, even before the stress of pregnancy makes the need for this nutrient much higher.

Folic acid is easily lost in preparation of foods. The vitamin is rapidly destroyed by heat. Canned foods may have lost up to 90 percent of their folic acid. It is sensitive to light, unstable when exposed to air and declines steadily in foods which are stored for long periods of time. Foods that contain the most folic acid are liver, wholewheat cereals and breads, legumes like dry beans, lentils and soybeans, bran, brewers yeast, nuts and seeds and all leafy green vegetables.

If, for any reason, you believe your diet does not give you enough of this nutrient or if you have any of the conditions mentioned above which might make your need for folic acid to be greater than average, by all means take a supplement and be sure to use a B12 supplement along with it, since the two work together very closely.

# CHAPTER 23

# Pantothenic Acid Fights Stress

ROGER J. WILLIAMS, PH.D., could be called the father of modern vitamin therapy. In his laboratory at the University of Texas he did more work than any other biologist on many vitamins, chiefly two of the B vitamins—pantothenic acid and folic acid. He gave both of them their names. He discovered pantothenic acid more than 50 years ago and proceeded on a lifetime of experiments, observations and theorizing until he accumulated a vast body of information about this vitamin.

He covered much of this research in his book *Physician's Handbook of Nutritional Science*. He states that this B vitamin is part of an enzyme system which is essential for all living organisms as well as many plants. He says, "These manufacturing chemicals (like pantothenic acid) are never found ready-packaged in ideal proportions for us or for any other organisms. Living with our nutritional environment and adapting to it is an exacting task worthy of our serious attention . . . in line with nature's plan we must strive and use our intelligence if we are to get a really good assortment for ourselves and our children."

In one experiment, Dr. Williams discovered the effect of this B vitamin on the production of normal young among his laboratory animals. Giving the pregnant animals 30 to 35 micrograms of this vitamin a day in addition to their usual nutritious chow resulted in 38 percent of normal births to the animals. Giving 40 to 45 micrograms per day produced

72 percent normal births and giving 50 micrograms produced 95 percent normal births in the experimental animals. In our country where the incidence of children who are defective in some way at birth is far above what it should be, these early experiments on animals are vitally significant.

Chickens suffer from "chick dermatitis" which Dr. Williams quickly cured with pantothenic acid. The unhealthy skin and feathers came back to health amost miraculously. This suggests that human beings who have trouble with hair and skin might have the sme experience. Dr. Williams said that the skin suffers first from malnutrition because its circulation does not supply it with copious nutrition. Also the mouth, tongue, lips and gums give evidence of malnutrition very early.

Looking for sources of this B vitamin, Dr. Williams discovered that royal jelly (food fed only to the queen bee by the worker bees) makes of this bee a queen who lives for several years and produces many thousands of fertile eggs. Feeding hens pantothenic acid improved the hatchability of their eggs. Giving it to rats and mice improved the size of their litters. Dr. Willliams believed that giving this B vitamin to pregnant women would improve the health of their children and lessen the incidence of birth deformities or mentally retarded children.

The following ailments have been reported in the presence of known deficiency in pantothenic acid: dermatitis and keratitis (a skin condition), ulcers in the digestive tract, intussusceptions (collapse of parts of the digestive tract), anemia, white hair, depigmentation of tooth enamel, sterility, congenital malformations, defects in the contractibility of the bowel, failure to produce antibodies which protect us from infections, hemorrhages in the adrenal glands, spinal cord disorders, dehydration, fatty liver, thymus gland disorders, kidney damage, heart damage, sudden death without warning, bone marrow deficiency, lack of white blood corpuscles, spinal curvatures, degeneration of the myelin sheaths of the nerves, uncoordinated gait, decreased longevity, allergies, headache, loss of memory and decreased resistance to stress.

Referring to this lengthy list of deficiency disorders, Dr. Williams said, "A careful consideration of these facts . . . leads us to recognize pantothenic acid deficiency as leading to not only a systemic disease but to a generalized disease of cells capable of damaging and incapacitating any and every structure in the entire body." This kind of disorder is different from any other he has ever seen. The deficiency might affect each of us differently. "No two individuals would be expected to suffer the same damage," he said.

In 1966 *Medical World News* reported on experiments in England where physicians were treating osteoarthritis with this B vitamin. They discovered that levels of this vitamin were far lower in arthritics than in healthy people. The lower the levels of the B vitamin, the more severe the symptoms. They injected the vitamin into their patients. When they got no results, they also injected royal jelly, the substance fed to the queen bee, thinking that another compound in royal jelly might cooperate with the B vitamin.

When they finally got encouraging results they added the amino acid cysteine to their injections. Sometimes results were slow in coming. No improvement for four to eight weeks. But "just when the patient is deciding that the cure is no good, the symptoms disappear overnight," said one of the physicians. The treatment had to be continued or the patients would relapse.

Some years ago a Japanese medical journal showed that there are decreasing levels of this vitamin in the blood of women as they grow older. K. Ishiguro reported in the *Tohoku Journal of Experimental Medicine,* May, 1972, that the major part of pantothenic acid in the body is found in red blood cells, in bound form—that is, the vitamin is not in free form but is bound chemically to other substances in the red blood cells.

He tested about 200 women living in a rural village in Japan. He found, he says, that there was little difference among the women so far as red blood cells are concerned. All the women appeared to have rather low levels of these important cells, as they do in our country, incidentally. But the vitamin that was bound to the red blood cells was lower in older women—chiefly those between the ages of 40 and 60 years. He believes that the body's mechanism for "binding" the vitamin into the cells may become deficient in later life, possibly because of some aspect of the menopause.

In 1981 *Medical Tribune* reported that a biochemist from the University of Pittsburgh has found that two vitamins are essential for the production and transportation in the body of antibodies—those compounds that help to protect us from infections. The two are pyridoxine (B6) and pantothenic acid.

In his book *Nutrition Against Disease,* Dr. Williams spoke of "supernutrition"—getting more than one seems to need of various nutrients for "superhealth." He believed that no plant or animal in nature actually has optimum nutrition. It is always possible to improve it using knowledge we have at present. The benefits for human beings might be limitless, for no human being is getting all he might need in the way of vitamins, minerals, trace minerals, proteins, essential fats and so on. If doctors could be persuaded to use "supernutrition" we might wipe out worldwide plagues, prevent the birth of damaged babies and bring a whole new concept of health and well-being into the world.

Dr. Williams' book *Nutrition Against Disease* is bulwarked with 81 pages of references for statements the author makes. It is impossible to fault or question any bit of information in this book just as it is impossible to call this distinguished scientist a crank or a faddist. You can safely use the information in this book to convince even the most confirmed skeptic of the power of nutrition against disease and the super-power of supernutrition. The official book *Recommended Dietary Allowances* states that probably 10 milligrams of pantothenic acid per day is about right for most of us. Dr. Williams recommended at least 15 milligrams.

Here are recommendations from other scientists and physicians who are using the concept of "megavitamin" therapy for many diseases. Abram Hoffer, Ph.D., M.D., a Canadian psychiatrist who uses these methods, says in his book *Ortho-molecular Nutrition* that he himself takes 100 to 300 milligrams of pantothenic acid daily as a "stress" formula, along with the same amount of thiamine, plus 200 to 800 units of vitamin E, 3,000 to 6,000 milligrams of niacin and the same amount of vitamin C along with certain minerals.

Emanuel Cheraskin, M.D., D.M.D., in his book *Psycho-dietetics* states that some psychiatrists who are treating schizophrenia give up to 12 grams of niacin daily, along with 12 grams of vitamin C, 200–500 milligrams of pyridoxine (B6), 400 to 1600 units of vitamin E and 200–600 milligrams of pantothenic acid.

Richard Passwater, Ph.D., says in his book *Supernutrition* that one's tissues might be saturated with pantothenic acid with a dose of 100 milligrams. Carl C. Pfeiffer, Ph.D., M.D., in his book *Mental and Elemental Nutrients* says that, at his Brain Bio Center in Princeton, N.J., he and his staff have given pantothenic acid in doses as high as 500 milligrams a day for treatment of various mental disorders. In extremely high doses, he says, teeth and joints may become sensitive.

John D. Kirschmann, Director of Nutrition Search, Inc., says in *Nutrition Almanac* that lack of pantothenic acid may be involved with anemia, low blood sugar, cystitis, fracture, epilepsy, insomnia, mental illness, multiple sclerosis, neuritis, cataracts, burning and tingling sensations, adrenal exhaustion, baldness, arthritis, gout, leg cramps, phlebitis, allergies, asthma, tuberculosis, muscular dystrophy, acne, psoriasis, gastritis, indigestion, alcoholism, and so on. He has collected this information from a wide variety of publications on nutrition.

Harvey Ross, M.D., in his book *Fighting Depression*, tells of giving 100 milligrams daily of pantothenic acid along with 500 milligrams of niacin and vitamin C and 100 milligrams of B6 in treating a schizophrenic boy. He also says that depression can be caused by simple deficiency in pantothenic acid. He describes his treatment of a drug addict who was depressed and had no appetite. Dr. Ross put him on a

## *Pantothenic Acid Content of Some Common Foods*

**(We give the milligram content of one serving, about 100 grams)**

| Food | Milligrams |
| --- | --- |
| Brains (all kinds) | 2.6 |
| Broccoli | 1.17 |
| Bulgur | 0.660 |
| Cabbage juice | 1.1 |
| Cashews | 1.3 |
| Cauliflower | 1 |
| Chicken | 1 |
| Chickpeas | 1.25 |
| Cottonseed flour | 4.320 |
| Eggs, whole | 1.6 |
| Filberts | 1.146 |
| Flounder | 0.850 |
| Heart | 3 |
| Kale | 1 |
| Kidneys | 4 |
| Lentils | 1.3 |
| Liver | 8 |
| Liverwurst | 2.7 |
| Mushrooms | 2.2 |
| Oatmeal | 1.4 |
| Peanuts | 2.8 |
| Peas, dry | 2 |
| Rice, Brown | 1.1 |
| Salmon | 1.3 |
| Sesame seed flour | 2.7 |
| Soybeans | 1.7 |
| Sunflower seeds | 1.4 |
| Turkey | 2.67 |
| Walnuts | 0.900 |
| Wheat bran | 2.9 |
| Wheat germ | 1.2 |
| Whey, dried | 4 |
| Yeast, brewer's | 12 |

diet to cure low blood sugar and added vitamin doses three times a day of 1,000 milligrams of niacin, and of vitamin C, plus 100 milligrams of pyridoxine and pantothenic acid, 400 units of vitamin E and one B complex supplement. He improved greatly.

Dr. Robert C. Atkins, M.D., prescribes for his patients various vitamin-mineral formulas in addition to a highly nourishing diet. His 1992 "sleep formula" includes 350 milligrams of GABA, 250 milligrams of inositol, 100 milligrams of niacinamide, 100 milligrams of calcium pantothenate, 60 milligrams of calcium carbonate, and 37.5 milligrams of magnesium carbonate. His anti-hypertension formula includes magnesium, inositol, garlic, B6 and 150 milligrams of pantothenic acid. His anti-arthritic formula includes 200 milligrams of pantothenic acid along with niacinamide, B6, vitamin C, vitamin E and a number of minerals. His immune-system formula includes 150 milligrams of pantothenic acid and his pre- and post-operative formula includes 200 milligrams of pantothenic acid.

Richest sources of this vitamin are: liver of all kinds, also brain, heart and kidney, eggs, herring, cod, wheat germ, bran, dried peas, peanuts. Medium sources are seafood, walnuts, meat, many vegetables, cheese. Lower amounts of the vitamin are found in many fruits and vegetables, almonds, oysters, lobster, shrimp and milk.

# CHAPTER 24

# Is Inositol the "Sleep Vitamin"?

DR. ROBERT ATKINS PRESCRIBES inositol as a sleeping pill. He says in his book *Dr. Atkins' Nutrition Breakthrough*, "Inositol, one of the B vitamins, is my first recommendation becuase it has proven so reliable in helping my patients to sleep. Most of them take one to three grams an hour or two before anticipated bedtime . . . Nutritional supplements work differently from pharmaceutical sleep inducers in an interesting way. Many patients who take barbiturates to sleep find that they need increasing doses as they become habituated to the drugs. In fact, many of *my* patients report that they can get by with less and less, eventually eliminating the supplements."

Dr. Atkins, a New York City cardiologist, also uses inositol to control anxiety. He says, "My favorite nutrients in treating anxiety are inositol, niacinamide, pantothenic acid, calcium, magnesium and GABA (gamma-aminobutyric acid)." He has also found that inositol is helpful in controlling abnormal heartbeats (arrhythmias) that often predict serious heart complications. In his basic formula for patients. Dr. Atkins recommends a total of 450 milligrams of inositol taken in divided doses, say, one third after each meal.

Treating his diabetic patients, Dr. Atkins says that this relative of the B vitamins may help the diabetic to avoid some of the neurological problems that go along with years of diabetes. "I prescribe two to six grams per day for those patients who have difficulty with neuropathy (nerve problems) or who have lost their knee or ankle reflexes," he says.

In his book Dr. Atkins tells of one patient with severe high blood pressure, taking two drugs for this and suffering from headache, loss of memory, depression and fatigue. He prescribed another drug to bring the pressure down as soon as possible, then prescribed a diet containing almost no carbohydrate, plus his basic vitamin-mineral formula in addition to one gram of pyridoxine and two grams of inositol every day. The patient's troubles cleared up and she took off unwanted weight.

Carl C. Pfeiffer, M.D., Ph.D. in his book *Mental and Elemental Nutrients* says that inositol is a lipotropic factor. This means it has a curative or preventive effect on fats, helps them to move normally, not getting deposited in the lining of arteries or the liver. Inositol and choline are both effective in this role. Dr. Pfeiffer says that, although a specific need for inositol in man has not been demonstrated, nor have specific deficiency symptoms, but . . . "its wide distribution in the body indicates an important role . . . Inositol is present in all tissues with the highest levels in the heart and brain . . . The spinal cord, nerves, brain and cerebral spinal fluid contain large amounts of inositol . . . It is also found in the aqueous humor of the eye."

"In mild hypertension," he says, "the use of one gram of inositol morning and night produce sedation and a gradual lowering of the blood pressure . . . Inositol is sedative and solves many insomnia and anxiety problems. Inositol may also reduce stress-elevated blood pressure." both Dr. Pfeiffer and Dr. Atkins report that inositol is an important ingredient of male semen. Sperm has 13 milligrams of vitamin C and 53 milligrams of inositol per 100 grams.

*Nutrition Almanac,* edited by John D. Kirschmann, states that inositol is "needed for the growth and survival of cells in bone marrow, eye membranes and the intestines. It is vital for hair growth and can prevent thinning hair and baldness. There is no known toxicity to inositol. He also recommends inositol for the following conditions: high cholesterol levels, stroke, constipation, dizziness, glaucoma, baldness, cirrhosis of the liver, asthma, gastritis, overweight and obesity.

At present inositol is not officially called a vitamin nor is it even mentioned as an essential nutrient in the official book *Recommended Dietary Allowances*. Dr. Roger J. Williams has said of inositol that just because this compound is manufactured in the human body is no reason to consider it unimportant. What happens, he asks, to someone who is just not manufacturing enough inositol to perform all the roles it has in the human body? It seems only prudent to take inositol in a supplement just to cover any such possibility.

E. Cheraskin, M.D., D.M.D., says in his book *Psychodietetics* that the ideal vitamin and mineral supplement should contain 100–500 milligrams of inositol which he calls "brain-cell nutrients." Perhaps the most important fact about inositol is that it, along with choline, is an important constituent of lecithin (less-i-thin) which is an ingredient of all body cells and of many highly nourishing foods we eat. In the *American Journal of Clinical Nutrition*, August, 1974, Charles Butterworth, M.D. and Dr. Carlos Krumdieck, M.D., Ph.D. discuss vitamin C and lecithin as most valuable aids in controlling hardening of the arteries. They report that, in a laboratory test tube, one part of lecithin added to one part of cholesterol, dissolves the cholesterol or emulsifies it, rendering it harmless. The authors say that it seems likely the lecithin in egg yolk would perform the same function, rendering the cholesterol harmless to arteries, liver and other parts of the body where accumulation of this fatty substance can cause such trouble. "It is our belief," they say, "that the available evidence clearly justifies, and indeed, calls for, studies on the effectiveness of these two substances—lecithin and vitamin C, for human beings."

At the time, Dr. Butterworth was Chairman of the American Medical Association Council on Foods and Nutrition. This being so, why do you suppose physicians are not, right now, recommending Dr. Butterworth's findings on lecithin to their heart and circulatory patients? Instead, led by the Heart Association, many physicians are cautioning patients against eating eggs and other foods rich in lecithin. It may be many years before the studies of Drs. Butterworth and Krumdieck are regarded as gospel. It may take many years of further study and debate before any official notice will be taken of the significance of these findings.

Why should the health seeker wait for all this to occur? There is no evidence that lecithin or vitamin C or inositol can be harmful. There is every indication they can all be very helpful. Lecithin is found in seed foods of all kinds— peanuts and peanut butter, soybeans, peas, lentils, nuts, wholegrains. It is available in many foods at your health food store, as is inositol. Inositol is available as a food supplement either alone or in combination with other related vitamins of the B complex.

# CHAPTER 25

# Choline for Preventing Brain Disorders

ALZHEIMER'S DISEASE IS a condition of dementia, usually developing in older folks, but sometimes occurring in quite young individuals. It involves loss of memory and deterioration of intellectual ability—the ability to read, write, calculate and use language. Other more bizarre symptoms may also develop. One Johns Hopkins specialist in this disease estimates that at least five percent of individuals over the age of 65 suffer from dementia and an additional 10 percent exhibit mild to moderate impairment of mental functions.

Dr. Joseph T. Coyle, the Johns Hopkins specialist, has stated that patients with this disease suffer loss of nerve cells that use a body-manufactured compound called acetylcholine—loss of 70 to 90 percent of these cells. Acetylcholine is necessary to carry nerve messages from one brain cell to another. Since choline is one ingredient of acetylcholine, some researchers studying Alzheimer's Disease are working with choline, the B vitamin relative, and a substance which contains lots of choline—lecithin.

Giving young volunteers drugs which destroy acetylcholine produces changes in these young people very similar to changes that occur in older folks. Animal studies have shown the same thing. A study at the National Institutes of Health involving young adults demonstrated that the memory of these people improved greatly when they were given choline. In another study ten elderly patients suffering from Alzheimer's Disease were given choline in large amounts—nine grams daily for two weeks. The mental ability of the subjects did not improve during this short test but the researchers state that some of the older folks seemed "less confused." They believe that a trial in younger folks whose disease has not progressed to a serious state might bring better results.

Two researchers at the Massachusetts Institute of Technology reported that eating a single meal containing lecithin increases significantly the concentration of choline in the brain and adrenal glands of laboratory animals. Several laboratories have been working on the effects of both choline and lecithin in therapy of patients with organic brain damage. Results are not dramatic in serious impairment of mental function, but much greater benefits are shown in those whose problems are less severe.

The 1978 edition of *Drugs in Current Use* lists choline as a "drug for treatment of cirrhosis of the liver and other liver disorders. Doses should not exceed six grams daily," the book says. Dr. Richard Wurtman was quoted in the *New York Times* in 1978 saying that his experiments have shown that choline in the diet goes directly into the brain. "It is taken up directly by the brain from the circulating blood and is used to make an important chemical transmitter of nerve signals—(acetylcholine). On an hour-to-hour basis the amount of the nerve signal transmitter in the brain seems to depend on how much choline-rich food the individual has eaten recently," he says. Dr. Wurtman says these facts mean that the composition of each meal will directly affect the synthesis of chemical signals in the brain.

Visiting a friend in a mental hospital or nursing home one is likely to observe more than a few cases of what doctors call "tardive dyskinesia," meaning disordered movements of arms and legs, as well as mouth, lips and tongue. The patient appears to be thrashing about uncontrollably. This condition is one of the side effects of certain "mood" drugs given to control hysteria, mania or depression. According to *Medical Tribune,* June 22, 1977, physicians have been able to control this terrible condition with choline—about 200 milligrams a day for every two pounds of weight. The patients in this test were between 36 and 80 years of age. Five of these continued to take the drugs while still taking the "mood" drug and the symptoms cleared up. Four other patients who had been taken off the tranquilizers previously also improved when choline was given. When the choline was discontinued some of the distressing symptoms returned.

Other things in one's lifestyle seem to be related to Alzheimer's Disease. Some tranquilizer drugs are known to cause loss of acetylcholine from brain tissues. Some over-the-counter drugs have the same effect—such drugs as pain killers, antihistamines and sleeping pills. Since many elderly people take these drugs frequently, it seems likely that they might be deficient in this important brain chemical because of the drugs. A study by the National Institutes of Health showed that about two-thirds of older folks surveyed reported using prescription drugs and 70 percent said they also use non-prescription drugs from the drug store, chiefly pain killers. Doesn't it seem possible that just taking too many drugs may be one important cause of Alzheimer's Disease?

Then, too, aluminum deposits are found in the brains of victims of this disease. This leads experts to theorize that this rather toxic metal may be part of the problem. It's present in many water supply systems, in many antacid drugs and, of course, in the metal cooking utensils we use.

As long ago as 1949 the *British Medical Journal* reported an experiment with rats in which total deficiency in choline brought about a kidney condition which caused high blood pressure. In 1962 the *Archives of Pathology* reported that choline deficiency in laboratory rats brought about severe heart and coronary artery lesions in a remarkably short time, along with high blood levels of cholesterol and fat. It seems that much further research should reveal many more health-giving attributes to this nutrient which we hope you will get enough of, either in food or in supplements or in lecithin.

Blepharospasm is a chronic, unremitting disorder in which

one or usually both eyelids close involuntarily. A severe case of this disorder is visually disabling. *The New England Journal of Medicine* in 1981 reported on the use of choline in treating this condition. The authors, from Toronto, report that taking choline every day—starting with a little more than two grams brought relief to three patients. Moving pictures, taken before and after, proved the results. One patient who had not left her home for three years because of this very troublesome disorder of her eyelids, found that, after taking 6.3 grams of choline daily she can now move about freely. The doctors suggest that this nutrient be tried before taking drugs for this condition.

The chief source of lecithin, hence choline, is the yolk of the egg—that part of the extremely nutritious egg which specialists of many kinds have warned us to eat in very limited amounts because of its cholesterol content. The next best source of choline and lecithin is probably liver and the cholesterol-haters have also warned us against this highly nutritious food because it, too, contains cholesterol.

The official book *Recommended Dietary Allowances* states that choline cannot be called exactly a vitamin, although it has many functions in the human body. It can be manufactured in the body, but only if enough B12, folic acid and methionine (an amino acid or link of protein) are present. No official RDA is listed.

Choline as such does not exist in food. It exists only as part of lecithin, chiefly in egg yolks, liver, soybeans and other nutritious foods. Most of the lecithin in health food stores is made from soybeans, since this is a less expensive source than eggs. It might be wise for all of us, especially those approaching middleage, to add both choline and lecithin to our diets. Lecithin is available in many forms at the health food store. You can take it in blender drinks, mixed with milk or fruit juice, or you can add it to soups, salads, or omelets, or mix it with your morning cereal. It's not the tastiest food in the world, so you may prefer to take it in capsules. We cannot recommend any dosage. It's food, not medicine. What may be just right for you may not be enough for someone else in your family depending upon the diets you eat. If you decide to take choline, be guided by the recommended dose on the label of the product you buy.

"The dietary links to Alzheimer's Disease have appeared in print since the 1930's," says Dr. Michael Weiner in *Reducing the Risk of Alzheimer's*. "Now, half a century later, we are taking notice of the self-destructive practices by means of which we have been quite literally poisoning ourselves and assaulting the one human organ for which there is no transplant remedy—the brain."

Throughout the book Dr. Weiner describes experiments in which the B vitamin choline or lecithin, of which choline is an ingredient, have been used successfully to treat Alzheimer's patients. He suggests that getting enough of these nutrients may help to prevent the disease. He mentions EPA, the fatty fish oil called eicosapentanoic acid, as a valuable nutrient for the brain and also helpful in preventing heart and circulatory disorders.

He lists thiamine (B1), pyridoxine (B6), niacin (B3), B12, folic acid, vitamin E, vitamin C and vitamin A as absolutely essential for sound nourishment which is apparently the key to preventing Alzheimer's Disease. Of minerals, he lists calcium and magnesium as the most important for combatting the entry of aluminum into our bodies and especially into our brains. He says, "Of the mineral nutrients that can help to prevent senile changes in the nervous system, the most important are zinc and magnesium." Selenium, which can be risky in large doses, is an antioxidant, hence very helpful, in small doses.

Of amino acids (links of protein) he recommends cystine because it contains sulfur which is helpful, glutamine which serves as a fuel to the brain, phenylalanine which helps to overcome depression and improve memory, and tyrosine which increases mental alertness. He also suggests how best to get all these essential nturients in an all-in-one tablet.

Physicians have found that the disordered nerve cells in the brains of Alzheimer's victims are loaded with the toxic metal aluminum. They don't know whether this is a side effect of the disease or the cause of the disease. So Dr. Weiner is concerned with our universal exposure to the metal in our environment, drugs and food. He is hopeful that calcium, magnesium and zinc, along with a number of vitamins and amino acids, can help us to overcome the toxic effects of the aluminum which seem to be evident in the brains of those unfortunate people with Alzheimer's Disease. He describes parts of the world where there is a great deal of aluminum in soil and water and almost no calcium or magnesium. In at least one such locality in Guam, mental disorders like Alzheimer's Disease have been widespread for many years. Raising the levels of calcium and magnesium in the diets of these people has all but eliminated these diseases.

"Alzheimer's Disease has not been around forever," Dr. Weiner says. "Nor have aluminum cans, foil or aluminum-saturated drugs, foods or drinks . . . the connection between this disease and aluminum and other nutritional factors is overwhelmingly strong." Dr. Weiner lists by brand name over-the-counter drugs which contain aluminum, giving the number of milligrams of this toxic metal which one would get in an average dose. These are chiefly antacids, buffered aspirins and drugs to fight diarrhea, as well as ulcer drugs and vaginal douches. Taking aspirin buffered with aluminum may result in getting up to 1,000 milligrams of aluminum a day, depending on the dosage.

Foods that contain aluminum are baking powders which are found in cake mixes, frozen doughs, self-rising flours, also processed cheeses. Some brands of household baking powders contain aluminum. Pickling salts contain aluminum used as a "firming" agent, so probably pickles of any kind should be avoided unless you know the source. One dill pickle, for example, may contain up to 10 milligrams of aluminum. A food additive called a "starch modifier" may contain aluminum, which suggests reading labels and avoiding those that list such products on their labels.

Aluminum cooking utensils must be abandoned, he says, since food and beverages cooked in them take up this metal in amounts that depend on the acidity of the food being cooked. He lists foods that are acid or alkaline, stating that either an acid or alkaline condition of the food means that it will absorb aluminum. It is estimated that Americans get from 22 to 38 milligrams of aluminum every day from all these sources. Although it has not been finally determined that it is the aluminum in the brain of the Alzheimer's Disease victim that causes the symptoms of dementia, the evidence is overwhelming that such is the case.

Says Dr. Weiner, "For those of us who wish to prevent this disease, the risk-reduction program offers a sound, scientific approach, readily enacted. For those suffering from this illness, the program outlined can do no harm. Instead, it offers a positive, inexpensive plan of action where little now exists."

# CHAPTER 26

# PABA Is a Good Sunscreen

THE B VITAMIN WITH the tongue-twister name, *Para-amino-benzoic acid,* is not listed as a vitamin in the official handbook *Recommended Dietary Allowances.* But its use in human nutrition has been long and interesting. Mostly it has been associated with skin welfare and graying hair. Nobody is quite sure why, or how it acts in the body.

We call it PABA for short. Drs. Bicknell and Prescott in their massive book, *The Vitamins in Medicine,* tell us that PABA is unique in that it is a vitamin within a vitamin. It seems that it is part of folic acid. When sulfanilamide, the antibiotic, first came into use in the 1940's, it was found that its chemical formula is very much like that of PABA. So when people or experimental animals were given the drug internally, the PABA in their intestines counteracted it, so that it became ineffective.

Early in research work with PABA, scientists discovered that, when they withheld it from the diet of laboratory animals, their hair became white. It was believed that PABA was essential for the synthesis of folic acid, another B vitamin, in the intestinal tract and the lack of folic acid was the real reason for the white hair.

At any rate, people with prematurely white hair wanted to know if lack of PABA was the reason for their loss of pigment and if they might be able to restore the color if they took PABA. One researcher claimed that he could restore lost hair color by giving massive doses of PABA over long periods of time.

# PABA IS A GOOD SUNSCREEN

Adelle Davis, in *Let's Get Well*, told us that she had seen many instances of gray hair which returned to its original color temporarily, but it quickly became gray again "unless one continues to eat yogurt, liver, yeast and wheat germ. Persons who take 5 milligrams of folic acid and 300 milligrams of PABA and pantothenic acid daily with some B vitamins from natural sources can usually prevent hair from graying and often restore its color."

The other field in which PABA has been recently shown to be almost a wonder drug is in the prevention of damage from sunburn. Way back in the 1940's scientists were finding they could prevent serious burns from the sun and from sunlamps by putting a PABA lotion on the exposed skin. And sure enough, it worked. We have no idea why it took so long for scientists to rediscover this important fact. That's the way things work out in the field of vitamin research. For years we got along with sunburn lotions which accomplished little or nothing.

In Spring of 1969 we began to get enthusiastic reports from scientists that they found PABA to be a "superior" sunscreen agent. The scientists from the University of Pennsylvania told the Society of Cosmetic Chemists that they were getting far better results using PABA lotion than any of the commonly available suntan lotions could give.

Then several Boston doctors developed another formula which they claimed would screen out the ultraviolet rays of the sun "to provide protection from sunburn, skin cancer and aging of the skin." The formula was effective whether you used it at the seashore, the desert or the mountains. They mixed the vitamin with ethyl alcohol and tested it on prisoners in Arizona under the hot, dry sunshine there. The formulas used and all the scientific information about the tests appeared in the *New England Journal of Medicine* for June 26, 1969.

Bicknell and Prescott describe many more experimental uses of PABA in diseases where skin problems are involved. It has been used in massive doses to treat lymphoblastoma cutis, lupus erythematosus, scleroderma, pemphigus, and dermatis herpetiformis. No one knows what causes any of these conditions or why PABA was effective in relieving them. But pictures in the book show clear improvement in the skin condition so long as the vitamin was being taken, and in massive doses.

Adelle Davis told us that PABA has also been used to treat vitiligo, the skin condition where pigment is lost, leaving large patches of entirely white skin. She told us that pantothenic acid has also been used in massive doses to bring the color back to these unsightly patches of skin. PABA applied in an ointment has produced good results.

Said Miss Davis, "I once told a 30-year-old woman with severe vitiligo that liver would probably help her more than any other food. A week later she joyously returned to show me that not a trace of it remained, but she had eaten ¼ pound of raw liver, frozen, diced and covered with catsup, at each meal. Several other persons have had the condition clear up slowly on a more appetizing diet."

In his book, *Dr. Atkins' Nutrition Breakthrough*, this New York cardiologist said he uses PABA for menopausal symptoms. He prescribes it, along with many other nutrients for arthritis, says it is his own personal favorite, which seems to be effective also in such connective tissue disorders as scleroderma, dermatomyositis and Peyronie's Disease. He says it has given his patients good results in combating stiffness. He prescribes as much as two or more grams a day.

In bringing down high levels of cholesterol he gives PABA along with large doses of vitamin C, quoting a Swedish physician who found, in a double-blind test, that the vitamin lowered cholesterol and triglyceride blood levels. Dr. Atkins himself takes his own basic daily formula every day, taking extra PABA if he's especially tired and large doses of vitamin A if a cold is coming on, plus one or two grams of vitamin C every two hours. His daily formula contains 1,200 milligrams of PABA. His formula is designed in such a way that he actually takes nine tablets, three after each meal, and the total content adds up to 1,200 milligrams of PABA.

H. L. Newbold, M.D. in his book *Mega-Nutrients for*

*Your Nerves,* mentions PABA in regard to graying hair, but says he has no firm proof that it can turn gray hair back to its natural color. However, he does believe that PABA is important for slowing the aging process. Ana Aslan, M.D. uses a certain form of novocaine injections to treat patients at her famed clinic in Romania. It seems that the chemical formula of novocaine and PABA are so close that the novocaine breaks down into PABA in the body.

PABA is a very useful nutrient that should be part of your supplements. The best food sources of PABA are those same foods in which all the other B vitamins are most abundant: meat (especially organ meats like liver), seeds of all kinds and wholegrain cereals of all kinds, nuts, leafy green vegetables, brewers yeast, wheat bran and germ.

# Vitamin C Is . . .

*Water-soluble,* meaning it cannot be stored for a long time in the body, but should be available in food or supplements every day.

*Responsible* for the health and maintenance of collagen in teeth, bones, cartilage, connective tissues, skin and the small blood vessels called capillaries, the healing of wounds, broken bones and burns, the detoxification of poisons (in the process of which the vitamin is destroyed) the maintenance of white blood corpuscles which fight infection, absorption of iron from the digestive tract, maintenance of the adrenal glands which protect us from stress.

*Present* in most abundance in fresh raw fruits and vegetables, chiefly the citrus fruits, strawberries, pineapple, guava, acerola cherries, rose hips, all members of the cabbage family, tomatoes, parsley, peppers, also liver.

*Safe* in very large amounts. Any vitamin C not needed is excreted harmlessly.

*Destroyed* by many chemicals, poisons, and other substances in today's world such as tobacco smoke.

*Official RDA* is 60 milligrams daily for adults, with a recommendation of at least 100 milligrams daily for regular cigarette smokers. Since individual needs may vary greatly and since individual exposure to poisons may vary greatly, one person's needs may not approximate those of another. All living organisms except human beings and several birds and animals make their own vitamin C in their livers. They manufacture very large amounts, especially when under stress.

*Available* in low or high potencies in individual supplements or one-a-day supplements.

# CHAPTER 27

# Linus Pauling Thinks Cancer May Be a Disease of Vitamin C Deficiency

PROFESSOR LINUS PAULING, probably the greatest biologist alive today and perhaps the greatest of all time, believes that cancer may turn out to be a disease of vitamin C deficiency. He made the announcement in June, 1976 on English radio. Dr. Pauling has been working for years with vitamin C in regard to many aspects of life and disease. He is in contact with other scientists and physicians in various parts of the world who are doing work along these lines.

He backed up his claim by referring to the work of a Scots physician which seems to show that large doses of vitamin C increase the average survival times of terminal cancer patients four-fold. And said Pauling, "vitamin C can sometimes produce quite dramatic remissions in advanced human cancer."

Pauling says that the first barrier to the malignant growth of a cancer is the ground substance between cells. Vitamin C is essential for maintaining the structural integrity of this material, hence the vitamin must be one of the body's best weapons for fighting cancer. Dr. Pauling believes that the best treatment for cancer is a judicious combination of medical methods that will eradicate the cancer mass: radiation therapy, surgery, chemotherapy, immunotherapy, plus "supportive measures prescribed in the short term to correct biochemical deficiencies, and in the long term to enhance natural resistance to any residual disease."

Cancer patients are known to be seriously depleted of vitamin C, said Pauling. Short term treatment should include vitamin C to correct this deficiency just as it includes supplemental iron to correct accompanying anemia. In the long-term view, said Pauling, vitamin C provides "a simple, safe, practical method of enhancing host resistance to malignant disease."

One of the best tests on which Pauling based his theory is the one conducted in a Scottish hospital by a surgeon who gave 10 grams of vitamin C daily—that's 10,000 milligrams—to terminal cancer patients who were "untreatable by any conventional method of therapy at the time of entry into supplemental ascorbate (vitamin C) as their only definitive form of medication." In other words, everything that could be done for these patients by orthodox medicine had already been done. Vitamin C was the only medication given them in their last weeks.

Pauling reported that there were many instances of relief of symptoms—reduced pain which permitted their doctor to discontinue sedatives. Their appetites returned. They had a renewed sense of well being. It seems that doctors are not especially interested in medicines that just make the patient feel better and many doctors apparently believe that vitamin C does indeed increase the general feeling of well being in many ill people. So, they asked, if that's all the vitamin does—what else is new?

What's new, said Pauling, is that results of the experiment seemed to indicate that these patients lived significantly longer than normal clinical expectations, considering how gravely ill they were. The Scots surgeon then got out records of 1,000 other cancer patients in the same hospital and compared them with the records of 100 patients to whom he had given vitamin C. He carefully matched each of his patients with 10 of those whose records were in hospital files. Matched patients must be the same age, same kind of tumor, same sex and, in the case of the 1,000 past patients, must have had no vitamin C treatment.

The results of this comparison showed clearly that the patients who got the vitamin C lived on the average four times longer than the original 10 patients to whom they were compared. Of the 100 patients treated with vitamin C, 15 survived longer than a year, compared to only 4 of the controls. Six terminal patients treated with vitamin C lived more than two years, compared to only 1 of the controls. Three of those treated with vitamin C lived for three years. None of those not so treated lived longer than 2½ years.

Of the five who survived more than one year, five are still alive including two who have lived for more than four years. Said the surgeon, "they should have died long ago." He said, too, that 8–10 percent of the patients who were "clearly dying of cancer and as a result of receiving nothing but ascorbic acid (vitamin C) show quite definite evidence of tumor regression and recovery. This is infinitely better than spontaneous regression. I have only seen three spontaneous regressions in my working lifetime."

Pauling believes that the material between cells must be kept healthy in order to prevent cancer. These cells are normally restrained from proliferating and running wild by a complex mechanism involving a substance called physiological hyaluronidase (PHI). Vitamin C is necessary for the production of this substance. It is destroyed in the process of building PHI. Given an adequate quantity of vitamin C, says Pauling, the body could presumably manufacture enough of this important substance to prevent cancer.

The effect of such a treatment would be to "disarm" the cancer cells. They would remain there, but further growth would stop. Perhaps ulcers would heal, pain, hemorrhaging, weakness, emaciation, malnutrition and all other distressing symptoms might be controlled. This explanation derives from what happens in scurvy, the disease of vitamin C deficiency. The substance between the cells breaks down, leading to tissue disruption, ulceration and hemorrhage—"identical to the local changes that occur in the immediate vicinity of neoplastic (cancerous) cells," says Pauling.

Breast cancer kills more American women than any other kind of cancer. In 1985 some 120,000 women were diagnosed as having breast cancer. According to an article in *The Journal of the American Medical Association,* more than one-third of women diagnosed with breast cancer will die from the spread of the cancer to other parts of the body despite conventional medical treatment.

In August, 1985 the Pauling Institute of Science and Medicine published in the prestigious *Proceedings of the National Academy of Sciences* an article on the effect of vitamin C on the incidence of spontaneous breast cancers in a specific strain of mice. These laboratory mice were bred over many years to be highly susceptible to breast cancer.

This three-year study, conducted by fourteen highly qualified members of the Institute's staff, was funded largely by the National Cancer Institute in Washington, a federal bureau interested in the prevention and/or treatment of cancer.

The Pauling study involved ten groups of mice, seven of which were given quite large amounts of vitamin C and three groups which received no vitamin C. Mice manufacture their own vitamin C in their bodies, which we human beings cannot do, so their food does not have to contain any vitamin C. So, without any vitamin C in their food and without any supplements, none of the mice got scurvy, as human beings would have, under similar circumstances.

On the basis of their inheritance over many generations, all the mice would be expected to develop breast cancer. However, the vitamin C given to the seven groups of mice prevented the early appearance of the cancer. Furthermore, the more vitamin C that was given to the mice, the later the cancers appeared. The mice that got quite large amounts of vitamin C fared much better in every way than those which got none.

The authors of the article referred to many studies showing depletion of vitamin C in the blood and tissues of cancer patients. They also referred to the essential role of vitamin

C in the normal function of the body's own immune system that helps to protect us from bacteria, viruses, foreign proteins and cancer cells. They mentioned, too, the fact that medical studies have confirmed the beneficial effects of the vitamin on patients with advanced cancer.

The authors also gave nine references to experiments by other scientists in which treatment with large doses of vitamin C was effective in delaying the appearance of various kinds of cancers or reducing the size of the cancers or prolonging the lives of the animals which had the cancers.

Other physicians, incidentally, have reported the beneficial effects of vitamin E in treating fibrocystic breast which involves lumps in the breast which may progress to cancers. Other physicians have found that deleting from the diet all foods and beverages that contain certain chemicals found in coffee, chocolate and cocoa can prevent the appearance of fibrocystic breast in women who are susceptible to it.

Several years ago the British journal *New Scientist*, reported research showing that, in thirty countries studied, those countries with the highest consumption of sugar also had the highest incidence of breast cancer. Those with the lowest sugar consumption had the lowest incidence of breast cancer. Perhaps there is a lesson here for all American women and especially those whose families have a history of this kind of cancer.

"Study Finds Vitamin C Ineffective on Cancer." Headlines like this appeared in newspapers early in January, 1985 when *The New England Journal of Medicine* published an article by six members of the Mayo Clinic staff stating in its conclusion that "it can be concluded that high-dose vitamin C therapy is not effective against advanced malignant disease regardless of whether the patient has had any prior chemotherapy."

On January 26, the Linus Pauling Institute issued a press release saying in part, "Dr. Linus Pauling, Professor Emeritus in Stanford University and a staff member of the Linus Pauling Institute . . . today charged physicians in the Mayo Clinic with issuing what he felt to be the false and misleading claim that they had repeated the work of Dr. Ewan Cameron, formerly head surgeon of Vale of Leven Hospital, Loch Lomondside, Scotland and now medical director of the Linus Pauling Institute . . . on the response of cancer patients to large doses of vitamin C . . .

"Dr. Pauling charged that the Mayo Clinic doctors had represented their investigation of the response of patients with advanced cancer to high doses of vitamin C as a repetition and check of similar studies reported earlier by Dr. Cameron and his associates whereas in fact it deviated greatly from the earlier study. He then proceeded to point out the various ways in which the Mayo Clinic experiment differed from the experience of Dr. Cameron in Scotland."

Among the differences were these. Dr. Cameron gave 10 grams of vitamin C daily to the cancer patients in his care from the time they began to take it until they died or until the present time, some of them for as much as 12 years. The Mayo Clinic patients received 10 grams of vitamin C for about two and a half months. None of the Mayo Clinic patients died while they were getting the vitamin C. Their deaths occurred only after the vitamin C had been stopped.

The press release went on to say that "An important point is that there is a rebound effect with vitamin C. Persons who take high doses of vitamin C for some time and then suddenly stop show a drop in the concentration of vitamin C in the blood to very low levels, such that some scientists have reported there is danger of developing scurvy . . . It is likely that some of the Mayo Clinic patients died as a result of the rebound effect when their high-dose vitamin C was taken away from them."

Pauling said further that there is no basis for the statement by the Mayo Clinic doctors that from their results it can be concluded that high-dose vitamin C therapy is not effective against advanced cancer. What they had shown instead was that vitamin C should not be given to cancer patients for a short period and then be withdrawn. The Mayo Clinic physicians had promised Pauling a copy of their report before it was published, for his criticism. They had not given this to him.

Said Pauling, "It is a tragedy that the Mayo Clinic study has been misrepresented by the investigators, with the cooperation of *The New England Journal of Medicine* in such a way as to prevent many cancer patients from benefitting by the intake of large doses of vitamin C as an adjunct to appropriate conventional therapy. With over 400,000 people in the United States dying of cancer each year, many tens of thousands would benefit from vitamin C according to the results obtained by Dr. Cameron, and probably a good many will be prevented from receiving this benefit because of the false and misleading statements in the . . . article and the editorial published in *The New England Journal of Medicine*."

Two Japanese studies of vitamin C therapy in terminal cancer patients showed that those who received large doses of vitamin C survived up to 15 times longer than those who got only small doses of the vitamin or none. Doses of vitamin C ranged from five to thirty grams daily. Average survival time for those getting four grams was 43 days. Those who got up to 30 grams daily survived more than 174 days. About ten percent of these lived much longer, one patient being still alive after 1,828 days of vitamin C therapy. A second patient was alive 2,080 days after a diagnosis of terminal cancer. Patients with cancer of the uterus responded best, with some surviving for 1,495 days. Three of the high vitamin C patients were clinically well when the report was made.

Furthermore, said the doctors, "In many cancer patients the administration of vitamin C seemed to improve the state of well-being as measured by improved appetite, increased mental alertness and decreased requirements for pain-killing drugs and other clinical criteria." A second experiment in another Japanese hospital showed similar effects as reported by the physician who was trying infusions of the vitamin through arteries directly into the region of the body around the cancer. These studies were reported in *Medical Tribune*, July 22, 1981.

Low doses of vitamin C can prevent or reverse the cell transformation which normally occurs after animal tissues are exposed in the laboratory to chemicals that cause cancer. Two physicians from the Children's Hospital in Los Angeles exposed such cells from embryo mice to such a chemical for 24 hours. Then one milligram of vitamin C was added to the test tube and stopped the transformation of the cells to cancer cells. Additional experiments showed that the vitamin can be added to the exposed cells as late as 23 days after exposure to the carcinogen and will still inhibit the cancerous transformation of the cells.

Dr. J. W. T. Dickerson, professor of biochemistry at the University of Surrey in England, stated that the vitamin can play a critical role in the treatment of cancer, because of its well known ability to preserve the body's defenses against disease and protection of the intercellular matrix. He said also that cancer patients have, generally, very low levels of vitamin C, suggesting that the patient's needs are increased in the various diseases known as cancer.

Dr. H. Ohsime of the International Agency for Research on Cancer in Lyon, France gave evidence that vitamin C prevents the formation of cancer-causing compounds (nitrosamines) in the stomach when nitrites combine with other compounds naturally in the digestive tract. He believes that the protective action of vitamin C might prevent both stomach and esophageal cancer.

Dr. T. K. Basu of the University of Surrey emphasizes that certain drugs impair the absorption of vitamin C. Aspirin, for example, may have this effect in those who take it for long periods of time—arthritics, perhaps.

Executive Health, December 1975 told of a study of 577 people all over the age of 50 which showed a death rate from all causes—mainly heart disease and cancer—which was two and a half times that of people who took some vitamin C. The protective power of the vitamin showed itself even though the amount of vitamin C taken every day was only 100 milligrams.

Melanoma is a form of skin cancer which may arise from

a previously harmless pigmented mole or birthmark or it may grow as a completely new cancer. It is a highly invasive tumor which spreads rapidly to lymph glands and circulatory system. If it is cut out before it has spread, it can usually be contained and the patient recovers completely. But once it has spread it is extremely difficult to remove or control. And it does not respond to radiation or drugs.

A team of French and American researchers reported that they used cultures of growing melanoma cells and treated them with vitamin C and copper. The vitamin C alone brought about a fifty percent destruction of the cancer cells. Adding a bit of copper compound increased the destruction of the cancer cells two-to five-fold.

The scientists believe that vitamin C and copper are incorporated into the skin cells because these nutrients are needed for the manufacture of the skin pigment melanin. They are harmless to non-cancerous cells which need this same pigment, but when they are taken up by the cancer cells they rapidly destroy them.

Today some physicians are using vitamin C to treat cancer with or without the usual "establishment" list of therapies: chemotherapy, radiation and surgery. These physicians have a hard time of it. Some hospitals will not permit doctors using vitamin C therapy to bring patients to their hospitals. If the vitamin C in massive doses must be given by intravenous therapy, this is not possible without hospitalization. Malpractice insurance firms frown on unorthodox medical therapy. If vitamin C is given and fails to cure the patient or even to bring about a feeling of well-being, the family may sue the doctor because he or she did not use just the three therapies approved by the medical establishment.

The best idea, of course, is to prevent cancer. Good nutrition helps. Eating a diet, every item of which contributes to your daily quota of protein, vitamins, minerals and trace minerals, helps to keep you healthy. This means avoiding all those products that contribute nothing or next to nothing nutritionally speaking—the "empty calorie" foods, we mean. Avoiding as much as possible all sources of cancer-causing chemicals and pollutants in your environment helps greatly. Cigarette smoke is one of the most damaging and the one most difficult to avoid.

Cancer of the urinary bladder appears to be an increasing threat as the toxins in our environment accumulate at a frightening pace and less and less is known about their potential for causing cancer. The body has defense mechanisms for disposing of some poisons. It eliminates them as rapidly as possible. One method is to excrete them in urine. So it seems possible that many of the poisons to which we are exposed daily find their way to the kidneys, then to the bladder for excretion.

Dr. Balfour M. Mount of the Department of Urology at the Royal Victoria Hospital and Department of Surgery at McGill University in Montreal tells in the *Canadian Medical Journal*, June 23, 1973 of a relationship between environmental poisons and bladder cancer in 1895 when a German physician tied the high incidence of bladder cancer among workers in the dye industry to the chemicals with which they were working. His discovery resulted in some laws to protect workers against such exposure.

We are told that there are at present some seven million new, manmade chemicals in the world. This information is from Chemical Abstracts Service, April 21, 1986. Some of these are undoubtedly in our environment and we are exposed to them although almost no testing has ever been done on their potential toxicity. In 1978 it was reported that about 63,000 such chemicals are in use. An additional 6,000 manmade chemicals were coming on the market every week at that time.

The Environmental Protection Agency announced around that time that they plan to test only 250 such chemicals every year, if they have the money, equipment and personnel, of course. It is obvious from these figures that a great many environmental chemicals have never been tested for their potential for causing cancer and the general public is never warned against their use.

Dr. Mount says that the incidence of bladder cancer in

smokers is about twice that of non-smokers and the prospects for recovery are much worse in those who continue to smoke than it is in non-smokers or in those who have stopped smoking. *New Scientist* (October 2, 1980) published a study saying, "Smoke from any source consists of minute particles suspended in a mixture of gases . . . a single cigarette produces about 5,000,000 particles . . . They are droplets of tar and consist of numerous chemicals; altogether there are about 3,000 different chemicals in cigarette smoke." The publication then listed about 20 different chemicals or groups of chemicals in cigarette smoke which are either carcinogens or cancer promoters.

There is also the possibility that smoking causes bladder cancer because of the ability of even one cigarette to lower vitamin C levels in both blood and urine. Dr. Mount says that sufficiently high levels of vitamin C can be obtained in the urine by taking 500 milligrams of vitamin C three times at intervals every day. He quotes Dr. Jorgen Schlegel of the Tulane Department of Urology who has been giving this advice to his bladder cancer patients for many years. Dr. Schlegel almost guarantees to his patients that there will be no recurrence of the cancer if they follow this prescription faithfully for life.

Dr. Irwin Stone in his book *The Healing Factor, Vitamin C Against Disease* defines smoking as "an intense form of concentrated individual air pollution . . . Carcinogenic poisons . . . are deposited on the tissues of the mouth, tongue, pharynx, bronchi and interior of the nose . . . a highly irritating form of local chemical stress which depletes the tissues of their stores of vitamin C." He recommends that the average non-smoker should be getting as much as five to 20 grams of vitamin C every day. A smoker should take three to five grams of vitamin C *more than that* for every pack of cigarettes he or she smokes. That's how terrible the danger from smoking is and that's how easy it is to give yourself at least some small protection against this poison.

Obviously, if you smoke, the best protection is to stop,

even if it means you must shut yourself in a room and go "cold turkey" as other drug addicts must. If you don't smoke, by all means do everything you can to avoid breathing the cigarette smoke of others, since this "passive smoking" has sometimes appeared to be even more harmful than the smoker encounters. If you are regularly exposed to cigarette smoke by all means give yourself whatever protection you can from lots of vitamin C taken at intervals during the day.

# CHAPTER 28

# Using Vitamin C in a Doctor's Practice Many Years Ago

DR. FREDERICK KLENNER PRACTICED in Reidsville, North Carolina. His reports on vitamin therapy for almost any disorder were not published in the slick, expensive professional journals published by universities and research centers. He did not report on farfetched experiments on rats which continue for three or four days. His work with vitamins began back in the 1940's.

In an issue of *The Journal of Applied Nutrition,* he told some of the following stories, all having to do with massive doses of vitamin C. He used it fearlessly. He reported no ill effects. He got improvement in just about any disorder he treated. He used vitamin C for many patients with aftereffects of severe virus infections. In 1953, he had a patient with viral pneumonia, unconscious, with a fever of more than 106 degrees. He gave her 140 grams of vitamin C intravenously over a period of 72 hours. By that time she was almost well.

He believed that stubborn aftereffects of viral infections are the cause of "crib deaths" that take the lives of so many apparently healthy infants. His theory agrees with that of another physician whose work we describe in another chapter. Dr. Klenner found there is a tragic lack of vitamin C in the blood of burn patients. He treated them by enclosing the burned parts in a heated cradle-like arrangement so that nothing touched the skin. No dressings. He used a three

217

percent vitamin C spray over the entire area, alternated with vitamin A and D ointment over the burn. He gave massive doses of vitamin C by mouth.

Dr. Klenner said all are victims of carbon monoxide, which is one of the most harmful elements in air pollution, especially car exhausts. For actual carbon monoxide poisoning he gave massive doses of vitamin C which seems able to separate the poison from the red blood cells which it is in the process of destroying.

He used vitamin C in massive doses in 300 consecutive pregnancies. Pregnancy is a stress and he gave vitamin C for all stresses. He believed failure to give this vitamin to pregnant women accounts almost to malpractice. His patients experienced no anemia. Leg cramps occurred in fewer than three percent and then only when the patient had run out of vitamin C. Abdominal marks (stretch marks) appeared on the abdomens of his patients infrequently and then usually when the women gained too much weight and took too little exercise. Labor was short and less painful. The perineum was "remarkably elastic" even 15 years later. No patients required catheterization. No infections, no cardiac stress, even though 22 of these women had rheumatic heart disease. One patient had been told by her doctor that another pregnancy would be fatal. Under Dr. Klenner's care she had two more babies, went back to teaching school and continued taking 10 grams of vitamin C daily.

After delivering a famous family of quadruplets, Dr. Klenner started all the babies on 50 milligrams of vitamin C the first day and increased the dosage as time went on. The ten children of another couple whose babies he delivered are all healthy and good looking and are referred to as "the vitamin C babies."

Dr. Klenner treated snake bite and insect bites with injected vitamin C. He believed that all diabetics should be taking massive doses of it. Lack of the vitamin is responsible for the slow healing of a diabetic's wounds, he said. The vitamin also helps the diabetic to make better use of insulin. It helps the liver to deal with carbohydrate foods. Sixty percent of

Dr. Klenner's diabetic patients could be controlled with only diet and vitamin C—as much as 10 grams daily. The other 40 percent needed less insulin and less oral medication if they were taking massive doses of the vitamin.

Dentists told Dr. Klenner that 500 milligrams of vitamin C prevent shock and weakness after tooth extractions. Klenner once watched an operation in which the intestines were weak and so "glued together" that any effort to separate them resulted in tearing them. The surgeon declared that the situation was hopeless and he closed the abdomen. Two grams of vitamin C were injected every hour for 48 hours, then four times a day. In one week the patient was discharged. "She has outlived her surgeon for many years," said Dr. Klenner.

He gave massive doses for mononucleosis. As a famous Tulane urologist did, he gave 1½ grams of vitamin C daily to prevent bladder cancer. Klenner believed that vitamin C is "the anti-cancer vitamin." Ascorbic acid will control myelocytic leukemia, provided 25 to 30 grams are taken orally each day, he said. He pointed out that many serious conditions are cured by giving five million to 100,000 million units of penicillin as an intravenous drip over four to six weeks. "How long must we wait," he asked, "for someone to start continuous ascorbic acid drip for two to three months, giving 100 to 300 grams each day for various malignant conditions?"

He treated overdoses of drugs with vitamin C. Also tetanus in combination with a drug. Two cases of trichinosis were treated with vitamin C and B vitamins. Corneal injury, chickenpox and sunburn were also treated with vitamin C. He treated alcoholics suffering from overdoses of Antabuse with vitamin C. He encountered doctors who used vitamin C to treat glaucoma, fever blisters, arthritis, shingles and poisoning from heavy metals like lead and cadmium. He found that vitamin C prevents the build-up of cholesterol in the blood. "Ten grams of vitamin C or more every day and then eat all the eggs you want!" he said.

Will massive doses of vitamin C cause kidney stones?

The urine of someone taking vitamin C will be so acid that formation of stones will be impossible, he found. And, since vitamin C induces ample urination, there is no chance that urine will collect and remain in the bladder—one of the possible causes of bladder and kidney stones. Dr. Klenner was not talking theoretically when he reported these matters. It is hard to question his good results and tell him he imagined them when he saw his patients frequently and knew their condition.

There seems to be no ulterior motive for him to use vitamin C as he did, if it does not perform as he said it did. Doctors who never cure any patients do not stay in business very long. Dr. Klenner was not selling vitamin C. He had no commercial reason for promoting its use.

In the January 1983 issue of *Executive Health* Dr. Linus Pauling told the story of Dr. Klenner, who became interested in the therapeutic capabilities of vitamin C early in his medical career. He had read a report by Dr. Claus Jungeblut of the College of Physicians and Surgeons saying that he had given polio to laboratory monkeys, then, with large doses of vitamin C, had prevented these animals from being paralyzed.

When a polio epidemic threatened Reidsville in 1949, Dr. Klenner began cautiously to inject vitamin C in the form of sodium ascorbate into his polio patients. He tested 60 patients with this disease. He first injected 1,000 to 2,000 milligrams, depending on age, giving the vitamin by intravenous or intramuscular injection. This dose was repeated every two hours for one day, then every six hours for the next two days. Every patient recovered uneventfully within three to five days. At that time, polio was a devastating disease for which there was no cure, leaving in its trail thousands of permanently crippled individuals.

In 1948 Dr. Klenner published an article reporting successful treatment of patients with viral pneumonia by injection of 2,000 to 4,000 milligrams of vitamin C a day. By 1949 he was giving as much as 15 to 20 grams (15,000 to 20,000 milligrams) of the vitamin, half of it by injection, half by mouth. In 1950, he reported that he had employed 80 grams of vitamin C per day for four days in two polio patients, half by injection, half by mouth. Both patients were cured.

In the 30 papers he published in medical journals since then, he described how he used vitamin C successfully, in very large doses, to treat viral pneumonia, polio, flu, measles, chickenpox, hepatitis, mononucleosis, puerperal sepsis, herpes zoster (shingles) and herpes simplex (cold sores). These are all viral diseases. Later, Dr. Klenner was recommending intravenous injections of 350 milligrams per kilogram of weight of the individual for any serious viral infection. This means about 25 grams of sodium ascorbate for a person weighing 150 pounds.

In 1951, Dr. Klenner said, "Many physicians refused to employ vitamin C in the amount suggested simply because it is counter to their fixed ideas of what is reasonable; but they do not refuse to try some new product being advertised by an alert drug firm. It is difficult for me to reconcile these two attitudes. On the other hand, many physicians who have been willing to try vitamin C against the virus of polio have attained the same striking results we reported. Scores of letters from practitioners here in the United States and Canada could be presented in evidence. In some instances, doctors have cured their own children of polio by giving vitamin C and in other cases doctors themselves have been cured."

Dr. Irwin Stone, in his book *The Healing Factor, Vitamin C Against Disease,* states that "the main value of Klenner's work is in showing that any active viral disease can be successfully brought under control with ascorbic acid if the proper large doses are used. He says, "It is inconceivable but true that Klenner's pioneering work has been almost completely ignored; no large scale tests have been made to explore the exciting possibilities of his provocative clinical results . . . Millions of dollars of research money have been spent in unsuccessful attempts to find a non-toxic effective virucide (killer of viruses) and all sorts of exotic chemicals have been tried. All the while, harmless, inexpensive and nontoxic ascorbic acid has been within easy reach of these investigators. It might prove to be the 'magic bullet' for the control of viral diseases."

Dr. Pauling said, "It is my own impression that this situation has not changed much in the years since Klenner made those observations. Many physicians still scoff at the idea that vitamin C in large or very large doses has value in controlling disease and this attitude seems to reflect their fixed ideas and their ignorance. On the other hand, many letters that my associate Dr. Ewan Cameron and I have received from physicians about their own observations and my own experience indicate that a larger and larger fraction of physicians is beginning to recognize the great value that vitamin C has in the control of infectious diseases, cancer and heart disease."

The final discouraging note on Dr. Klenner is that the local hospital finally refused to allow him to bring his patients there because of his use of vitamin C in treating them. Speaking of cancer, Dr. Klenner said, "Who can say what 100 grams or 300 grams given intravenously for several months might accomplish in cancer! The potential is so great and the employment so elementary that only the illiterate will continue to deny its use."

If you are interested in following the suggestions of Dr. Pauling, Dr. Klenner and Dr. Cathcart in regard to massive doses of vitamin C, there is no reason why you should not. Taking as much as four grams of vitamin C every day in divided doses, preferably with meals, sounds like a good idea. Don't just gulp down a handful of vitamin C tablets in the morning and forget about them the rest of the day. This vitamin is water soluble. Whatever you do not need is excreted in about four hours. So taking your vitamin C with each meal should provide you with enough to flood your tissues with it and perhaps add greatly to the health of every part of your body.

# CHAPTER 29

# Vitamin C and the Health of the Heart

THE JANUARY 1978 ISSUE of *Executive Health* published an article by Linus Pauling, Ph.D. on "Vitamin C and Heart Disease." Discussing the current fascination with the theory that it's cholesterol-rich foods that cause heart disease, Dr. Pauling presented some 25 references to authoritative medical and scientific journals, most showing that the amount of cholesterol in the diet has little effect on incidence of heart disease and deaths from heart attacks, even though a high cholesterol level in the blood is often related to such conditions.

There are two kinds of cholesterol—high density lipoprotein (HDL) and low density lipoprotein (LDL). The first appears to be highly beneficial and tends to prevent heart problems. The second, LDL, is destructive and tends to bring about heart problems. Both contain cholesterol. This relation between HDL and cholesterol and heart disease had been reported as long ago as 1951, said Pauling, but had been ignored. Thus the problem of cholesterol becomes complicated: decreased incidence of heart disease is correlated to some extent with a decreased level of LDL cholesterol and to a greater extent with an increased level of HDL cholesterol.

Pauling quotes Dr. Mark Altschule as saying, in regard to many past experiments and observations, "They do not support the currently popular theory that high blood cholesterol is a 'risk factor' in heart disease." "It is necessary, of course," says Pauling, "that physicians be conservative, but the medical authorities should not close their eyes to new evidence for twenty years."

Dr. Pauling then considers the accumulating evidence that deficiency in vitamin C may indeed be very important in causing our modern heart problems. He discusses the role of vitamin C in protecting and rebuilding collagen, the "glue" that holds us together. Lack of vitamin C might be the cause of the plaques that form on the inner walls of arteries (hardening of the arteries) which cut down the flow of blood to and from the heart. He describes a review of this evidence by C. Krumdieck and C. E. Butterworth which appeared in *The American Journal of Clinical Nutrition*, August, 1974. It dealt with the interactions of vitamin C, cholesterol and lecithin in preventing this condition. Dr. Krumdieck and Dr. Butterworth are professors at the University of Alabama and Dr. Butterworth was, at the time, chairman of the American Medical Association's Council on Foods and Nutrition.

The *Journal* article stated "A rather large volume of literature supports the hypothesis that vitamin C decreased susceptibility to vascular (blood vessel) injury. There is also evidence that both vitamin C and the unsaturated lecithins (in food) participate in the mobilization and excretion of cholesterol . . . It is our belief that the available evidence clearly justifies and indeed calls for a carefully controlled evaluation of the effects of vitamin C and the lecithins on atherosclerosis (hardening of the arteries)."

The Alabama scientists describe a 1944 experiment in which ten young healthy volunteers were put on a diet in which there was no vitamin C. Two of them suddenly developed serious heart complications, with pain in the chest, heart murmurs and partial heart block. The experiment was terminated at once, to prevent death, although neither of the volunteers had, as yet, shown any symptoms of scurvy, the disease of vitamin C deficiency.

Captains of old sailing ships, hundreds of years ago, used to describe sudden deaths of young sailors who gasped, clutched at their throats and chests and died within moments—

surely an apt description of a modern heart attack. Scurvy killed many thousands of sailors in those days since no foods containing vitamin C were available on long sea voyages, so the crew got none of this vitamin.

The Spring, 1984 issue of the Linus Pauling Institute of Science and Medicine *Newsletter* takes up the subject of vitamin C and heart health, pointing out that a new study in *The Journal of Human Nutrition* seems to demonstrate the validity of the earlier studies. This 1981 study involved 13 men (average age 77 years) and 12 women (average age 87 years). Six of the men and five of the women had coronary heart disease—the condition that is responsible for most modern deaths from heart conditions. The other volunteers showed no evidence of this disease. Each patient was given one gram (1,000 milligrams) of vitamin C orally each day for six weeks.

Initial levels of HDL were lower and levels of triglycerides (another kind of fats) were higher in the heart patients than in the healthy volunteers. That was to be expected if theories on these two fatty compounds are sound. But, after only six weeks of vitamin C treatment, the HDL levels (the beneficial kind of fats) became higher in the heart patients so that they corresponded with those of the healthy volunteers. The authors of the article stated, "Latent ascorbic acid deficiency may be one of several risk factors contributing to the present epidemic of ischemic heart disease in the western world."

It also seems evident that a vitamin C intake of at least one gram a day, taken preferably in two or more doses, will lower the probability of developing coronary heart disease. It is also interesting to note that the white blood cells of 15 of the 25 heart patients showed lower than normal levels of vitamin C, but after six weeks of taking the vitamin the white blood cell levels came up to normal. White blood cells are protection against bacteria, viruses, foreign proteins and other enemies which assail our bodies.

In his *Executive Health* article Dr. Pauling pointed out that cigarette smokers have low levels of vitamin C in their blood and says, "part of the damage done to their hearts' health by smoking may be attributed to the destruction of their vitamin C by the toxic substances in the inhaled smoke." By now we know that cigarette smoke is not the only poison to which most of us are exposed continually. There are air pollutants, water pollutants, myriad chemicals in food and beverages, drugs, both over-the-counter and prescription, sedentary lives and many other modern environmental threats in which vitamin C may play a protective role.

In an article published originally in *Chemical and Engineering News* in 1974, Dr. Pauling stated, "I believe that it is possible by rather simple means, especially nutritional, to increase the length of life expectancy for young people and middleaged people (and, to some extent, perhaps, old people) by about 20 years. Not only can that life expectancy be increased, I believe, but also the length of the period of well-being can be increased by the same amount or perhaps even a little longer, because it is likely that, as long as the process of aging goes on, the process of deterioration that culminates in death will proceed more rapidly at a late age than an earlier one."

"There's one other nutritional orthomolecular treatment that I'll mention," he continued, "This is a negative one involving sugar—sucrose. John Yudkin was professor of biochemistry at the University of London some years ago and he published a paper on his research on sucrose in relation to heart disease. He studied the incidence of heart disease as a function of the amount of sugar ingested, and he concluded that people who take 120 pounds of sugar per year have six times the chance at a given age of coming down with coronary heart disease as people who take 60 pounds per year or less. Those who take 150 pounds or more a year have 15 times the chance at a given age of developing coronary heart disease as those who take 60 pounds or less."

Dr. Pauling recounts an experiment in a state correctional school with 18 volunteers locked in a ward and fed a carefully controlled diet consisting of all the essential amino acids (proteins), a small amount of fat, all the vitamins and minerals in recommended amounts and glucose (pure sugar) as the only carbohydrate. The scientists in charge measured 26 clinical characteristics and found that they all stayed the same when the prisoners went from the prison diet over to his chemically determined diet—except one. The blood cholesterol levels of the volunteers dropped from 207 to 155 average within a month.

After a few months the prisoners complained about the taste of the food so the scientist replaced one quarter of the glucose with sucrose (table sugar)—no other changes—and blood cholesterol levels went back to the original high level. "It's the sugar that's the culprit," says Dr. Pauling. "I believe that if people were to avoid sucrose (table sugar) hardly ever a spoon from the sugarbowl onto anything, avoid sweet desserts, except when you're a guest somewhere, avoid buying foods that say 'sugar' as one of the contents—they could cut down on the incidence of disease and increase life expectancy. Take a fair amount of vitamins. Stop smoking cigarettes and you'll have a longer and happier life—more vim and vigor and a better time altogether."

Diabetes is one disorder in which circulatory disorders are usually present and may be the eventual cause of death. Is it possible that deficiency in vitamin C may be the cause of diabetes or that such a deficiency may have some bearing on the course of diabetes and its effects on the body? New studies from Vanderbilt University and Guy's Hospital in England seem to show compelling evidence of such a relationship.

Dr. George V. Mann, Associate Professor of Biochemistry and Medicine at Vanderbilt believes that, in the future, massive doses of vitamin C may be used along with insulin to prevent or delay the circulatory complications of diabetes. This includes hardening of the arteries and the disorders that may follow in brains, in heart and blood vessels, in kidneys, in eyes and in many other organs of the body.

Insulin is required for the transport of vitamin C into cells of certain tissues. Diabetics may lack insulin. Therefore, it seems possible that this vitamin is not transported into these cells, resulting in a kind of local scurvy. Vitamin C is needed for the manufacture of collagen, the body "glue" that holds cells together. When it is not present in ample amounts, tissues tend to fall apart, resulting in cataracts, hemorrhages and many artery disorders.

Dr. Mann theorizes that possibly the same mechanism that transports blood sugar through the cell walls also carries vitamin C. In diabetics blood sugar levels are too high, so the mechanism may not be able to transport vitamin C at the same time. Old people as well as diabetics tend to have high blood sugar levels. Giving both groups large doses of vitamin C may force the vitamin into the tissues, even though the body's transportation system may be defective.

Isn't it possible, Dr. Mann theorizes, that the circulatory disorders and cataracts of old age are the results of a diminishing insulin effect? True, these groups do not generally have the classic symptoms of deficiency in vitamin C or scurvy, possibly because they have enough insulin and vitamin C to reach certain cells. But the cells that need insulin and vitamin C the most may be left in a deficient state.

In his laboratory, Dr. Mann discovered that in the concentrations of blood sugar which diabetics often have—up to 800 milligrams per cent—the sugar does indeed stop off the transportation of vitamin C into the cells. The next step, experimentally, is to put diabetic animals on diets deficient in vitamin C to test the degree of harm to circulatory systems, eyes and so on.

What do diabetic specialists say about Dr. Mann's theory? The Director of Education at the Joslin Diabetes Foundation thought it is interesting. He doesn't want diabetics trying immense amounts of vitamin C right away, he says, but surely we should have more research along these lines.

Dr. Harold Rifkin of Montefiore Hospital in New York agrees that the idea should be studied further. He also warns that diabetics taking large doses of vitamin C may find that their urine tests are off, for somehow the vitamin gives false negative tests for diabetics and false positive tests for non-diabetics. Presumably, this occurs because the chemical structure of glucose which is blood sugar (C6 H 12 06) and vitamin C (C6 H8 06) are similar enough that tests do not discriminate between them.

A team of British investigators, working independently, announced in *Medical World News,* April 1974 that there is a complex relationship between insulin, glucose and vitamin C metabolism. Dr. W. J. H. Butterfield of Guy's Hospital and his colleagues found that non-diabetics who were given an injection of insulin showed a significant increase in vitamin C in surrounding tissues. So it's possible, he thinks, that lack of sufficient vitamin C in the diet may reduce the sensitivity of tissues to insulin, thus reducing the body's production of insulin. This would eventually cause diabetes. Obesity causes diabetes by increasing the amount of insulin needed by tissues to dispose of the accumulated glucose or blood sugar.

Using a complicated testing system which they developed, the doctors injected insulin and found a release of vitamin C in every non-diabetic person tested and an increased output of the vitamin after the injection. The diabetics, on the other hand, showed no effect on their vitamin C levels, but did show the definite and expected results in blood sugar uptake.

The British physicians intend to continue their investigations, especially the part vitamin C may play in retinopathy—disorders of the retina of the eye which are frequent complications of diabetes. Their research was reported in *Perspectives in Biology and Medicine,* Winter, 1974.

Another bit of vitamin C research described in *Atherosclerosis,* Volume 19, 1974, states that the cholesterol level of the blood, the liver and the heart artery decreased when vitamin C was given to laboratory rats along with methionine, one of the links of protein. Levels of another kind of blood fat, triglycerides, also decreased in the heart artery and liver. Vitamin C alone brought about some decrease, though not as much as the two substances together. It is noteworthy that rats make their own vitamin C. They were apparently not making enough in their livers to lower the levels of fats in the blood. So additional vitamin C and the amino acid brought about this healthful change.

Diabetics who take large daily doses of vitamin C must be very conscious of the effect this substance may have on their urine tests for sugar. A false test may result in giving a dose of insulin that is too large or too small with drastic results. There is nothing harmful to the diabetic about taking large doses of the vitamin. The warning here applies only to days when the diabetic is going to have a test for sugar in the urine. It's best to omit the usual vitamin C dose before going for such a test. Or if you test your urine at home, it's best to omit your vitamin C doses perhaps for several days before making the test. Levels of blood sugar are not affected by the large doses of vitamin C—just the urine tests. For non-diabetics there is no reason not to take large doses of vitamin C which may perhaps protect you against ever succumbing to this very serious chronic disease.

In *Circulation,* a professional journal, November 1961, research on vitamin C in the treatment of hardening of the arteries in the Soviet Union was reviewed by Ernest Simonson, M.D. and Ancel Keys, Ph.D. The experiments described by the Russians showed clearly that vitamin C prevents hardening of the arteries and other circulatory disorders in laboratory animals. The American authors say, "The great contributions of the pioneering work in Russia on hardening of the arteries are obvious to all, and we may be sure that valuable research will continue in that country."

In 1967 *Medical World News* (April 14) commented on the work of Dr. Boris Sokoloff and his associates in Florida who found, working with rabbits having very high levels of cholesterol, that large repeated doses of vitamin C lowered blood levels of cholesterol and triglycerides, resulting in fewer plaques inside arteries which are the symptoms of artery hardening. They also tested 60 human volunteers with serious disorders of fat metabolism and some with heart trouble as well and found that vitamin C in large doses lowered levels of the harmful triglycerides.

# VITAMIN C AND THE HEALTH OF THE HEART

Dr. Sherry Lewin of London Northeast Polytech believes that vitamin C is much more effective if taken in smaller doses at intervals throughout the day, rather than taking only one or two larger doses. He also suggests taking it with a glass of citrus juice. In *New Scientist*, November 29, 1973 he wrote of having cured his own case of angina with large doses of vitamin C. Dr. Lewin wrote a classical book on the subject of vitamin C. We list it in our bibliography.

Here is evidence from over 30 years ago showing that vitamin C in large enough doses is powerful against the diseases that kill more Americans than any other. Why have we ignored this evidence all these years, when vitamin C, even in very large doses, is completely harmless?

# CHAPTER 30

# Vitamin C and Mental Health

A NEW ZEALAND PHYSICIAN, Dr. Michael H. Briggs, reported in a letter to the editor of the *British Medical Journal* that patients in mental hospitals often suffer from chronic lack of vitamin C because of poor dietary habits. They cannot be coaxed to eat enough fresh raw foods which are our best source of this vitamin. He has found there is another reason why they are short on vitamin C. Mental patients may have an overabundance of copper in their blood which is very destructive of vitamin C. As excitement or mental disturbances occur in mental patients, levels of copper rise in their blood, and levels of vitamin C decline. Dr. Briggs believes the copper-vitamin C situation may result in chronic deficiency in the vitamin.

A British psychiatrist, too, has been using vitamin C in treatment of mental patients. Dr. G. Milner's interest was aroused when he read of research indicating that anxiety and excitement tend to destroy the body's store of vitamin C. He found that schizophrenia patients have lower levels than average of vitamin C in their blood even though they are getting "average" amounts of the vitamin in their food.

Dr. Milner calls a condition of fatigue and depression, irritability and vague ill health "subscurvy." it is not a full-blown case of scurvy, but it is an indication that levels of vitamin C are low in any such patient. He set up an experiment in a mental hospital in England with the cooperation of the medical staff. Some of the forty male volunteers had been in the hospital for as long as 45 years.

Dr. Milner found that 12 of the men already had symptoms of scurvy which no one had thought to be very important. Milner gave 20 of the volunteers one gram of vitamin C daily in a liquid preparation while the second 20 patients got only some flavored water. No one, including doctors, nurses and patients, knew which group got the vitamin C. All patients were given tests to determine their frame of mind—whether paranoid, depressed, manic and so on. Nurses and doctors also made notes of the individual patients' emotional state from day to day.

When the test was completed, Dr. Milner found that the patients taking the vitamin C had improved considerably, according to all the tests and reports of those caring for them. He believes that these people have a far greater need for this vitamin than the rest of us, since they became seriously deficient even though they were eating a diet in which, presumably, there was enough vitamin C.

A letter to the *British Medical Journal*, May 12, 1962 reported on a Canadian doctor's experience with a patient suffering from schizophrenia. Dr. Abram Hoffer treated her with one gram (1,000 milligrams) of vitamin C every hour for 48 hours. At the end of this time she was mentally well. She remained so for six months, when she died from an unrelated disease.

H. L. Newbold, M.D. wrote in *Meganutrients for Your Nerves* of an experiment at California's Stanford University where Dr. Linus Pauling conducted a series of "loading tests," financed by the National Institutes of Health. By "loading tests" we mean that extremely large doses of vitamin C were given to the volunteers. When doses as high as 40 grams (40,000 milligrams) were given to schizophrenics, little or none of it was excreted in urine, which seemed to indicate that seriously mentally ill patients needed more than one thousand times the amount recommended as a daily requirement. Similar loading tests with other vitamins produced similar results. Pauling concluded that many people suffering from schizophrenia require many times the normal amounts of vitamins in their enzyme systems.

Dr. Newbold also said of vitamin C, "You always hear of vitamin C that it is good for bleeding gums. It is true that if gums are bleeding because of scurvy vitamin C will correct the problem. But vitamin C, as all other vitamins and minerals, is used by every cell in the body. If you have scurvy you will have much more to worry about than bleeding gums. You will be tired and depressed. Wounds will heal poorly. If the condition lasts long enough (and to a profound enough degree) you will die."

Dr. E. Cheraskin, in his book *The Vitamin C Connection* stated that "Mother Nature seems to have recognized nerve cells' special need for vitamin C, for the level of ascorbic acid is considerably higher in cerebrospinal fluid than in blood plasma . . . Vitamin C's concentration in the brain exceeds that in any other organ except the adrenal glands." He says, too, that Dr. Humphry Osmond, a research psychiatrist, and Dr. Hoffer of Canada describe vitamin C as a "natural internal tranquilizer." It counteracts anxiety. In fact, these researchers contend that weight for weight, ascorbic acid "is as active as haldol"—a major tranquilizer which is given to help people cope with the stress of modern life.

Tranquilizer drugs have a tendency to addict the people who take them. Once they get "hooked" it's hard for them to give up these drugs. However it's much easier if these addicted people are given plenty of vitamin C, because the vitamin itself acts as a tranquilizer. Dr. Cheraskin described an experiment in Bristol, England where 57 severely retarded men had been taking tranquilizers for an average of six and a half years. Leaving other prescribed drugs unchanged, Dr. J. Jancar replaced, tablet for tablet of the tranquilizer drugs with 50 milligram tablets of vitamin C. Then for three months the vitamin C was gradually withdrawn and finally more than half the volunteers could do without the tranquilizers entirely.

# VITAMIN C AND MENTAL HEALTH

Researchers from the National Council on Drug Abuse and the Methadone Maintenance Institute of Chicago announced that vitamin C relieves three side effects of Methadone: constipation, reduced libido and restless sleep. With a daily administration of 3,000 milligrams of vitamin C other annoying side effects of the drug Methadone were also eliminated.

Working in the San Francisco Drug Treatment Program, two researchers used vitamin C in massive doses along with other vitamins, minerals and protein supplements to treat drug-withdrawal symptoms. All 227 volunteers had a complete physical exam and testified to a long list of symptoms: runny eyes and nose, sweating, chills, muscular aches and pains, diarrhea, abdominal cramps, drug craving, loss of appetite, sleeping difficulties. Those who took vitamin C had the best results in terms of withdrawal symptoms. Dr. Cheraskin says he does not believe that research should be confined to drug users. Why not try it as well with smokers, overeaters, heavy drinkers and other addicts!

# CHAPTER 31

# Scurvy in Old Folks and Vitamin C

SCURVY, THE DISEASE OF total deficiency in vitamin C, has been known since 1515 B.C. Today, those most at risk from scurvy are, generally speaking, babies fed commercial formulas, military personnel eating dried rations and elderly people living on grossly deficient diets. *Nutrition Reviews* told of a healthy male volunteer at the University of Iowa School of Medicine who was put on an otherwise nutritious diet containing no vitamin C for only 90 days.

Here are some of the symptoms which developed: hyperkeratosis (horny projections on the skin), hemorrhages in various organs, black and blue spots, eye hemorrhages, arthritis, fluid retention, aches and pains, lassitude and weakness, a dry mouth and dry eyes, enlarged salivary glands and destructive changes in hair and gums—in only 90 days!

The researchers reversed all these disagreeable and dangerous symptoms within 116 days during which the volunteer was given only six and a half milligrams of vitamin C daily. It must have been a hard and painful five months but the young man survived. We suppose the researchers were trying to discover just how even this small an amount of vitamin C can prevent the worst ravages of scurvy.

The *Nutrition Reviews* article continued with a discussion of the frequency with which scurvy is found in the elderly, especially in those living alone. They tend to abandon ordinary meal preparation, says the author. They live on small amounts of "easy foods" like milk, soup and bread and this can lead to scurvy, since none of these foods contains any vitamin C.

A story taken from the *Journal of the American Medical Association*, in 1977 described a woman brought to a California hospital who had been bleeding internally over the years. The doctors operated on her to stop the bleeding in her abdominal cavity. Several years later she returned with the same problem and another operation was performed. Again and again this procedure was performed until the woman had been given a total of seven operations over several years and a number of her organs had been removed. One member of the staff asked her what she generally ate. She told him. She seldom ate any fruits or vegetables. The doctors gave her massive doses of vitamin C and all her symptoms disappeared. She remained well so long as she continued to take the supplements and all her old symptoms returned when she discontinued them.

The older generation of Americans is the fastest growing segment of our population. We do not know how many of them live alone and spend little time or money on nourishing meals. There is no way to know how many of them are taken to hospitals with mysterious symptoms like the individuals described above, so expensive tests are performed and a great deal of trouble is taken in trying to diagnose the problems, apparently without anyone ever asking the patient what he or she eats and how often. It's certainly a rare physician who has ever suspected scurvy in a patient in a modern hospital. But it's there, all right.

A 72-year-old man, living alone, was admitted to a hospital in Oxford, England with symptoms of increasing lack of appetite, great distress in his digestive tract and chest pain. During the previous year he had become much weaker, easily fatigued and had lost about 28 pounds. Six weeks earlier he had had sudden attacks of chest pain followed by cough and breathlessness. One month earlier he vomited blood and found bright red blood in his stool. He bruised easily. He had also experienced seizures for several years past, consisting of loss of consciousness, twitching of limbs and incontinence, preceded by a feeling of great abdominal discomfort and depression.

The doctors gave the patient lots of tests and found, they thought, an ulcer or stomach cancer. They decided to operate. They asked him what he usually ate. Bread, milk and various kinds of soups, he said—a not uncommon diet for an elderly man living alone. The doctors put him on a diet to relieve the obvious symptoms of scurvy, the disease of vitamin C deficiency—bruising easily, for example. He was given a high protein diet and 1,000 milligrams of vitamin C every day for two weeks, then 150 milligrams a day for the next month.

Following this treatment, said *Nutrition Reviews,* May, 1983, the patient continued to improve. He cast aside the air of lassitude, gained weight and began to relish his meals. His skin hemorrhages rapidly decreased and no new ones appeared. The blood disappeared from the feces. Liver function tests were negative. The epilepsy was satisfactorily controlled. The patient was discharged after eight weeks of hospitalization and when subsequently seen this patient was well.

At a symposium on vitamin C in 1986 Stuart C. Hartz, Sc.D. reported on Vitamin C and Blood Lipoproteins in an Elderly Population which showed that vitamin C has a beneficial effect on the blood fats in elderly people, specifically by raising levels of the helpful fat called High Density Lipoprotein. He pointed out that, as we age, levels of this helpful compound tend to decrease. Vitamin C can reverse this tendency.

As long ago as 1965 *The Journal of the American Geriatrics* Society reported on giving three grams of vitamin C daily along with large doses of the B vitamins to old folks suffering from such poor circulation that their feet were always cold. Other patients had patches of gangrene and skin discoloration due to circulatory difficulties. In every case, relief was obtained.

In 1967 Dr. J. Shafer, a Glasgow physician, was called to attend two patients with "florid scurvy"—that is, advanced cases of this disorder which has only one cause—lack of vitamin C. Significant heart trouble was diagnosed on the basis of tests. After only one week in which they were given large doses of vitamin C the two patients had no heart symptoms at all.

"In view of the present prevalence of malnutrition among the elderly," Dr. Shafer said in *The Lancet,* he was concerned about the possibility that just plain lack of vitamin C was being generally diagnosed as heart trouble. Is it possible, he asked, that we are treating these people for heart trouble when all they need is a good strong dose of vitamin C? He said that scurvy is "not an uncommon disorder." It occurs mostly among old folks who live alone, those who have peculiar ideas about what to eat and those who have diseases of the digestive tract which necessitate elimination of foods rich in vitamin C.

He used the term "doctor-caused" scurvy when the disorder occurs in patients who have restricted their diets on the advice of their doctors and where the doctor does not provide them with a vitamin C supplement. If you have been told, for example, to eliminate from your meals all fresh fruits and vegetables, this is just about the surest way to develop a full-blown case of scurvy. If the physician has not enough knowledge of nutrition to prescribe a heavy daily dose of vitamin C, the patient will likely show up with many new symptoms which the doctor will not recognize as "scurvy," since most doctors believe this disease was wiped out 300 years ago.

Is it possible, Dr. Shafer asks in *The Lancet,* that large doses of vitamin C act like a drug in calming the hearts of scurvy victims. He reminds his readers that if vitamin C is given with digitalis (a powerful heart drug) it prevents or minimizes the changes in heart action which the drug brings on and allows the patient to continue to take the drug with fewer unpleasant side effects.

Another physician, Carl F. Shaffer in the *American Journal of Clinical Nutrition,* January 1970, summarized the beneficial effects of vitamin C on the circulatory health of older folks like this. He said that the main function of vitamin C is to help in the manufacture of collagen. One aspect of hardening of the arteries is the various processes that go on around that formation of collagen in the lining of the arteries. Hardening of the arteries can be produced in laboratory animals with normal blood levels of cholesterol and no fatty deposits on the inside of their arteries. You just withhold vitamin C. Deficiency in vitamin C is much more common among older folks and they are the ones who suffer most from hardening of the arteries, heart attacks and other circulatory troubles.

# CHAPTER 32

# Vitamin C and the Health
# of the Eyes

CATARACTS ARE ONE of the leading causes of loss of sight and total blindness in our country. It is astonishing that so little work has been done on the great importance of vitamin C to the health of the eyes. Fluids in the healthy human eye contain relatively enormous amounts of vitamin C, 30 to 50 times the amount of the vitamin found in the blood. This suggests that this vitamin must play an important role in eye health.

At a 1980 seminar for science writers, Dr. Shambhu D. Varma, director of eye research at the University of Maryland, presented evidence that vitamin C may help to prevent the kind of cataract that is believed to be caused by light. Light shining into the eyes can trigger a photo-chemical reaction that produces a chemical which has been shown to be damaging to the eye lens.

This damaging substance is superoxide, he said, a breakdown product of oxygen. Dr. Varma has discovered in experiments that vitamin C destroys this harmful enzyme. Vitamin C is well known as an antioxidant—that is, a helpful compound which counteracts the harmful breakdown products of fat, when fat is oxidized or rendered rancid by oxygen. Vitamin E also has the capacity to act as an antioxidant.

Dr. Varma said that light as a cause of cataracts has been under investigation for only about a decade. His work does not *prove* that superoxide causes cataracts, nor does it *prove*

241

that vitamin C protects against the enzyme. But it does suggest a relationship between light cataracts and getting enough vitamin C as well as eating a highly nutritious diet, is certainly warranted, he believes.

Cataracts in diabetics are six times more common than in non-diabetics. They are believed to be caused by large amounts of a sugar solution called sorbitol which accumulates in the eyes of diabetics. It occurs here only when blood sugar levels are raised to certain heights, which happens often in diabetics.

Dr. Varma has been working on ways to destroy the enzyme that produces the sorbitol from blood sugar. He has found that flavonoids are effective in animal experiments where they can block production of the enzyme and prevent cataracts from forming. The flavonoids are given to the animals in the form of eye drops. These are not available for human use, Dr. Varma said, and will not be for a number of years.

Certain flavonoids are substances that accompany vitamin C in fruits, berries and vegetables. So it seems reasonable that they would cooperate with the vitamin in many helpful body processes. Many vitamin C supplements also contain bioflavonoids, or they may be taken in supplements separately. The one named rutin is the one frequently used. We do not know whether these are the kind of bioflavonoids used by the Maryland physician, nor do we know if they would be effective taken orally. But there is no harm in trying them orally along with the vitamin C. They are wholly beneficial and without any possible damaging side effects.

In Irwin Stone's fine book *The Healing Factor, Vitamin C Against Disease,* he told of Royal Air Force experiments in 1941 in which doctors gave vitamin C for inflammations of the cornea, a condition which probably reduces the amount of the vitamin in the eye. The researchers reported that large doses of vitamin C are necessary "to flood the bloodstream with excess of the vitamin." In 1946, several other researchers confirmed this report. They gave one and a half grams of vitamin C daily to heal deep corneal ulcers. In 1939, several doctors got good results in 90 percent of cataract patients treated with only two series of daily injections of 150 to 1,000 milligrams of the vitamin. These doctors were treating "incipient" cataracts, meaning that they were just beginning to form and had not yet caused much destruction of sight.

A Detroit physician in 1939 gave large doses of vitamin C by mouth to patients with senile cataract. He got improvement in 60 percent of the group, mostly within the first two weeks of treatment. He believed that the benefits were due to clearing of other parts of the eye, the blood vessels of the retina and the optic nerve. All these parts of the eye apparently need large amounts of vitamin C.

In 1952 an ophthalmologist reported excellent results treating incipient cataracts with about one gram of vitamin C daily, along with a diet that emphasized fresh fruits and vegetables AND NO SUGAR. In a number of his 450 patients, he revealed, cataracts did not progress for a period of eleven years during the vitamin C treatment. Dr. Stone mentioned that vitamin C may be used as an eye wash in the form of a sodium ascorbate solution. Sodium ascorbate is available in crystal or powdered form. Just a pinch of this powder in a three-ounce paper cup and stirred around produces a solution that can easily be used as an eye wash.

Throughout the literature on cataract one cannot escape the fact that diabetes and related disorders are closely interwoven with the occurrence of cataracts. If you wish to escape cataract as you grow older the first order of business is to sharply restrict the amount of sugar you eat, finally eliminating it entirely and making fresh fruits your only source of sugar. It's easy, once you begin to add fiber in the form of bran and other fiber-rich foods to your meals. They are so filling that you have no empty stomach growling away between meals, so there is little craving to eat something sweet. Several of the B vitamins and vitamin A are also known to be essential for eye health, so you should make certain you are getting enough of these and a great deal more of vitamin C. If a cataract has already been found in your eye, perhaps you can prevent it from progressing further by simply taking these simple dietary precautions.

Ben C. Lane, an optometrist, has found, he said in a paper titled "Ocular Hypertension Triggered by Stimulus to Accommodation and Deficit Nutriture" that vitamin C is extremely important for preventing glaucoma, the eye disease which brings high intraocular pressure that threatens blindness if not controlled. He has found that this pressure increases as levels of vitamin C in the blood decrease. The trace mineral chromium works with the vitamin, he says. Perfectly fitted reading glasses are also important in preventing glaucoma. If the eye muscles fail to focus the eyes for close work the body raises pressure within the eye to compensate.

In his book, *The Healing Factor, Vitamin C Against Disease,* Dr. Irwin Stone told of biochemists in 1962 who found 12 separate biochemical processes that go on inside your eye which involve vitamin C. He says that, since 1930, biochemists have known that vitamin C is found in the eye in much higher levels than in the blood or many other body tissues. He also tells of a number of cases in which eye pressure was reduced in glaucoma with oral doses as high as 2,000 milligrams while in other cases intravenous injections of the vitamin as high as 70 grams were given. They reduced pressure in the eye quickly.

# CHAPTER 33

# Vitamin C and Ankylosing Spondylitis

ACCORDING TO the *Merck Manual,* 12th edition, ankylosing spondylitis (Marie-Strümpell Disease) is "a chronic, progressive disease of the small joints of the spine separable as an entity from rheumatoid arthritis on genetic, epidemiological, pathological, clinical, serologic and therapeutic grounds . . . neither aspirin nor phenylbutazone (butazolidin) can cure or arrest the progressive ankylosis (stiffness of the spine)."

Statistics reveal that one out of every 330 adult men suffer from ankylosing spondylitis. Army doctors have found that it is a frequent cause of backache in soldiers.

In 1964 Norman Cousins, long-time editor of the prestigious *Saturday Review,* flew home from a lengthy, tiring and frustrating trip abroad. His slight fever and general achiness rapidly developed into a stiff neck and back and great difficulty in moving arms, hands, fingers and legs. His doctor hospitalized him when his sedimentation rate reached 80 mm per hour. The sedimentation rate is the rate at which red blood cells settle out of anticoagulated blood. It may indicate an inflammatory condition, an infection or a cancer.

The doctors decided Mr. Cousins had a very serious collagen disease. This category includes all the arthritic diseases. As the crippling disease progressed, leaving him unable to turn over in bed, the doctors told him he was suffering from ankylosing spondylitis. Spondylitis is inflammation of the vertebrae. Ankylosing means stiffening or locking in place. The patient was faced with eventually being totally unable to move.

Mr. Cousins' doctors told him he had one chance in 500 of recovering; one specialist said he had never personally seen a recovery from as serious a case as this. Mr. Cousins was being given a number of pain killers for the agonizing pain he was suffering. Associates at the *Saturday Review* researched these drugs and reported to him the highly toxic side effects he might expect. Butazolidin and aspirin were the two he was most worried about, for the doctors prescribed massive doses of both these drugs. A test showed that he was allergic to all of them. He was covered with hives and "felt as though my skin was being chewed up by millions of red ants."

Mr. Cousins decided he would stop taking the drugs and somehow get well on his own. His wide reading had acquainted him with many theories on the power of the mind over illness. He knew how terribly destructive to health negative emotions, hopelessness and anxiety can be. He decided he would turn his thoughts to getting well and abandon all negative thinking. He started a program of reading books on humor and laughter and watched comic films sent in by a friend.

Then he remembered his reading about vitamin C. He asked himself, "Couldn't it combat inflammation? Did vitamin C act directly or did it serve as a starter for the body's endocrine (gland) system—in particular, the adrenal glands? Was it possible, I asked myself, that ascorbic acid had a vital role to play in 'feeding' the adrenal glands?"

He had also read that arthritics seem to be deficient in vitamin C. He thought perhaps this might be because the body uses up its supply of vitamin C in fighting the breakdown of collagen which is the connective tissue damaged in these diseases. Fortunately, his doctor was a long-time friend who had a completely open mind about his treatment and was willing to try anything Cousins suggested.

He told his doctor he wanted to take massive doses of

vitamin C. His doctor said he thought there might be danger of kidney damage. Cousins was willing to take the risk. The doctor told him that the largest dose of vitamin C ever given in that hospital was three grams (3,000 milligrams) injected into muscle.

Cousins speculated that "introducing the ascorbic acid directly into the bloodstream might make more efficient use of the vitamin, but I wondered about the body's ability to utilize a sudden massive infusion. I knew that one of the great advantages of vitamin C is that the body takes only the amount necessary for its purposes and excretes the rest . . . I wondered whether a better procedure than injection would be to administer the ascorbic acid through slow intravenous drip over a period of three or four hours. In this way we could go far beyond the three grams. My hope was to start at 10 grams and then increase the dose daily until we reached 25 grams (25,000 milligrams)."

His doctor was astonished at the suggestion. Again he said he was afraid of kidney damage as well as damage to veins subjected for so long to an intravenous drip. "He said he knew of no data to support the assumption that the body could handle 25 grams over a four-hour period, other than by excreting it rapidly through the urine," says Cousins.

They tested the patient's blood and started the intravenous drip, administering 10 grams the first day. Within four hours the blood test showed a 9-point improvement.

"Seldom had I known such elation," said Cousins. "The ascorbic acid was working. So was laughter. The combination was cutting heavily into whatever poison was attacking the connective tissue. The fever was receding and the pulse was no longer racing."

They increased the amount of vitamin C a little every day until, by the end of the week, Cousins was getting 25 grams in an intravenous drip. By this time he was off all drugs and sleeping pills and was sleeping naturally. By the end of the eighth day he was able to move his thumbs without pain. The blood tests continued to improve. Two weeks later he was able to go south to bathe in the warm ocean. He could stand by himself, walk, even jog a bit. For many months he had pain and stiffness when he lifted his arms, his fingers were less skillful than he wished when he played the organ, he sometimes had difficulty turning his head. But this presumably incurable disease had been conquered without drugs.

Seven years later, in 1971, he found in *The Lancet*, a British medical journal, a study of how aspirin destroys vitamin C in the human body. This, apparently, is one reason why arthritics are generally deficient in the vitamin, since aspirin is the commonest drug used for arthritic pain. "It was no surprise, then," says Cousins, "That I had been able to absorb such massive amounts of ascorbic acid without kidney or other complications."

Norman Cousins' account of his victory over this crippling disease appeared in the conservative *New England Journal of Medicine* for December 23, 1976. In the latter part of his article he speculates on the possibility that vitamin C may have acted as a placebo in his case. A placebo is a pill or treatment which contains nothing of any medical value. But often the patient feels better, believing that the pill is powerful. He believed in vitamin C so thoroughly, he says, that perhaps it was his belief rather than any biological action of the vitamin which brought his blood corpuscles back to normal and took the stiffness from his spine. He discusses the place of placebos in medical treatment and suggests that much more research should be done along these lines.

He describes his visit to the clinic of Dr. Anna Aslan in Rumania, who told him she believes there is a direct connection between a strong will to live and chemical balances in the brain. She thinks that the will to live stimulates the entire glandular system, thus possibly bringing about "cures" that are otherwise inexplicable. Of course, Dr. Aslan also used a drug of the novocaine family which breaks down into a B vitamin inside the body. And she gave immense amounts of tender, loving care, security, hope, encouragement and praise to patients in her geriatric (old folks) clinic.

Dr. F. J. Ingelfinger, the distinguished editor of the *New*

*England Journal of Medicine,* wrote an editorial in the same issue as the Cousins article, trying to analyze the incident. He reminded his physician readers that miraculous, unexplained cures take place sometimes in medicine and that complaints about overwhelming the patient with drugs "are as ancient as the drugs themselves."

"Of greatest interest—at least to me," said Dr. Ingelfinger, "is the nature of Mr. Cousins' processes of reasoning as he cures himself by willpower, laughter, vitamin C and self placebotion . . . here is an astute, perceptive, articulate and distinguished layman who takes his treatment away from the medical establishment and wins out." How does it happen, then, that his doctors were not as familiar as Mr. Cousins was with the possibility of cure from willpower, laughter and the action of vitamin C, whether real or imagined?

"Well," says Dr. Ingelfinger, "when a patient's condition involves 'a serious collagen illness,' 'adrenal exhaustion,' polypharmacy (lots of drugs), the advantages of a high-fiber diet, and 'allergy tests' for drugs, medical fallibility, perplexity and controversy could hardly be greater; and the latest medical-journal articles on such clinical topics range from pure bunkum to results of experiments that are scientifically unexceptionable but still do no more than nibble away at the margins of vast expanses of ignorance . . . at present, it is not possible for the medical establishment, any more than for Mr. Cousins, to speak with confidence about collagen disorders, their protean (variable) manifestations and their often unpredictable course."

We are sorry to say we think this is a cop-out, Dr. Ingelfinger. The incident Mr. Cousins describes happened in 1964. In the ensuing 28 years, so far as we can determine, not a single physician made any attempt to use an intravenous drip of vitamin C for arthritic diseases—whether for its real or imagined value. Mr. Cousins reported no side effects. Such a treatment could have done no harm to the thousands, perhaps hundreds of thousands, of agonized patients who have suffered from this condition in those 28 years. Why has not the medical profession, or the National Institute of Health, or the Arthritis

Foundation *or somebody* in charge of something experimented further with this harmless therapy, just to see whether they might be able to ease a little pain and stiffness, even if they cannot work the complete miracle Mr. Cousins reported?

Cousins himself said he did not make the story public earlier because he did not want to raise false hopes in other sufferers from these diseases. But every treatment given to a victim of a chronic arthritic disease raises false hopes. Aspirin may control the pain for a while. Then the patient can't tolerate any more aspirin. Butazolidin controls the pain but the side effects may be far more devastating than the disease. So the drug must be discontinued. Cortisone, used to ease pain in many other arthritic diseases, is fraught with perils, including the eventual total destruction of the body's bones. Why would it be unethical to "raise false hopes" by giving the patient a completely harmless treatment?

As Mr. Cousins pointed out plaintively, someone in a hospital is always sticking needles into patients for one purpose or another. Intravenous administration of drugs is quite common. Why, then, not try intravenous administration of a harmless vitamin? We cannot help but feel that the answer has nothing to do with the confusion of the medical profession over methods of treatment of collagen diseases. It has to do rather with the fact that most doctors learn what they know of medical therapy from drug salesmen. No drug salesmen are selling vitamin C. It can't be patented. It costs next to nothing. No money-hungry drug company wants to bother with it.

Several letters from physicians were later published in the *New England Journal of Medicine*. They spoke only of the value of "placebo," laughter and "the will to live." They said that any effect of the vitamin C was that Cousins had faith in it. "We ought to do more studies of 'the placebo effect,'" they said. Not a single physician indicated that he believed the massive vitamin C injections had any effect.

But the letters that came to Norman Cousins were different, he said in an article in *Saturday Review* for February 18, 1978. He said that most of the letters indicated "evidence of an open attitude by doctors to new or unconventional approaches to the treatment of serious disease. There was abundant support for the measures that had figured in my own recovery—a well-developed will to live, laughter and large intravenous doses of sodium ascorbate (one form of vitamin C). Far from resenting the intrusion of a layman into problems of diagnosis and therapy, the doctors who wrote in response to the article warmly endorsed the idea of a patient's partnership with his physician in search for a cure."

He told two stories of laymen who got in touch with him which would be unbelievable except that most of us have had similar experiences with doctors. One, a lawyer with a 4-year old daughter dying of viral encephalitis, asked his doctor about giving the child vitamin C in massive doses. The doctor told him this was nonsense and he didn't welcome instructions from a layman.

So the lawyer bought a pound of powdered sodium ascorbate (which has a slightly salty taste, but not a sour taste). He asked the doctor if he might give his little girl some ice cream. The doctor said certainly. So the next day the little girl got a dish of ice cream laced with 10 grams (10,000 milligrams) of vitamin C. The next day the dose of vitamin C was larger, and the next larger still. The child continued to eat the ice cream. Two weeks later she was well enough to be removed from the oxygen tent. She was completely recovered when the lawyer last reported to Cousins. He had been giving her 25 grams (25,000 milligrams) of sodium ascorbate in her ice cream every day without the doctor's knowledge.

A Boston woman phoned Cousins about her husband, a terminal cancer patient who had been through the standard treatment—radiation, surgery and chemotherapy. She was very concerned about his condition. Cousins said he could not offer any advice since he was a layman, but he told her of the experiments of Dr. Ewan Cameron of Scotland, who had been giving terminal cancer patients large doses of vitamin C as their only treatment and comparing their condition to

251

that of other similar patients getting orthodox treatment. There is no question that the patients treated with vitamin C have less pain, can conduct their lives almost normally, and most of them, live much longer pain-free lives than the patients not so treated.

The woman asked her doctor about giving vitamin C to her husband. He answered with a "quack, quack" and told her the entire business was tommyrot. She and her husband severed their relationship with their doctor, although he was a longtime friend. The cancer patient moved home from the hospital and has gained some ground. "His appetite has improved; and so has his will to live," says Cousins. "He has already had a few more months of life than seemed possible only a short time ago."

Many of the 3,000 physicians who wrote to Cousins spoke of the value of faith in one's doctor and one's treatment, and speculated that it was Cousins' will to live, rather than the vitamin C which caused his almost miraculous recovery. But some of the 3,000 physicians said "don't you believe it was just faith and the will to live which worked this miracle." Two Illinois researchers told him their extensive research had showed the effects of vitamin C on red blood cells which apparently restores the body's "balance" or "homeostasis."

Said Cousins, "One can understand the apprehensions of the medical profession about the absurd notion that vitamins are the answer to any illness. Yet it is also true that some doctors have fostered the equally erroneous idea that the average supermarket shopping basket is insurance against any nutritional deficiency. Considering the preservatives, coloring agents, additives, and sugar overload in many processed foods, the pronouncement of the White House Conference on Food, Nutrition and Health in 1969 seems highly pertinent; namely, that one of the great failures in the education of medical students is the absence of adequate instruction in nutrition. . . . It is worth calling attention to the current practice of many British hospitals of administering intravenous doses of ascorbic acid instead of antibiotics as a routine postoperative procedure in guarding against infection.''

Ten years after his collagen disease was pronounced incurable by specialists in a leading New York hospital, Cousins met on the street one of the doctors involved in the prognosis. He gave him such a vigorous handshake that the physician winced and asked him to let go. ''He said he could tell from my handshake that he didn't have to ask about my health, but he was eager to hear about my recovery.''

We suggest a 10-gun salute for Norman Cousins, who has the courage to take on the entire medical establishment and coax from about 3,000 of its members the acknowledgment that laymen should play a large part in deciding on their own treatment, that all of the modern gadgetry of the hospital is useless without faith in the doctor and the treatment he is giving.

Said Cousins, ''Hundreds of letters from doctors . . . reflected the view that no medication they could give their patients is as potent as the state of mind that a patient brings to his or her own illness. In this sense, they said, the most valuable service a physician can provide to a patient is helping him mobilize all the resources of mind and body in order to maximize his own recuperative and healing potentialities.''

Along with, of course, the judicious use of good nutrition and the preventive and healing powers of those mysterious food elements our doctors know almost nothing about—vitamins and minerals.

For some reason which we have never been able to understand, Mr. Cousins stopped talking in public about his experience with intravenous vitamin C. Before his death in 1990 from cardiac arrest, he wrote and spoke at length about the benefits of an optimistic frame of mind when one is ill, but somehow forgot that the intravenous vitamin C was perhaps the largest item of cure in his bout with a very serious disease.

# CHAPTER 34

# Vitamin C Counteracts
# Many Poisons

SCIENTISTS HAVE KNOWN for years that fish use vitamin C
for proper bone growth and to increase their tolerance to
environmental stresses. Yet they never knew exactly how
this occurred. Now they do, and the discovery may help
biologists to better combat the effects of pollution on fish,
according to an announcement from the federal Fish and
Wildlife Department in June, 1976.

Biologists at the National Fisheries Research Laboratory
in Columbia, Missouri first learned of the mechanism while
studying channel catfish that were affected by the insecticide
toxaphene, widely used on cotton crops in the South where
channel catfish are also raised commercially.

About six years earlier catfish grown in fish farms in
that area were developing a curvature of the spine that, in
extreme cases, broke the fish's back and stunted growth as
much as one third. Scientists linked this condition to toxaphene residues in the water. Concentrations as low as 37
parts *per trillion* in the water were found to have serious
long-term effects on catfish.

One primary use of vitamin C by the fish is to aid in the
formation of collagen, as it is in human beings. Collagen
is the "glue" that literally holds us together. Calcium and
phosphorus are deposited around and within this collagen
framework forming a skeleton. If too little vitamin C is present, the mineral content can be decreased, making the back-

bone brittle and finally snapping it, which can result in internal bleeding.

Vitamin C is also an essential nutrient of the liver as it is in human beings. The liver detoxifies poisonous substances in the environment. Without it, fish cannot respond as well or adapt to stresses. Most of the vitamin C which the fish manufactures for itself is diverted to the liver under these circumstances and the bones and collagen suffer from deficiency. Since fish farming is a profitable industry in that part of the country, vitamin C is now being included in commercially prepared fish food for the catfish. It protects them completely from "The Broken Back Syndrome."

So here we have a creature which manufactures its own vitamin C. But, faced with just one water pollutant which is quite poisonous, its store of vitamin C is quickly exhausted and the skeleton of the fish deteriorates. We can only suppose that the same thing happens to a human being when he or she is exposed to an environmental poison. But human beings can't manufacture their own vitamin C. They must get all of it from their diets. Doesn't it seem likely that the same thing happens to human beings when they are exposed to environmental poisons?

Why, then, should they not be encouraged to add vitamin C supplements to their meals and snacks, as the vitamin C was added to the fish food? How is it possible that many nutrition "experts" still say that no modern American ever needs to take a vitamin supplement if he or she is eating a "well-rounded diet"? A need for far greater amounts of at least this one vitamin is evident considering that all of us are exposed, every day of our lives, to many pollutants suspected of being able to harm us greatly even at low doses. The fish were exposed to only one and look at the effects it had! And how quickly the additional vitamin C repaired the damage!

# CHAPTER 35

# The Wonder Drug Interferon and Vitamin C

ON MARCH 31, 1980 the cover of *Time* magazine featured a new drug called interferon. *Medical World News* for February, 1980 called interferon "a research triumph that might revolutionize medicine." *Time* all but predicted that cancer could indeed be conquered by this miracle drug which is manufactured by the body itself! The only problem is that the body makes such small amounts of this compound that some other source of interferon must be found before laboratory scientists can experiment with animal or human cancers.

Until recently the only source of interferon was leucocytes—the white blood cells which the scientists took from discarded flesh left from surgery. Each cell produces such infinitely small amounts of interferon that making a "drug" from these cells requires expensive work—so expensive that treating only one cancer patient with interferon produced this way would cost about $40,000. To put it another way, one pound of this mysterious substance might cost from 10 to 20 billion dollars!

As news of the potential for fighting cancer and viral diseases spread through the scientific world, drug company executives began to dream of huge profits and began to invest many millions in research and manufacturing plants to produce this wonder drug as soon as methods were refined. The American Cancer Society and the National Cancer Institute began to pour money by the millions into this research which promised that so many people could get so rich by patenting and producing the drug that would finally conquer cancer.

Meanwhile, in California, Dr. Irwin Stone, a biochemist, was speaking before an Ascorbate Update Seminar. He was speaking about interferon. He said, "In interferon therapy the main problems are the high prohibitive costs of exogenous (made outside the body) human interferon and its lack of availability in sufficient quantities. This is due to the difficulties in preparing and purifying it from such rare raw material as human white blood cells or cultures derived from them." He pointed out that all the cancer patients and all victims of viral diseases are suffering from subclinical scurvy. If they had corrected this condition by getting enough vitamin C before the interferon was administered, they could probably have produced enough interferon in their own bodies so that they would not have needed this expensive drug.

He said that the ability of blood cells to engulf and destroy viruses and other harmful invaders of the body depends on their content of vitamin C. Interferon has been found effective against viral diseases, different kinds of cancer, the collagen diseases like arthritis, the autoimmune diseases like multiple sclerosis, also bacterial infections and in the topical treatment of eye infections. Dr. Stone said that vitamin C in massive doses may stimulate the body's own production of interferon. This would explain the great success many physicians have in using vitamin C this way against all diseases involving viruses and bacteria.

"What could be simpler, safer and less expensive than giving patients megadoses of ascorbate and letting them produce their own interferon inside their own bodies," he asked. "Toxicity is not a problem because doses of up to 200 grams a day are commonplace and 300 grams of sodium ascorbate have been used intravenously without untoward side effects. Using doses of ascorbate in this range usually clears serious viral disease infections, such as viral encephalitis, viral pneumonia, herpes, hepatitis and many more within three days. A couple of Japanese hospitals routinely use 10 grams of ascorbate a day on their blood-transfused patients to act as a prophylactic (preventive) against hepatitis. They have reduced the incidence of transfusion hepatitis from about seven percent to practically zero.''

If indeed it turns out that vitamin C in massive doses causes the body to produce its own interferon, which then protects against viral diseases and cancer, it seems unlikely that the medical and scientific establishment will accept this simple, sane and reasonable solution to so many health problems. The infinitely complex and expensive machinery that has already been set into motion to produce interferon as a drug (and a very profitable drug) will just continue to expand even if the interferon produced this way turns out to be inferior and dangerous. This is the way the modern drug industry works.

Vitamin C is a simple compound that occurs in food and in the human body. It cannot be patented or sold for astronomical amounts. It is available everywhere without a doctor's prescription. Government bureaus continue to support with huge research grants any research on "drugs" as such—compounds that will make immense profits for the drug industry. Research money for investigating the possibility of a vitamin being just as effective as a drug is unavailable from such sources. Even as illustrious a scientist as Dr. Pauling tried seven times to get a grant from the National Institutes of Health for studies on vitamin C and was rejected each time. He finally got a modest sum for studies on breast cancer which we report on in another chapter of this book.

# CHAPTER 36

# An Orthopedic Surgeon
# Prescribes Vitamin C

In 1981 a California physician, Robert F. Cathcart, III made nutritional history by publishing in *The Journal of Orthomolecular Psychiatry* an account of his use in treating patients with massive—really massive—doses of vitamin C. Dr. Cathcart is a world-famous orthopedic surgeon whose hip prosthesis is being used in surgery in many parts of the world. He suffered from colds and hay fever and tried vitamin C for relief which he was surprised to find came very quickly. He began to use the vitamin in treating patients. By 1981 he had successfully treated 9,000 patients using this nutrient in massive doses.

Writing in the Linus Pauling Institute of Science and Medicine *Newsletter*, Fall, 1978, Dr. Linus Pauling described what he means by "orthomolecular medicine"—the achievement of and preservation of good health and the prevention and treatment of disease by regulating the concentration of molecules that are normally present in the human body. Important orthomolecular substances are the vitamins, especially vitamin C.

The rest of the *Newsletter* concerns Dr. Cathcart, who uses vitamin C in extremely large daily doses to cure viral diseases. In an interview for the journal *Chemtech*, quoted by Pauling, Dr. Cathcart described his methods of treatment which involve doses of vitamin C taken at intervals during the day. When he was asked about possible danger of such

259

high doses he replied, "If a patient who is accustomed to high vitamin C intake is hospitalized or otherwise comes under the care of certain physicians, the physician may cut off the vitamin C . . . and do it just when the patient needs it most."

When he was asked about vitamin C and the common cold, Cathcart replied, "I think that a person who has no really good reason to take vitamin C, no immediate illness, should probably do as Pauling says and take somewhere around four grams a day. People with allergies may find that they are more comfortable with higher amounts. I'm the last person in the world to maintain that you will never get a cold if you're taking maintenance doses of vitamin C. I get occasional colds, but I can block the symptoms with vitamin C. I never cease to be amazed at the number of patients who report to me that they used to get colds all the time and never get them since they began taking vitamin C . . . I take 10 to 15 grams a day, first, because I used to have hay fever—vitamin C takes care of hay fever nicely in about two-thirds of all cases—and second, because there is evidence that it (vitamin C) reduces cholesterol and thus helps to prevent atherosclerosis (hardening of the arteries). Third, I believe that vitamin C contributes to prevention of some cancers."

The interviewer from *ChemTech* asked Dr. Cathcart if he had published his findings about vitamin C in medical journals. He replied, "No, but I've tried. My manuscripts were rejected." "What did the referees say?" asked the interviewer. "Usually in professional journals experts are asked to pass on each paper received, then forward the comments to the author. Is that the practice in medical journals?" Dr. Cathcart replied, "In my case the manuscripts were just flat out refused."

The inquirer asked if it might have something to do with an establishment protecting itself. Cathcart replied, "I really believe that the doctors involved in these decisions don't believe this is true." Said the interviewer, "In other words you think they are saying that this qualified physician who has an international reputation for his hip prosthesis has made all this up. Colds, flu, hepatitis, mononucleosis, diseases a second year medical student could recognize with high probability—they don't *believe* this?'' ''Yes,'' said Dr. Cathcart, ''They think I'm deceiving myself somehow.''

Dr. Cathcart has found that massive doses of vitamin C can be used in many diseases and the patient will show evidence of not needing so much vitamin C by getting diarrhea. Dr. Cathcart calls this ''bowel tolerance.'' As the patient improves and need for vitamin C becomes less, his body announces this fact by producing mild diarrhea. Here are some of the diseases which Dr. Cathcart has treated with vitamin C in many thousands of patients.

*Ankylosing Spondylitis and Rheumatoid Arthritis.* Bowel tolerance is increased by each of these painful, crippling diseases, says Dr. Cathcart. Clinical response to massive doses of vitamin C varies. Sometimes there is remission of the disease. Sometimes not. ''I would advise the patient's increased need for ascorbate to be met regardless,'' he says. *Herpes, Cold Sores, Genital Lesions, Shingles.* Acute herpes infections are usually improved with doses of vitamin C to bowel tolerance—that is until diarrhea appears. However, recurrences are common. Zinc in combination with vitamin C is more effective in this condition.

*Crib Deaths.* Dr. Cathcart, along with a number of other specialists, believes that crib deaths are caused by sudden depletion of the body's vitamin C. The induced deficiency in some vital regulatory center kills the child, he says, and ''I have never heard of a crib death in an infant saturated with ascorbate.''

*Maintenance doses.* Dr. Cathcart advises his patients to take vitamin C in doses that are not quite high enough to cause diarrhea—as daily doses. Some patients report that their sinus trouble clears. Others report euphoria. In such cases, reduce the dose to a comfortable level—that is, no more diarrhea. About four grams (4,000 milligrams) a day, taken in divided doses, is just about right for most of us, he has found. If special stress is encountered, then raise the dose to 10,000 milligrams. At the slightest hint of a threatening viral disease increase the size and frequency of the dose. He also says, "Avoiding all sugar and processed foods will prove valuable if the patient's goal is almost complete prevention of viral diseases."

What are some possible complications? Kidney stones? In Dr. Cathcart's experience, vitamin C does not cause kidney stones, *but probably prevents them*. The few patients complaining of canker sores with small doses of vitamin C usually do not have such problems with large "bowel tolerance" doses. Patients with canker sores also need more vitamin E.

Dr. Cathcart says further that small doses of vitamin C may cause a few "nuisance complaints," but large doses taken to fight an infection are tolerated because of the body's great need at these times. He has found that large doses taken daily reduce the incidence of gouty arthritis. There is no evidence, he says, that vitamin C destroys vitamin B12.

Dr. Cathcart warns that sudden withdrawal of the vitamin, after a long period of taking massive doses, may invite colds, allergies and so on. Maintenance doses of four grams daily do not seem to cause this dependency. The major problem is an emergency hospitalization. Suddenly withdrawing the vitamin at a time when the body's needs are greater than ever may have serious consequences. He believes that such conditions may be so serious that people taking large doses of the vitamin daily should carry warning notices to this effect in their wallets or in a Medic Alert type of bracelet. Many doctors scoff at the idea of taking vitamins. But any conscientious physician, told that the patient needs continuing large doses of vitamin C daily, should certainly not refuse to give it in the hospital.

Dr. Cathcart is a highly experienced physician and surgeon. He has no financial interest in vitamin C. He is risking disapproval from his medical colleagues by demonstrating that this simple, harmless, inexpensive nutrient can be used in place of, or as an adjunct to, possibly destructive and dangerous drugs. If his use of vitamin C produced no improvement in any of his patients, he could be faced with malpractice suits of immense proportions.

He has discovered that the sicker the patient is (with whatever condition) the more vitamin C he or she can take, by mouth, without any side effects in the way of diarrhea. He said, "At least 80 percent of adult patients will tolerate 10 to 15 grams (10,000 milligrams to 15,000 milligrams) in fine crystals in one half a cup of water in four divided doses per 24 hours without having diarrhea. The astonishing finding is that almost all patients will absorb far greater amounts without having diarrhea, when ill. This increased tolerance is somewhat proportional to the toxicity of the disease being treated. Tolerance is increased some by stress (anxiety, exercise, heat, cold, etc.)."

Some of his patients have been taking up to 200 grams a day every 24 hours without any distress. "It was found," he said, "that the maximum relief of symptoms, the most shortening of the course of the disease and the greatest reduction in complications could be obtained by oral doses just below the point causing diarrhea . . . Apparently there is an almost unbelievable and unappreciated potential draw by diseased tissues on ascorbic acid (vitamin C) . . . In the cases of systemic viral infections, it is often more important to properly estimate what "gram" disease it is and persuade the patient to take adequate doses than to know what virus is being treated.

"True, under these circumstances, large amounts of the vitamin will be lost in the urine. But this is necessary to push adequate amounts of ascorbate into the tissues at the very seat of the disease and maintain full vitamin C functions . . . Also large amounts of vitamin C in the urine will prevent many bladder and kidney infections."

Here are some examples of other disorders Dr. Cathcart has treated and the amounts of vitamin C needed. *Mononucleosis*. A woman librarian with mono "claimed to have taken two heaping tablespoons of crystalline vitamin C every two hours, consuming a full pound of ascorbic acid in two days. She felt mostly well in three or four days, although she had to continue about 20 to 30 grams a day for about two months." *Viral Hepatitis*. This is one of the easiest diseases for vitamin C to cure, he says. Since the disease itself often causes diarrhea, this makes it difficult to decide exactly how high the doses should be. He gives 40 to 100 grams of the vitamin and says that stools and urine return to normal within two to three days.

*Gastroenteritis*. This disease may require 60 to 150 grams of vitamin C to block the symptoms. Vitamin C could be used in conjunction with whatever antibiotic is given. They work together. *Candida Infections*. These occur less frequently in patients taking antibiotics if large doses of vitamin C are used at the same time. It seems to have little effect on the disease itself, but it helps to ease the stress caused by this disorder.

*Trauma and Surgery*. Swelling and pain are remarkably reduced when massive doses of vitamin C are given to "bowel tolerance"—that is, up to the point where diarrhea appears. In major surgery the vitamin should be given in the form of sodium ascorbate intravenously. Most doctors know how to do this, he says, and most hospitals have the equipment. *Allergies and Hay Fever*. Usually are benefitted by vitamin C. Sometimes Dr. Cathcart adds pantothenic acid and vitamin B6.

*Back Pain from Disc Disease*. One gram of vitamin C a day has been found to reduce the incidence of necessary surgery. Much larger doses (to bowel tolerance) can often lessen the difficulties with pain-killing drugs. "It is not the total answer for back pain patients, however," Dr. Cathcart says.

# CHAPTER 37

# Nutritional Help for AIDS Patients?

THE DISEASE AIDS (Acquired Immune Deficiency Syndrome) is now known to be a worldwide epidemic which, if uncontrolled, some specialists predict, will kill millions of people by the end of the century. The body's immune system consists of many defenses including antibodies (those compounds manufactured by the body when one is immunized against a disease—polio, for example). The small amount of viral or bacterial stuff in the vaccine is enough to create in the body those antibodies that can protect against this particular disease. So the individual, thus vaccinated, is immune to this disease for a specified time after the inoculation.

Many blood compounds, many glands and many nutrients are also involved in "immunity"—a general term for the protective network that guards us against germs, viruses, poisons and toxins of all kinds. What happens, then, when suddenly *all* these defenses disappear and there seems to be not a single body compound that is capable of acting against life-threatening invaders of any kind? Such is the condition of victims of AIDS. The entire immune system has collapsed. These people are subject to attack by any bacteria, virus, fungal disease or poison that they encounter. Physicians now know that there must be something in the blood of these people which suppresses the immune system. Totally.

In *American Health*, May–June, 1983, an article by a

researcher at Rockefeller University, Jeffrey Laurence, M.D., recounts stories of a number of AIDS victims who have come to the hospital where he was working on cancer research. One of the AIDS patients, a young man, showed all the symptoms of premature senility known as Alzheimer's Disease. More and more patients with AIDS showed up behaving very strangely, going to work, sitting and doing nothing all day. When they died, an autopsy showed that their brains had shrunk and atrophied.

Dr. Laurence, at an early date, decided that a virus of some kind was responsible for the disease, then, in the summer of 1981, he saw what he describes as "something no one had ever seen before." It wasn't a virus or a bacterium or a parasite, but a sure sign something unusual had been there: "a huge immunological imprint . . . a chemical suppressing the immune system 1,000 times more powerful than any similar chemical can do. This extraordinary potent 'suppressor factor' . . . suggested AIDS was unlike any other kind of infection . . .

"I began simply taking chemicals off the shelf and throwing them into test tubes to see whether they would block the suppression. I tried anything known to affect the immune system . . . Nothing. I tried antibodies against interferon, the antiviral substance . . . Nothing." Then he began to put amino acids (links of protein) and vitamins into his test tubes along with the mysterious compound that is so powerful against the immune system. He tried alanine, an amino acid, vitamin C and vitamin E. He says, "put . . . these in high enough doses in a test tube *and they block the suppressor factor so that cells have a normal immune response.*" Then he decided that these nutrients could not be used against AIDS because they would have to be given in such large doses that they would be toxic. He said, "The vitamin C equivalent in man of the dose that works in the test tube is 10 to 20 grams a day, far too toxic."

He seems to have either not read or not believed the wealth of scientific material concerning massive doses of vitamin C and their harmlessness, as well as the safety of vitamin E and amino acids. A number of physicians throughout the country read Dr. Laurence's article and began at once to treat their AIDS patients with the nutrients he mentioned, adding other nutrients as needed and putting their patients on diets that nourished them completely.

They found that conservative medical journals would not print their articles or letters on the subject. Dr. Robert Cathcart of California wrote several articles on his theory of treating AIDS with massive doses of vitamins. He said, in part, in *Medical Hypotheses,* vol. 14, pages 423–433, 1984, "My previous experience with the utilization of ascorbic acid in the treatment of viral diseases led me to hypothesize that ascorbate would be of value in the treatment of AIDS . . . Preliminary clinical evidence is that massive doses of ascorbate (50 to 200 grams per 24 hours) can suppress the symptoms of the disease and can markedly reduce the tendency for secondary infections. In combination with usual treatments for the secondary infections, large doses of ascorbate will often produce a clinical remission which shows every evidence of being prolonged if treatment is continued."

In the article Dr. Cathcart continues to describe treatment with vitamin C and other therapies, for the benefit of physicians reading the article who are treating AIDS patients. Dr. Cathcart also has the following suggestions for preventing AIDS. He says, "Morishige has demonstrated the effectiveness of ascorbate in preventing hepatitis B from blood transfusions. A similarity exists between AIDS and hepatitis B. It has been my experience that patients treated with large doses of ascorbate during the acute phase of hepatitis will not develop chronic hepatitis. My experience with herpes simplex infections (cold sores) has been the same. Although ascorbate is helpful to a degree with chronic viral infections, it is in the treatment of acute viral diseases that it is most effective.

"It is on this basis that I recommend that all persons who fear exposure to AIDS and certainly anyone receiving blood transfusions or other blood products which could in the most remote way have been obtained from an AIDS carrier, be put on bowel tolerance doses of ascorbate.''

He says also, ''Ascorbate does ameliorate the AID syndrome to a significant degree. I want to emphasize, however, the absolute necessity of massive doses. Additionally, one must avoid and treat opportunistic infections. Multiple infections, lack of understanding in the use of (vitamin) C, or inability to tolerate the doses prescribed, all result in a poor prognosis. The success of treatments with ascorbate entirely depends on consistent administration of (vitamin) C sufficient to neutralize the free radicals produced by the various diseases.'' Free radicals are destructive substances formed in cells which can be destroyed by vitamin C or vitamin E, in massive doses.

A letter to me from the Director of the National Institute of Allergy and Infectious Diseases at the National Institute of Health, dated August 23, 1983 said, in part, ''We are well aware of the literature on vitamin C and infections. Dr. Robert Edelman, a member of my staff and Chief of the Clinical and Epidemiological Studies Branch of the Institute has been in contact with some of our Institute-supported research and with Dr. Cathcart regarding ascorbic acid and AIDS . . .''

Since then no statement concerning the potential value of vitamin C along with other nutritional support in the treatment of AIDS has ever been made by anyone from the medical establishment, so far as I can discover, and I watch news reports and medical journals constantly for any such statements.

Apparently a number of AIDS victims in some cities are using vitamin C and other nutritional support either with the cooperation of their broad-minded physicians, or on their own, or in spite of their physicians. In the years that have intervened since the above letter was written, officials of the medical and federal establishment have made many statements and have appeared many times on television to assure the American public that AIDS is indeed a worldwide epidemic of major proportions and that they are doing all they can to produce, at some future date, a drug that will cure the disease or a vaccine that will prevent it. They estimate that such helpful events may be possible within five years or ten years, according to which specialist is speaking. Meanwhile, fatalities continue to mount at an alarming rate.

# CHAPTER 38

# Treating AIDS with Vitamin C

AT A PRESS CONFERENCE on successful treatment of Acquired Immune Deficiency Syndrome (AIDS) Dr. Robert E. Cathcart, III of Los Altos, California made the following statement which was released to the press. The date was May 12, 1987.

Since early 1983, I have treated more than 200 AIDS and AIDS infected patients with large doses of ascorbic acid along with other nutrients and a diet essentially eliminating junk food. These treatments have not resulted in a cure for AIDS but have, on the average, doubled life expectancy, and considerably ameliorated the symptoms resulting in less disability until shortly before death. They have also considerably reduced the expense of treating the AIDS patient due to the reduction of necessary hospital care. One patient has survived six years; another four years. Six patients seem to have stabilized the loss of T-helper cells for two to three years.

My treatment of AIDS patients and the resulting findings of the amelioration of symptoms is based on previous findings (starting in 1969 and involving over 13,000 patients) that ascorbic acid administered in massive doses can cure acute viral diseases such as the common cold, mononucleosis, acute hepatitis, influenza, measles, mumps, chicken pox, etc.; control persistent viral infections such as herpes and chronic hepatitis; and, more recently, the treatment of chronic Epstein-Barr infections and chronic HBLV infections. Additionally,

270

ascorbate in massive doses can be used in conjunction with antibiotics to synergistically treat bacterial infections markedly reducing the time required to treat the infection, virtually eliminating complications, and preventing allergic reactions to the antibiotics. Ascorbate in massive doses will almost completely eliminate allergic reactions to antibiotics and is very helpful in the treatment of allergies such as hay fever and asthma. Ascorbate will assist the body in rapidly healing wounds and surgical incisions, reducing the pain, swelling, and chances of infection.

Ascorbate accomplishes all this because in massive doses it acts as a *free radical scavenger*. While man, monkeys, and guinea pigs do not make ascorbate themselves, all the other mammals and many other animals do so. The major function of the large amount of ascorbate that these other animals manufacture is for the purpose of scavenging free radicals. Ascorbate is the reason that a four-legged animal can eat filthy things off the ground without getting sick, that they have a relatively high resistance to infections, and that their wounds heal so rapidly.

The fact that the higher primates have lost the ability to produce ascorbate but have not lost the ability to utilize it as a free radical scavenger, has resulted in the major problem that whenever humans become infected, injured, or have some allergic reaction, free radicals are produced which burn up the ascorbate in the involved tissues or even throughout the body generally, and result in a condition I call *acute induced scurvy*. In this condition there is no vitamin C left in the tissues involved for such vital functions as mobilization of white cells, phagocytosis by white cells, making of interferon, making of collagen, and many other non-controversial housekeeping functions of vitamin C. It is easy to see why in this state of acute induced scurvy many infections become chronic, wounds heal slowly, and secondary complications frequently result. It also appears that free radicals, and the resulting depletion of ascorbate in the tissues, have something to do with arming of antibodies and causing undesired allergic reactions.

271

The magnitude of this potential use of ascorbate as a free radical scavenger increases dramatically with increased toxicity in illness. I discovered in 1969, that the sicker a patient is, the more ascorbic acid can be ingested without it producing diarrhea. The ascorbic acid which is utilized and drawn off the gastrointestinal tract does not reach the rectum and therefore does not produce diarrhea. A healthy adult who is tolerant to ascorbic acid can take from 10 to 20 grams of ascorbic acid per 24 hours without it producing diarrhea. That same person with a mild cold can take 30 to 60 grams per 24 hours; with a severe cold, 100 grams; with an influenza, 150 grams; and with mononucleosis or viral pneumonia sometimes over 200 grams per 24 hours (almost a half a pound). This increased tolerance with illness was astonishing and reflected the utilization of ascorbate as a free radical scavenger in the body in these toxic conditions.

Many people, attempting to treat a cold, have been unsuccessful because insufficient amounts of ascorbic acid were used. I call a cold, toxic enough to allow you to take 100 grams per 24 hours before diarrhea is produced, *a 100 gram cold*. A 20 gram cold can easily be treated with 2 grams an hour but patients do not usually seek assistance from a physician unless they have at least a 60 to 75 gram cold. Two grams an hour will not cure these severe colds but 60 to 75 grams per 24 hours will. You do not send a boy in to do a man's job. This is a major problem that physicians have had in attempting to treat colds and other severe infections they are called on to treat.

Ascorbate does not cure AIDS, but it can ameliorate symptoms considerably. The most fundamental injury to patients by the AIDS infection is the destruction of the T-helper cells. These T-helper cells are perhaps the most important cells of the immune system in that they direct many of the most vital functions of the immune system. Without T-helper cells the patient becomes susceptible to secondary infections and cancer. The normal T-helper cell count is greater than $400/mm^3$. When the T-helper cell count drops below 50 or $20/mm^3$ there is little that can be done and septicemia and death become unavoidable. However, many patients with AIDS die of complications before the T-helper cells drop to these disastrous levels. The chances of these premature deaths are reduced considerably by the proper use of ascorbate.

One particular use of ascorbate has been in the treatment of pneumocystis carinii pneumonia (PCP). PCP is the leading cause of death in AIDS patients. While the parasite causing the disease, pneumocystis carinii, is killed by several antibiotics, a major problem is the extremely high incidence of allergic reactions to the antibiotics used. This high incidence of allergic reactions to antibiotics administered when the patient is profoundly ill is due to the large number of free radicals arming the antibodies which then cause the allergic reactions. The reason so many people become allergic to antibiotics is because they take them when they are sick. Massive doses of ascorbate will disarm the unwanted antibodies and at the same time augment the immune system's attack on the parasite.

A current thought is that the AIDS virus multiplies in the T-helper cell when the T-helper cell is activated. This is a dilemma when one considers whether to "stimulate" the immune system. Ascorbate, by making short work of colds and other minor infections, and by reducing the duration and complications of major infections, reduces the activation of T-helper cells and thereby slows the multiplication of viruses.

By reducing the duration, severity and complications of secondary infections before the T-helper cell count drops disastrously low, prolonged debilitation, hospitalizations, expenses, etc. are markedly reduced. The final death period is more sudden with less suffering. Unfortunately, one of the reasons for sudden death in AIDS patients who have sustained themselves for a more prolonged period of time with massive doses of ascorbate, is that when that ascorbate is withdrawn in the hospital, death ensues rapidly. A patient maintained on massive doses of ascorbate must not have the ascorbate withdrawn in a period of great toxicity.

273

# CHAPTER 39

# Vitamin C Against Dangerous Drugs

RESEARCHERS AT THE Preclinical Psychopharmacology Laboratory at Indiana University have studied Haldol (Haloperidol), a drug for treating psychoses or mental illness. This is a powerful drug with many potential side effects that may be worse than the original disease for which it is given. Here they are: drowsiness, jaundice, anemias, raised or lowered blood pressure, abnormal heart beat, heart attack, faintness or dizziness, spasms of the neck muscles, rolling back of the eyes, convulsions, difficulty in swallowing and symptoms associated with Parkinson's Disease. It may cause an unusual increase in psychotic symptoms, paranoid reactions, fatigue, lethargy, restlessness, hyperactivity, confusion, bizarre dreams, insomnia, depression, euphoria, itching, swelling, sensitivity to light, and so on for almost a whole page in any manual of drugs.

The Indiana researchers gave vitamin C along with the drug and found that the vitamin improved the helpfulness of the drug. They don't know how or why the vitamin achieves this effect, but they are suggesting that the vitamin should be used along with the drug to see if a smaller amount of the drug might be needed. Using smaller amounts of the drug would probably prevent some of its most serious side effects. The same may be true of many other prescription drugs.

In *Medical Tribune*, August 20, 1986 Dr. Linus Pauling

writes of experiments performed by E. Cameron and G. Baird who used sodium ascorbate in the treatment of morphine withdrawal in patients being treated for cancer. They used 10 grams a day. In *Medical Tribune,* December 15, 1982, Robert F. Cathcart, III, M.D. wrote on the quandry facing physicians who want to control fever in children but do not want them to risk increased incidence of Reye's Syndrome which often afflicts children given high doses of aspirin. Give the children vitamin C, said Dr. Cathcart, a 25% solution of 2cc to 4cc of sodium ascorbate (without preservatives) given intramuscularly to infants will usually have a dramatic effect on elevated temperature.

"Since some of the symptoms of aspirin toxicity are perhaps not coincidentally some of the symptoms of ascorbate deficiency, it may be that aspirin increases the body's utilization of ascorbate. Perhaps it is an accumulatively induced deficiency of ascorbate which has something to do with the increased incidence of Reye's Syndrome in profoundly ill children administered aspirin," said Dr. Cathcart.

Daily doses of vitamin C might help to protect some alcohol users from the liver damage that years of drinking can cause, researcher Vincent Zannoni said at a vitamin C symposium in October, 1986. He is professor of pharmacology at the University of Michigan Medical School. Guinea pigs given massive doses of vitamin C can resist fat buildup in their livers which can otherwise lead to cirrhosis. An experiment in human beings showed the same effect. Dr. Zannoni suggests 5,000 milligrams a day and suggests this much for those people who drink up to the equivalent of three beers a day.

Dr. Herbert Sprince of Jefferson Medical College has found that vitamin C protects the body against a substance which develops in the bodies of those who drink alcohol and also smoke cigarettes. It's called acetaldehyde. Dr. Sprince gave large doses of vitamin C along with the B vitamin thiamine and found that it gave some protection from lung diseases, alcoholic heart disease and alcoholic degeneration of the brain.

Two California scientists reported in 1980 that they had remarkable success in treating drug addicts with nutritional therapy. The account of their work appeared in *The Journal of Orthomolecular Psychiatry*. Dr. Irwin Stone and Dr. Alfred F. Libby believe that addicts suffer from deficiencies in both vitamin C and high quality protein. They have found, they say, that addiction produces in its victims acute scurvy symptoms along with deficiency in many other nutrients as well.

The Methadone treatment for addiction merely substitutes a legal drug for an illegal one, they say, just continuing the severe biochemical stress contributing to their illness. The two scientists decided to treat both the lack of protein and the lack of all nutritional elements involved in the deficiency disease from which drug addicts appear to be suffering. The treatment is inexpensive, nontoxic, uses no drugs or narcotics and is entirely "orthomolecular"—the word coined by Dr. Linus Pauling which means supplying to the body the optimum amount of nutritional material, especially substances normally present in the human body, rather than drugs.

The two California researchers say their treatment was rapidly effective in bringing good health to the addicts they treated. They began with immense doses of vitamin C in the form of sodium ascorbate. This is not so acidic as plain ascorbic acid, so is less likely to cause upset stomach in immense doses. They sometimes gave 25 to 85 grams (25,000 milligrams to 85,000 milligrams) a day, along with massive doses of other vitamins, minerals and protein in an easily assimilated form.

Under this treatment, they say, the heroin or Methadone can be discontinued and no withdrawal symptoms are encountered. If the addict later takes a "fix," it is immediately detoxified and no "high" is produced. It is like an injection of plain water. There is great improvement in addicts, they say. In a few days, appetite returns and they eat well. They have restful sleep and the constipation which Methadone brings is relieved. After about four to six days, the dosages of nutrients are reduced to "holding levels."

In 30 addicts tested in this pilot study results were excellent in all cases. It appears that this simple, non-toxic, inexpensive procedure should serve as a basis for large scale testing to develop a new program for freeing addicts from their addiction. In drug overdosage, sodium ascorbate can be a lifesaver, they tell us. Unconscious over-dosed addicts are given the sodium ascorbate intravenously while those able to swallow can be given the same amount in a glass of milk. Sodium ascorbate does not have the sharp acid taste of ascorbic acid. It has a faint salty taste, nothing more.

This remedy is not just for heroin addicts, say Stone and Libby. It is non-specific and works with all drugs, so no time need be wasted in identifying the drug whose overdose brought the addict to the clinic. Say the authors, "We speculate on ascorbate's action as due to the high levels of sodium ascorbate in the brain as competing for and displacing the narcotic from the opiate receptor sites. If this be the case, then it might be possible to use this phenomenon to quickly bring them out of anesthesia."

If one adds up all the misery in drug addiction: the suffering, the degradation, the crime, the jail sentences, the destruction of careers, families and personality and the deaths, it is difficult to think of anything that holds greater promise than this harmless, inexpensive treatment which would bring the addict back to health without withdrawal symptoms and give him or her the chance to start a new life, well-buttressed with nutritional aid that practically guarantees no return to a drug-oriented life. The person who is well-nourished—truly well-nourished—has no need for drugs, does not feel any craving for them.

Perhaps best of all is the fact that the former addict will be able to take his "medicine" home with him and will not have to depend on visits to his doctor's office. The "medicine" consists only of harmless vitamins, minerals and protein. So long as he or she takes them, along with a good, nourishing diet at mealtime, there seems to be little chance that a return to addiction could occur.

# CHAPTER 40

# Vitamin C Helps You to Absorb Iron

IRON IS ONE dietary mineral most of us know something about. We have seen commercials speaking of "tired blood" which means, we suppose, too little iron in the blood to perform all those important functions which iron performs. We know that not getting enough iron is likely to lead to one kind of anemia—with weakness, fatigue and defective functioning of many body processes.

Generally speaking, nutritionists believe that most men and boys get enough iron with meals, especially if they eat plenty of meat and eggs, both of which are good sources. Children are more likely to be short on iron because rapid growth demands more blood, and women of childbearing age, because they lose considerable blood each month in menstrual periods.

One problem with maintaining enough iron in your blood is the problem of absorbing it. Although many vegetarian foods contain iron it is not absorbed very well from these foods—not as well as it is absorbed from meat, seafood and eggs. Dark green leafy vegetables like spinach are good sources, as are real wholegrains, wheat germ and wheat bran. Liver is the best source, along with other organ meats.

But how can you be sure all the iron you get at meals is absorbed? One way is to get some vitamin C at the same meal as the iron. Two University of Kansas blood specialists discovered recently that taking 100 milligrams of vitamin

C with each meal that contains meat increases the absorption of the iron by nearly 40 percent. Taking 100 milligrams of vitamin C with vegetarian meals results in absorbing three times more iron than you would absorb without the vitamin C. Dr. Sean R. Lynch of Kansas University told a New York Academy of Sciences Symposium in October, 1986 that the total intake of iron from food is less important than the availability of that iron. If the iron is not absorbed, it's wasted.

As long ago as the 1950's, scientists were discovering that iron is more completely absorbed at meals where citrus fruits (rich in vitamin C) are eaten. In one study orange juice containing 40–50 milligrams of vitamin C was added to a meal of bread, butter, jam and an egg labelled with iron. The absorption of the iron jumped from 3.7 percent to 10.4 percent when orange juice was added to the meal. When orange juice along with 70 milligrams of vitamin C was added to a breakfast of two whole wheat rolls and coffee, iron absorption went up by two and a half times.

Dr. Lynch believes that the vitamin C forms a chelate (that is, a very strong bond or combination) with the iron in the acid environment of the stomach—a combination so strong it remains soluble when the food enters into the alkaline environment of the intestines. This effect takes place only if vitamin C is present in the meal, not if it is taken before the meal. This suggests that it's a good idea always to take your supplements *with* a meal so that they may play their normal role of helping to process the food. If this is impossible because you are "eating out" or a frequent guest at banquets or something of the sort, then take your supplements just after you eat. You need that vitamin C to help absorb the iron in the meal.

At the same symposium, a Swedish physician from the Department of Medicine, Sahlgren Hospital, University of Gotenberg, stated that each main meal should preferably contain 24–50 milligrams of vitamin C and even more. The balance of evidence, said he, indicates that vitamin C has a key physiological role in iron absorption.

279

So the best idea is to eat a wide variety of foods at every meal. A sandwich of bread and meat or cheese contains no vitamin C. Adding just one or two pieces of fruit supplies it. A dinner of meat and custard pie contains no vitamin C. Adding a big salad and a fruit cup for dessert provides vitamin C to make certain the iron in the meat is absorbed.

The tea-and-toast and processed cereal meals eaten by so many older folks may contain so little iron that symptoms of pallor, fatigue, listlessness, faintness and sometimes breathlessness may appear. Your doctor is the only person who can diagnose iron deficiency and iron deficiency anemia. It is easy to correct such anemia by eating plenty of foods that are rich in iron and using a good source of vitamin C or a supplement at the same meal.

# CHAPTER 41

# Two Challenging Books by Linus Pauling

In 1979 the eminent Linus Pauling, Ph.D., twice a Nobel Laureate, authored a book with Ewan Cameron, M.D., of Scotland. The book is *Cancer and Vitamin C, a Discussion of the Nature, Causes, Prevention and Treatment of Cancer with Special Reference to the Value of Vitamin C*. Dr. Cameron is the physician who treated terminal cancer patients at his hospital in Scotland with 10,000 milligrams daily of vitamin C.

These patients were "untreatable" by any conventional method of treatment, so vitamin C was their own only definitive form of medication. Everything that could be done for these patients by orthodox medicine had been done. Dr. Cameron found that pain was relieved. The appetites of the patients returned. They had a renewed sense of well-being. They lived on the average four times longer than similar patients treated with orthodox therapies. Of the 100 patients treated with vitamin C, 15 survived longer than a year, compared to only four of the "controls." Three of those treated with vitamin C lived for three years. Of the five who survived more than one year, five were still alive in 1979, including two who lived for four years longer.

The book by Pauling and Cameron cannot possibly be called "faddist or biased." The authors begin with a description of what cancer is, what causes it and what forms it takes. They devote one chapter to the orthodox treatment of cancer: surgery, radiotherapy, chemotherapy (drugs), hormones and immunotherapy. Their judgments are moderate and fair. They give credit where it is due. Drug therapy, in some kinds of cancer, has progressed to the point where, the authors say, "we can talk of a cure in acute leukemias of children, and Hodgkins Disease."

They devote one chapter to "unorthodox" cancer treatment—Krebiozen, Laetrile, the Gerson treatment, and so on. They point out, for example, that the Gerson treatment, using large amounts of fresh raw juices, contains large amounts of vitamin C, vitamin A, the B vitamins, minerals and other nutrients that may have been largely responsible for its success in some patients.

One section of the book is devoted to theories as to exactly how treatment with vitamin C may bring a cure or regression of the cancer and how it can overcome the pain, weakness, lack of appetite and loss of weight which weaken the terminal cancer patients and contribute to the final fatal outcome.

Greatly over-simplified, their theory is that this vitamin, in large enough amounts, strengthens the resistance of the patient to the attacking cancer cells and, by toughening the intercellular cement, prevents the cancer cells from metastasizing or, as Cameron and Pauling put it, the vitamin is "walling off the tumor in a dense network of fibrous tissue."

Part five of the book recounts the experiments of Dr. Cameron in his hospital in Scotland. Case histories of a number of his patients are discussed in detail. In other chapters the authors go into great detail on exactly what can be expected from the vitamin in preventing and treating various diseases and why it is effective. They answer criticism of megadoses of the vitamin fairly and honestly. They include information for physicians to use in treating patients with vitamin C either orally or intravenously.

In the several very helpful appendices there is general information about cancer, an explanation of the various drugs used, a discussion of nutrition and the essential nutrients, explanations of the various surgical terms and a glossary of all unfamiliar medical and scientific terms used in the book.

# TWO CHALLENGING BOOKS BY LINUS PAULING

The book is *Cancer and Vitamin C, a Discussion of the Nature, Causes, Prevention and Treatment of Cancer with Special Reference to the Value of Vitamin C.* It is available from the Linus Pauling Institute of Science and Medicine at 440 Page Mill Road, Palo Alto, California 94306. A paperback edition is available from Warner Books, New York City.

In 1986, Pauling published another book, *How to Live Longer and Feel Better,* this time in paperback. In this most recent challenge to the medical establishment, Pauling wades in where angels fear to tread and says he believes that the establishment is barking up the wrong tree when they pinpoint fats and cholesterol as the cause of our epidemic of heart and circulatory disease. It's our overconsumption of sugar, he says, that's doing the damage.

In 1968 Pauling shocked the scientific world with his article in the prestigious *Science* publication, introducing the idea of "orthomolecular" medicine—that is, using certain nutrients in much larger amounts than is customary to satisfy the excessive need for these nutrients at various sites in the body. The brain is the most sensitive of all human organs to its molecular composition, he says. It may suffer from deficiency in certain nutrients—a sort of cerebral scurvy. Massive doses of vitamin C, the B vitamins and certain other nutrients can satisfy this need and alleviate many psychological problems.

The immune system depends largely on vitamin C and other nutrients, he says, for its ability to destroy invaders like viruses, bacteria, foreign proteins and poisons. By taking large enough amounts of vitamin C most people can prevent colds and flu or shorten their duration.

This book has chapters on allergies, circulatory disorders, arthritis, disorders of the eye, the ear and the mouth, all in relation to various nutrients including vitamin C, and their healthfulness in alleviating unpleasant and dangerous disease conditions. Nowhere does Pauling guarantee a "miracle cure" of any disease. The book, with 463 references in the bibliography, demonstrates instead what can be done to improve health with nutritional therapies and a commonsense way of eating and living.

A surprising number of American physicians are using these ideas in treating cancer as well as many other diseases. Pauling estimates that one percent of all American physicians may be using similar ideas in treatment of patients. He says, "I believe that, in general, the treatment of disease by the use of substances, such as ascorbic acid that are normally present in the human body and are required for life, is to be preferred to treatment by the use of powerful synthetic substances or plant products, which may, and usually do, have undesirable side effects."

The author's qualifications are extraordinary and unique. At his 85th birthday celebration in 1986, he was hailed in these words by a CalTech chemistry professor. "In my opinion, I think, in everybody's judgment, Linus Pauling is the greatest chemist of the 20th century." Seven hundred distinguished guests attended the gathering. Pauling has published 600 scientific papers and 12 books and received two Nobel prizes. He is known internationally for his creative genius in biochemistry, his courage in presenting new and controversial concepts and defending them against those who challenge them. His latest book was a triumph. Although his publishers promoted the book extensively with review copies sent to the media along with a magnificent and expensive biography and summary of Pauling's career, although he appeared on TV in many cities, the book was almost totally ignored by the scientific community. To the best of my knowledge, no medical or scientific journal in our country published a review of it.

*New Scientist*, published in England, said this, in part, in their review, "It is incredible that, 15 years after he first ventured into the field with his book on *Vitamin C and the Common Cold*, Pauling has neither been silenced by contradictory evidence nor hailed as a prophet. The fact of the matter appears to be, as he suggests, that the biomedical professions don't want his theories but have no arguments against them. Whether ultimately he's right or wrong in his theories, the controversy looks perfect material for the philosophers of science as an example of the futility of trying to break out of a still viable paradigm (the biomedical professions)."

# CHAPTER 42

# A Book on Cancer Therapy by Nutritional Means

ANOTHER EXCELLENT BOOK on the subject of cancer is titled *Vitamin C Against Cancer* by H. L. Newbold, M.D., of New York City.

The opening pages of the book detail the case history of a well-known New York woman with terminal lung cancer— one of the most difficult kinds of cancer to treat with any form of therapy. She had been taking chemotherapy and radiation. The side effects were so devastating that she told Dr. Newbold that, if he could not help her, she would kill herself.

Dr. Newbold did not tell her to abandon the treatment she was taking. He did offer to give her nutrition therapy and vitamin C treatment. She agreed. It began. Dr. Newbold gave her vitamin C intravenously along with minerals and trace minerals. Several days later, so much progress had been made that the intravenous vitamin C was stopped. She continued to take vitamin C by mouth until she was taking 36 grams daily in divided doses.

She returned to the medical men at the hospital and told them she had discontinued all chemotherapy. They told her she would be back by the end of the month begging for more drugs. Instead she went back a month later and the doctors could find no evidence of cancer. This patient tells her own story in her own words in the second chapter of the book.

Now, sensibly, Dr. Newbold does not, on the basis of this one extraordinary case, tell you throughout the rest of the book that vitamin C can cure all cancers in everybody. Instead, he starts with the facts uncovered by Dr. Linus Pauling, Dr. Ewan Cameron, Dr. Irwin Stone, Dr. William Saccoman, Dr. Archie Kalokerinos and many others, devoting a chapter to each one.

Each chapter is a recorded account of Newbold's interview with each man, word for word. You are told how many cancer patients each man has dealt with, what the results have been in general, what the failures have been. You hear from the man himself in his own words why he decided to try this treatment, what nutritional treatment he uses along with it, how many patients also had chemotherapy and/or radiation.

Dr. Newbold then interviewed a prominent advocate of chemotherapy and an advocate of radiation treatment of cancer. You read here the exact words of each man, defending his specialty. Then there is a chapter detailing the words of a biostatistician who works in the cancer field who believes that chemotherapy has made little progress against cancer except in three types: acute leukemia in children, the lymphomas, and early breast cancer.

More interviews follow, pro and con. Dr. Newbold speaks to the reader as if he or she had just been diagnosed as a cancer victim. Where to turn? What to think? Who is most knowledgeable in this complex field? Is there really any hope through chemotherapy? Should you agree to radiation therapy? Dr. Newbold gives full and frank information on both sides of every question.

The last half of the book is a discussion of nutrition in general and nutrition as it applies to the cancer patient. The author gives explicit instructions for administering vitamin C intravenously, although this, of course, can be done only by a physician. He encourages the reader who wants to try this therapy to give the book to his or her doctor so that the doctor will have full information on exactly how to apply this revolutionary new technique—treating possibly terminal cancer with massive doses of a vitamin!

We can almost hear our readers exclaim as they read this review. "But where can we find doctors who will agree to give us this kind of treatment?" Once again, Dr. Newbold has anticipated your question. He explains patiently how it happens that most American doctors are reluctant to engage in something as revolutionary as this. Shop around for a doctor who will agree to the vitamin C treatment, he says. Probably a young doctor is most likely to listen to you, and read the book. Perhaps it may be an older, more mellow one who is "secure enough to admit he doesn't know everything."

Even if there were no mention of cancer, the provocative information on nutrition in this book would make it worth buying. Newbold has startling recommendations for what you should eat every day just to stay healthy. He has tested his ideas, he says, on thousands of patients and he knows, without any double-blind tests, that his kind of diet produces good health. We think his diet program is unnecessarily restrictive, but we are perfectly willing to agree that nobody can go wrong by following it to the letter, meals and diet supplements as well.

One of the most original of his theories is that our craving for sweets stems from the ancient period in pre-history when our ancestors lost the liver enzyme that allowed them to produce their own vitamin C in their bodies and made it necessary for them (and us) to get all our daily supply from food. Vitamin C occurs in nature mostly in fruits. Fruits contain sugar. So those ancient ancestors of ours who had the most dependable "sweet tooth" are the ones who sought out fruits and berries most zealously and thus avoided dying from scurvy, the disease of vitamin C deficiency.

To this day, says Newbold, we still have our craving for sweets, but what we are really seeking is vitamin C, for that's how our "sweet tooths" developed. In modern supermarkets almost every food contains sugar in varying amounts, some of them far, far sweeter than any fruit. So we eat them to satisfy our craving for sweets. But there is no vitamin C in most of these sweet foods.

Speaking of a cancer patient who ate large amounts of sweets, "I strongly suspect," says Newbold, "that the patient's urgent desire for sweets was due to his body's trying to get more vitamin C. He was starving for it. Nature urged him to eat sweets, but to nature sweets means fruits and hence vitamin C. Instead, he ate sugar sweets and only depleted his body all the more of vitamins and minerals."

We are sure you will enjoy the friendly style of this book, the thorough information it gives you on many aspects of the group of diseases called cancer and the hope it will give you that you and your family may be able to prevent this terrible disease by planning your diets and diet supplements wisely. Your doctor should welcome a book on this subject, for it offers him hope of a new, harmless, beneficial therapy for cancer when every other therapy has failed.

# CHAPTER 43

# Three Specialists Write a Book on Vitamin C

THE AUTHORS OF a book, *The Vitamin C Connection*, are E. Cheraskin, M.D., D.M.D., W. Marshall Ringsdorf, D.M.D. and Emily L. Sisley, Ph.D. Drs. Cheraskin and Ringsdorf have been for many years with the University of Alabama. They write of the importance of the immune system which is our protection against enemies such as viruses and bacteria. Histamine is a body substance often called out in response to many kinds of stress such as infections. Vitamin C is a natural anti-histamine which suggests its many helpful qualities for asthmatics and allergics.

In a chapter on sugar and diabetes the Alabama authors relate some astonishing experiments on the helpful effects of vitamin C in controlling blood sugar levels. The use of vitamin C for terminal cancer patients has been told many times. The book describes these uses for prolonging survival rates, easing pain and producing a feeling of well being, even in terminal patients.

Drs. Cheraskin and Ringsdorf are both specialists in the field of dentistry. Their chapter on mouth health is enlightening. In regard to bleeding gums they quote two authorities who say that "investigations of actual cases have in every instance shown a deficiency in (vitamin C) and saturation with ascorbic acid has never failed to effect a cure."

Glaucoma, the eye condition that causes most blindness in our country, is another condition which responds well to massive doses of vitamin C. The authors tell of a clinic in Rome, Italy where as much as 35,000 milligrams of vitamin C, given in a single dose, decreased pressure in the affected eye within two hours! Chinese doctors have also reported dramatic decreases in pressure in the eyeball within minutes when vitamin C was given intravenously.

In a chapter on the beneficial effects of vitamin C supplementation on mental health, the authors include a comparison of a minor tranquilizer drug and vitamin C. They list 131 lines of small type in the *Physicians' Desk Reference* on this drug covering contradictions, warnings, psychological and physiological dependence, warnings of use in pregnancy, management of overdoses, precautions and adverse reactions of JUST THIS ONE MINOR TRANQUILIZER—all the reasons why it must be given with great care and the expectation of very serious side effects.

Of vitamin C which is probably far more effective in maintaining a healthy outlook on life, our authors say, "in not one reference guide we know of is there even a single contraindication, warning, precaution or note about dependence, overdose, adverse reactions or any problem in pregnancy." They later describe successful effects of vitamin C in curing addiction to drugs and alleviating withdrawal symptoms.

They recount the story of Norman Cousins' successful recovery from a serious paralyzing illness when he insisted on getting intravenous vitamin C in massive doses. Cousins himself told the story of a lawyer who wanted his little daughter to be given vitamin C for viral encephalitis. When the doctors refused to do this, the lawyer mixed at least 10,000 milligrams of vitamin C powder in his daughter's ice cream every day. She recovered.

When a University of Minnesota physician found that patients at a dialysis center developed severe anemia, he examined the water being used for dialysis and found it contained chlorine. He added vitamin C to the water and neutralized the harmful effects of the chlorine. He now recommends putting vitamin C in your drinking water if it is heavily chlorinated. Only a tiny amount of the vitamin is needed to neutralize the chlorine.

What about the so-called terrible consequences of taking too much vitamin C? The Alabama authors take up the sensational stuff on side effects that has appeared in newspaper columns and magazines. They carefully explain the fallacies in all these cautions. No, massive doses of vitamin C do not cause kidney stones. Part of the evidence that they don't lies in the files of hundreds of physicians who have been prescribing vitamin C for up to 40 years of practice. Infertility? No evidence. Diarrhea? Substituting sodium ascorbate for all or part of the ascorbic acid will alleviate such a problem. Sodium ascorbate can be given in immense amounts by intravenous drip—quite safely.

Other excellent suggestions in this book tell you how best to determine your own vitamin C needs and how to manage this if you smoke or have other personal habits or occupations that may necessitate more than average amounts of vitamin C. The authors also give excellent recommendations for a healthful diet to accompany your vitamin C supplement. The bibliography of journals and books occupies 44 pages. If *The Vitamin C Connection* did not revolutionize the practice of medicine and preventive medicine in our country, it's only because doctors have not read it. It's all there for the reading.

# CHAPTER 44

# An Early Book on the Powers of Vitamin C

DR. IRWIN STONE IS the author of a book *The Healing Factor— Vitamin C Against Disease* in which he deals with almost every plague with which modern industrialized human beings are afflicted. In alphabetical order they are: aging, allergies, asthma and hay fever, arthritis and rheumatism, bacterial infections, cancer, colds, diabetes and its opposite—hypoglycemia or low blood sugar, eye disorders like glaucoma and cataract, heart and circulatory disorders, kidney and bladder diseases, mental illness, poisoning by chemicals and metals like lead, cadmium and mercury, pollution and smoking, ulcers, viral diseases, and wounds.

There is convincing evidence in the book that all these conditions may improve by the simple addition to one's food supplements of massive doses of vitamin C. The evidence comes from animal and human experiments. Much of the research was done in early years after the discovery and synthesis of vitamin C when the official cynical viewpoint on vitamins had not as yet developed. There was, instead, great enthusiasm for trying many kinds of experiments with this newly acquired substance which is completely harmless and apparently so powerful in its action on the body.

The largest part of Dr. Stone's testimony on vitamin C is involved with its function in relation to collagen, the physiological "cement" that holds us together. Vitamin C is the essential ingredient of collagen. "Collagen is the body's

293

most important structural substance." It is the ground substance, or cement, that supports and holds the tissues and organs together. It is the substance in the bones that provides the toughness and flexibility and prevents brittleness. Without it the body would just disintegrate or dissolve away.

"It comprises about one-third of the body's total weight of protein and is the most extensive tissue system. It is the substance that strengthens the arteries and veins, supports the muscles, toughens the ligaments and bones, supplies the scar tissue for healing wounds and keeps the youthful skin tissues soft, firm, supple and wrinkle-free.

"When ascorbic acid (vitamin C) is lacking, it is the disturbance in collagen formation that causes the fearful effects of scurvy—the brittle bones that fracture on the slightest impact, the weakened arteries that rupture and hemorrhage, the incapacitating muscle weakness, the affected joints that are too painful to move, the teeth that fall out, and the wounds and sores that never heal. Suboptimal amounts of ascorbic acid over prolonged periods during the early and middle years, by its effect of producing poor quality collagen, may be the factor in later life that causes the high incidence of arthritis and joint diseases, broken hips, and heart and vascular diseases that cause sudden death, and the strokes that bring on senility. Collagen is intimately connected with the entire aging process," says Dr. Stone.

Let's talk in detail about just one chapter in the book—cancer, the disease whose very name strikes terror in the heart of anyone alive in modern America. Over half a million people develop cancer every year in this country. More than 280,000 will die of it next year. More than 700,000 people are under treatment for cancer at any given time. At present the official, orthodox treatment involves radiation, surgery or drug therapy.

Dr. Stone reminds us that any of these three methods of treatment present the body with intense biological stress. This depletes the patient's body of vitamin C. When rats, which manufacture their own vitamin C, are exposed to can-

cer-producing substances, they immediately begin to manufacture vast amounts of vitamin C as protection. Dr. Stone
tells us of experiments in which guinea pigs were exposed
to cancer-causing substances. These which were given ample
amounts of vitamin C developed the disease later than animals
on vitamin C deficient diets. Guinea pigs, like man, do not
make their own vitamin C. They must get it in food.

Dr. Stone quotes National Cancer Institute scientists as
saying that vitamin C destroys cancer cells, that it is harmless
to animals in extremely large doses—which would correspond
to 350 milligrams of the vitamin for a human being. And,
finally, they say, "In our view, the future of effective cancer
chemotherapy will not rest on the use of host-toxic compounds
now so widely employed but upon virtually host nontoxic
compounds that are lethal to cancer cells, of which ascorbate
(vitamin C) . . . represents an excellent prototype example."

Then, says Dr. Stone, in the screening program that has
gone on at the National Cancer Institute for many years to
find new cancer-killing substances, vitamin C has been "by-
passed, excluded from consideration, and never tested for
its cancer-killing properties. The reason given for not screening ascorbic acid is even more fantastic—ascorbic acid was
too non-toxic to fit into their program!"

Then follow four pages of evidence of the effectiveness
of vitamin C in cases of cancer, and the power of vitamin
C against some cancer-causing agents, the very inadequate
amounts of the vitamin that have been used in most unsuccessful trials and finally one astonishing story of a 71-year-old
man with leukemia who took up to 42 grams of vitamin C
daily "because he felt better when he took these large doses."
Whenever, at his doctor's insistence, he stopped taking the
vitamin, his symptoms returned. They disappeared when he
once again began the vitamin therapy.

Dr. Stone asks, "If megascorbic (large doses of vitamin
C) therapy could do so much for an aged leukemic with so
many other complications, what could it do for the young,
uncomplicated leukemic? The answer to this question could

be obtained easily and each day lost may mean more lives wasted. At the present time, millions of dollars are spent in screening all sorts of poisonous chemicals for use in leukemia, while a harmless substance like ascorbic acid, with so much potential, lies around neglected and ignored.''

# CHAPTER 45

# A Miscellany on Vitamin C

IN 1981 *The Journal of the American Medical Association* published an article on the excellent effects of vitamin C on gum health. The author described an experiment at the National Institute of Dental Health using monkeys which, like human beings, cannot make their own vitamin C but must get it from food. Those monkeys given diets in which vitamin C was very low soon showed inflammation of the gum tissues and greater gum pocket depth than those animals which got plenty of the vitamin.

After 23 weeks the animals deficient in vitamin C showed reduction in white blood cells which are essential for protection against germs of all kinds as well as fungal infections. The animals getting enough vitamin C had no such problems. In this article the conservative AMA finally announced that enough vitamin C is indeed essential for gum health. It's taken many many years of research and the use of other methods of fighting gum disease for official medicine to realize that the many thousands of people who died of scurvy over past centuries first became ill with festering, bleeding gums, loose teeth and a mouth so painful the scurvy victim could hardly eat. Scurvy is the disease of vitamin C deficiency.

Since people in times past who had scurvy "wheezed," a Connecticut physician, E. Neil Schachter, tested a group of patients with asthma which came on whenever they exercised. They pedalled on a bicycle-like device until they were tired or until their heart beat exceeded 170 per minute. Dr.

Schacter then tested their breathing in terms of how much they could breathe in and breathe out. These figures declined by about 30 percent from the expected normal. He then gave each of the men 500 milligrams of vitamin C before testing, then tested them again on the machine. They showed 15 percent less trouble breathing.

In 1974 an Australian physician, Archie Kalokerinos, M.D., working with Aborigine children, discovered that one of every two children in that locality was doomed to die in infancy. Looking for a possible reason, he found that these children were all getting far too little vitamin C and that their most serious illnesses came during the season when they were getting immunizations.

In other parts of the world when monkeys (which also do not make their own vitamin C) are given immunizations, so many of them die that they are now given vitamin C before the injections are given and mortality is far less. Dr. Kalokerinos began to give vitamin C to the children under his care before their immunizations were given. Mortality dropped to zero.

In his book on the subject, *Every Second Child,* he says, "If it was known that the diet included . . . 30 milligrams of vitamin C a day then there seemed to be no reason for concern . . . Much had been written about this vital subject and an enormous amount of research had been done. One leading research institute after another had clearly demonstrated that under conditions of stress, infection and injury, there was an increased utilization of vitamin C and 30 milligrams a day may not be sufficient to cope with the demand."

All the babies who were brought to this physician were given vitamin C and mortality dropped to zero. Usually children had no symptoms of vitamin C deficiency. Just the same, the additional vitamin, given before the immunizations were given, saved the lives of countless Australian babies.

At the Department of Health and Human Services in Washington where billions of dollars of tax money are spent every year improving vaccines and otherwise attempting to keep disease under control, no mention is made of vitamin C in preventing disease. Usually anyone who uses the word vitamin C is politely ushered out the door, patted on the head and told to go home and forget this faddist nonsense. Annually, many American children are injured or totally incapacitated by reactions to immunizations. We, the taxpayers, pay the astronomical costs of compensation for damages and care of the injured children. Giving vitamin C *before* the vaccine is given costs pennies and might be able to save the lives and health of many infants. One can only wonder how much the powerful drug lobby has to do with this situation.

In 1983 *Chemical and Engineering News* reported on the work of Earl B. Dawson and colleagues at the University of Texas Medical Branch in Galveston. Dr. Dawson said that 35 men working in the petroleum industry were found to have defective sperm—sperm unable to fertilize the female egg cells. Testing the men for vitamin C, the scientists found they were all very deficient in this nutrient. When they were given only 1,000 milligrams of the vitamin every day, the condition was corrected and normal sperm appeared, *after only one week of vitamin therapy*. The scientists have found that employees of similar industries in South Africa routinely receive a daily vitamin C supplement to maintain body levels of this nutrient.

*The Lancet* in 1968 published an article on using vitamin C for prickly heat. Children who were given the vitamin every day for two weeks improved and got rid of their rashes. In 1966 *Science News* reported that rats given tetanus toxin were given vitamin C which prevented death. The studies were done in India.

*The New England Journal of Medicine,* August 24, 1972 printed a letter from Edward Poser, M.D. of Chicago who said he had given patients very large doses of vitamin C without any problems with kidney stones. One patient had cataracts. Four grams of vitamin C daily resulted in cleared lenses within four months. This patient refused to give up his usual vitamin C doses so he kept on taking it for 13 years. Over that time there were no side effects of any kind.

Five British physicians reported in *The Lancet,* September

7, 1974 on the use of vitamin C for preventing and treating pressure sores in bedfast patients. In the group of patients who got the vitamin there was a reduction of 80 percent in the pressure-sore area.

In *The Lancet,* October 12, 1974 Abram Hoffer, M.D. protested the point of view that any vitamin C in the urine should be considered "wasted." One often hears from those who deplore the use of megavitamin therapy that the individuals using it have "expensive urine." Said Dr. Hoffer, "The question is not whether it is wasted, but whether it is effective. When there is general consensus that a substance is therapeutic, there is little discussion of waste. But with ascorbic acid there is no such consensus. Many physicians equate consensus with efficacy. This often delays for many years the proper examination of a new therapeutic idea because consensus may require up to 40 years."

Replying to a previous article suggesting that large doses of vitamin C might bring about infertility in women, Dr. Hoffer reported in *The Lancet,* November 17, 1973 that he had, at that time, given over 3,000 patients massive doses of vitamin C over a 20-year period and had not seen any occasions of scurvy when the high doses were lowered. He had not seen any withdrawal symptoms of any kind. He had not seen any increase in incidence of collagen diseases or oxalate kidney stones. He had not seen any decrease in fertility among his patients.

Dr. Jerome J. DeCosse, professor of surgery at the Medical College of Wisconsin, used vitamin C to treat intestinal polyps—three grams daily for up to 13 months. In 1974, researchers from Northern Arizona University and Loma Linda University School of Medicine put guinea pigs on diets with no vitamin C. A second group was given just enough of the vitamin to prevent scurvy, but no more. The third group was given 100 times more vitamin C than is needed to prevent scurvy in these animals. The health of the mouth tissues improved in direct proportion to the amount of vitamin C the animals received.

In *The New England Journal of Medicine,* January 3,

1974 physicians at a boarding school reported on giving some of the 641 children at school massive doses of vitamin C over a period of 14 weeks. Those children who got the vitamin had fewer incidents of all kinds of "disability," as well as colds, than those who got placebos. "Significantly more children on vitamin C had no sick days observed in the . . . survey," said the physicians.

At a symposium on vitamin C in 1981 Linus Pauling stated that he advocated megadoses of vitamin C to treat and prevent cancer. Ten grams of vitamin C daily (10,000 milligrams) "would insure a 10 percent decrease in age mortality for cancer patients and a 50 percent decreased incidence of cancer among normal population." At the same symposium Dr. Alton Ochsner of the Ochsner Clinic in New Orleans said that 45 years earlier he had started giving vitamin C when he found contaminated wounds that would not heal. As little as 1,000 milligrams started the healing process almost immediately, he said.

"Today," he said, "we give a few grams a day to all surgical patients . . . The good thing about vitamin C: you can't give too much." Dr. Pauling also recommended using vitamin C along with whatever chemotherapy or other therapy is being used to treat cancer. It works as well as chemotherapy, he said, and there is some evidence that it combats the negative side effects of the drugs given to cancer patients.

Vitamin C prevents liver damage. *The Journal of the National Cancer Institute* reported in April, 1973 that laboratory mice, given chemicals known to produce liver cancer, did not get the cancer when they were given vitamin C. Mice manufacture their own vitamin C, but under these circumstances, they obviously needed much more. Dr. T. S. Wilson at Barncoose Hospital in Redruth, England studied the vitamin C levels of older people admitted to his hospital, then recorded what course their health took. In every case those with higher levels of vitamin C in their blood lived longer than those with lesser amounts of the vitamin.

In 1981 researchers at the University of Rochester School of Medicine took white blood cells from volunteers and infected them with influenza virus. They then added vitamin C to some of the cells and not to others. In those which had the vitamin C the normal function of the white blood cells—fighting invaders—was strengthened. In the cells to which no vitamin C was added no such protective effect took place.

*Medical World News,* June 21, 1968 told of Dr. Jorgen Schlegel, chairman of Tulane University's urology department, who advised his patients who have had bladder cancer to take plenty of vitamin C and the condition will not return. He prescribed 1,500 milligrams a day for preventing the reappearance of the tumors. He also recommended vitamin C for all smokers. The aim, he says, is to exceed the body's requirements for the vitamin so that it will spill out into the urine, so that precancerous compounds will not develop in the bladder.

The results of a study of 50 young guinea pigs—an animal that, like man, lacks the ability to synthesize vitamin C—suggests that the need for the vitamin in *young* human beings for good health and development is probably at least 20 times higher than the accepted RDA. In the case of human children this would come to 1,500 milligrams daily. Said the researcher at the Linus Pauling Institute of Science and Medicine, "The burden of proof must now shift to the medical scientists who are really concerned about the health and physical condition of young people to show that considerations that apply to young guinea pigs do not apply to young people."

Dr. Emanuel Cheraskin wrote in the *International Journal for Vitamin and Nutrition Research* in 1973 that 527 dentists and their wives were studied in terms of daily reported vitamin C consumption and colds or other respiratory disorders. The evidence collected over a period of several years showed that taking the vitamin daily did indeed discourage the appearance of colds and other respiratory disorders.

In 1981 the Linus Pauling Institute performed an experiment on skin cancer, vitamin C and vitamin E. Hairless mice were used, because they are very susceptible to skin cancer when exposed to the ultraviolet light of the sun. The mice were given either vitamin C or vitamin E and exposed to sunlight for a period of 15 weeks. Some of the mice began to develop malignant tumors shortly after the end of this period. The mice given vitamin E enjoyed almost no protection from the sun, but the vitamin C had a very great protective effect on the mice which were given this vitamin.

In the *Journal of Orthomolecular Psychiatry*, Third Quarter, 1976 Dr. Irwin Stone told the story of research by Dr. Dean Burk and his colleagues who were then at the National Cancer Institute. It was published in the professional journal *Oncology*. The article said, "The present study shows that ascorbate is highly toxic or lethal to Ehrlich ascites carcinoma cells in vitro (in a test tube) . . . the great advantage that ascorbate possesses as potential anticancer agent is that it is, like penicillin, remarkably nontoxic to normal body tissues and may be administered to animals in extremely large doses (up to five or more grams per kilogram). . ."

Dr. Stone comments, "Let me remind you that five grams of vitamin C per kilogram for a 150-pound adult amounts to 350 grams or 350,000 milligrams, over three-quarters of a pound." The NCI researchers said further they believed the future of cancer therapy rests not in drugs so toxic they harm the cancer victim as well as the cancer cells, but in products which are lethal to cancer cells but harmless to healthy cells, like vitamin C. Since that time history has not shown that this prediction came true, at least so far as the National Cancer Institute is concerned.

A relatively low vitamin C intake may predispose women to develop cervical dysplasia, often a forerunner to cancer. A study was done at the Albert Einstein College of Medicine and reported in *Medical Tribune*, January 12, 1983. It showed that in women with a daily intake of vitamin C of less than 30 milligrams, there was a sevenfold increase in the risk of this condition. Carotene (the plant form of vitamin A) was also studied and found to be protective against this cervical condition.

Sjorgren's Syndrome (pronounced "Shogren") is also

called "dry eye" or "dry mouth." Both conditions are apparently becoming quite common these days especially among older folks. *The New England Journal of Medicine* reported on May 14, 1970 that five men, deprived of vitamin C until they developed scurvy, also developed Sjogren's syndrome. This is defined in a medical dictionary as a condition which features dry eyes and conjunctivitis, also dry mouth and throat, inflammation and crusting of the nose, enlargement of salivary glands and arthritis. The men with scurvy also had dry skin, excessive hair loss, dental decay and recurrent breakdown of dental restorations.

In 1981 *Medical Tribune* reported on a Japanese trial giving large doses of vitamin C to terminal cancer patients. Those who got the vitamin C survived 1½ to 15 times longer than other patients who got none. The vitamin also decreased their pain and improved appetite and mental alertness. Three of the patients treated with massive doses of vitamin C were still alive at the time the report was made, "clinically well with no significant progression or regression of their tumors," said Dr. Akira Murata of Saga University, Japan. A smaller study conducted at another Japanese hospital showed similar results.

Said Linus Pauling, Ph.D. in the Spring, 1981 issue of the Linus Pauling Institute newsletter, "During the last year I have been asked by a good number of people to comment on the statement that taking large doses of vitamin C causes crystals of this vitamin to appear in the kidney and other tissues of the human body. Dr. Pauling referred to a 1979 article in *The New England Journal of Medicine* concerning kidney stones in a condition called systinosis. The *Journal* incident described a child with this condition given vitamin C in an effort to see if it might help. It did not.

Dr. Pauling theorized that, if the vitamin had been given as sodium ascorbate or calcium ascorbate, the crystals of cystine might not have formed. He explained in detail all the body mechanisms that produced the effect. Individuals with this disease need to have alkaline urine to prevent crystals of cystine from forming. Vitamin C itself produces acid urine.

Dr. Pauling pointed out that very few people have this disorder and, when they are identified they should take vitamin C as sodium ascorbate or calcium ascorbate.

Incidentally, Dr. Pauling (twice a Nobel Laureate) was turned down eight times by the National Cancer Institute in his efforts to get a financial grant for a two-year study of vitamin C in preventing the growth of breast cancer in mice. The chairman of the advisory committee who finally recommended the grant said, "Pauling, after all, is one of the most eminent scientists of our age. When a man like that gets turned down by the NIH Study Section it's clearly of more than routine interest."

The Winter, 1983 newsletter from the Linus Pauling Institute in California described studies by Dr. Constance Tsao who gave five healthy volunteers eating a "well-balanced" diet while she measured the amount of calcium in their urine when they were taking no vitamin supplements and when they were taking 10 grams of vitamin C daily. All the volunteers showed an increase in the amount of vitamin C in the urine when they were taking 10 grams.

The study was planned to see whether amounts of calcium sufficient to create kidney stones were excreted depending on the amount of vitamin C being taken. There was no significant change in the calcium excreted when the volunteers were taking no vitamin C and when they were taking 10 grams. Dr. Tsao also says that other scientists have found that large doses of vitamin C may slightly reduce the amount of calcium excreted. Another study reported in *The American Journal of Clinical Nutrition* found that large doses of vitamin C had no effect on the amount of calcium excreted. Kidney stones are more likely to occur in people who excrete large amounts of calcium.

Dr. Cathcart of California has given massive doses of vitamin C to many thousands of patients and says that he has never seen a kidney stone in any of these patients. Dr. Irwin Stone in his book on vitamin C says that large doses of vitamin C are the best possible insurance *against* many diseases of the bladder and kidney. As long ago as 1969 scientists discovered that large doses of vitamin C—large enough to produce a rise in the level of vitamin C in the urine—will prevent the development of bladder cancer. Tulane University scientists who presented this evidence said that a daily intake of one and a half grams of vitamin C spaced in three doses throughout the day should be taken by individuals who "due to age, cigarette smoking or other factors, may be prone to bladder tumor formation." Dr. Stone in his book gives many references to studies showing that formation of urinary, salivary and gall bladder stones may, indeed, be due to deficiency in vitamin C.

*Executive Health,* March, 1987, reported on a study at the University of Bergen Institute of Hygiene and Social Medicine, in which Drs. S. E. Vollset and E. Bjalke studied the diets of almost 17,000 Norwegians for more than eleven years and found that 438 died of stroke. The death rate proved to be significantly lower among those with larger intakes of fruits and vegetables.

In 1983 a similar study in England showed that eating fresh fruits and vegetables may prevent strokes. *The Lancet* pointed out that high blood pressure is one very common cause of strokes, as is cigarette smoking. Incidence of stroke has decreased in England and in our country possibly because of more interest in healthful eating, an increase in the intake of vitamin C and a decrease in the amount of salt that is being used. Too much salt is believed to be partially responsible for high blood pressure.

The British study showed a sharp decrease in numbers of stroke where more vitamin C and vitamin C-rich foods are being eaten. The editorial pointed out that fresh fruits and vegetables, rich in vitamin C, also contain other nutrients that are probably valuable in preventing strokes—fiber, for example. Low levels of fiber in the diet have been associated with high blood pressure. It's true, too, that fruits and vegetables are low in salt and high in potassium which tends to counteract the unhealthful effects of using too much salt.

So adding lots of fresh fruits and vegetables, as many

raw as possible, to your diet will add to your daily intake of vitamin C, as well as many other essential nutrients. Eat some raw vegetables at every meal in salads, finger-salads or cole slaw. Use lots of fruits for dessert and snacks rather than sugary goodies.

# CHAPTER 46

# How Much Vitamin C Do You Need?

IN THE YEARS SINCE massive doses of vitamin C have been prescribed by many physicians in this country and abroad, those researchers who, for some reason, dislike the idea that just plain vitamins can treat or prevent illness have been telling us we're all wasting our money. Their belittling, disparaging comments suggest that all vitamin C over a dose of perhaps 30 to 100 milligrams is excreted almost immediately in the urine so all we "faddists" are doing, say these detractors, is to create very expensive urine for ourselves.

At the same time they tell us that vitamin C may bring us harm. They never explain just how this perfectly natural substance, which plays many important roles in the human body, could harm us if indeed it is all excreted within a few hours! Harmful compounds are almost always substances that are stored in the body, accumulating until the total amount overwhelms us.

Those researchers who regularly use vitamin C in very large amounts continually look for some evidence of harm from the vitamin and have never been able to find any. The detractors, too, have never been able to produce any verified cases where large doses of vitamin C have brought anything but benefit.

We have a significant record of tests done in a school for mentally disturbed patients who were getting extremely large amounts of vitamin C. Four physicians from this Virginia school wrote in *The Journal of Orthomolecular Psychiatry,* Volume 5, Number 1 about their careful tests to determine exactly how much vitamin C is excreted in urine.

Ninety-one patients getting from four to 48 grams of vitamin C daily were tested. (This is 4,000 to 48,000 milligrams of the vitamin.) Thirty-one of these patients were excreting vitamin C. Sixty of them were not. This means, we must assume, that these 60 sick people needed this much vitamin C daily or perhaps needed even more than this, since the vitamin was doing its job in their cells and was consumed in the process.

Four months later these same patients were tested again. Of 99 tests, 20 patients were excreting vitamin C. The other 79 patients apparently needed this much vitamin C or perhaps more. Later tests turned up the fact that about one-fourth of the patients were excreting vitamin C. Later, 149 new patients were admitted to the school. Urine tests showed not a particle of vitamin C in the urine of any of these. Doesn't this demonstrate clearly that these individuals were not getting anywhere near the amount of the vitamin they needed? Could this not be, as many orthomolecular psychiatrists believe, one of the causes of their mental and emotional illness—just lack of enough vitamin C to make up for the great stress caused by the illness?

While these tests were going on, the researchers also tested school personnel—nurses, doctors and administrators. Of 25 samples of urine taken, 10 showed vitamin C. Six did not. So at least six of these supposedly well individuals were not getting enough vitamin C to be able to spare any to excrete in their urine.

How about the supposedly great danger of large doses of vitamin C? In this situation all patients were being observed constantly. Tests were being given and symptoms checked daily. Of the entire population of patients, getting an average of nine grams of vitamin C daily, not a single symptom of any ill effect could be found. The "average" figure of nine grams means, of course, that many of the patients were getting much higher doses. Eighteen staff members have been taking from six to 18 grams of vitamin C daily for many years. None of them has noticed any ill effects.

Say the authors, "The psychiatric patient is under high stress and obviously requires very large doses of ascorbic acid. The long-term supplementation of ascorbic acid is apparently a very low risk regimen."

All living creatures except human beings, guinea pigs and a few other creatures including the great apes, make their own vitamin C. When they are under stress, they manufacture lots more vitamin C than when not under stress. Dr. Irwin Stone has found that the laboratory rat manufactures 1,800 milligrams of vitamin C per day. Under stress this creature manufactures as much as 15,200 milligrams of vitamin C per day. A mouse manufactures up to 19,250 milligrams daily, a rabbit 15,820, a goat 13,300, a dog or a cat 2,800. Human beings? Not a single milligram. They must get all the vitamin C they need from food. Or supplements.

Since a goat may weigh as much as a 150-pound human being, Dr. Linus Pauling points out that it's reasonable to assume that a human being weighing 150 pounds needs about what a goat needs—13,000 milligrams of vitamin C daily for good health. Since animals under stress manufacture even more vitamin C to fight the stress, there is every indication that human beings need more vitamin C when *they* are under stress.

It is an impossible task for any human being to count on 13,000 or more milligrams of vitamin C to counteract stress, if he has nothing but diet from which to get his vitamin C. It must come from supplements. Dr. Mark Levine, research associate in the Laboratory Cell Biology and Genetics of the National Institute of Diabetes, Digestive and Kidney Diseases, is quoted in *Medical Tribune*, May 7, 1986 as saying that science still cannot tell how much of the vitamin is the "right amount" for optimal health for a human being.

In five years of research Dr. Levine and his colleagues have determined that the guinea pig, for example, needs, to prevent scurvy, 1½ milligrams per kilogram of weight (that's about two pounds of weight). But that same guinea pig needs up to 16 milligrams per kilogram of weight to maintain growth and health, reproductive capability, wound healing and general good health. This is ten times as much as is required to prevent scurvy in this little animal.

Veterinarians have no trouble prescribing vitamin C in vast amounts for their four-footed patients. In a recent syndicated column Dr. Michael Fox, an internationally known veterinarian and humanitarian, replied to a reader whose cat suffered from a "blocked bladder." Dr. Fox recommended one gram (1,000 milligrams) of vitamin C daily to "keep the urine acidified." Also, he said, make the cat drink plenty of water, even if it means feeding salt to make the cat thirsty. One gram of vitamin C is an enormous dose for a creature as small as a cat. A human being weighing 150 pounds might need 10 times the amount needed for a 15-pound cat.

A letter to the editor of *New Scientist,* May 8, 1986 from a British veterinarian proposed treating breast cancer in elderly dogs with vitamin C in large doses. He says, "As a veterinarian who has long been aware of the efficacy of vitamin C . . . I am disgusted . . . to read of the attempts by so many members of the medical profession to bury their heads in the sand whenever vitamin therapy is proposed. This means they are denying a possible remedy to their patients."

He goes on to say that dogs, of course, manufacture their own vitamin C. But, he says, possibly this process breaks down in old age and the old dog is certainly not capable of manufacturing enough vitamin C to prevent cancer. Why not, he suggests, study the effects of massive doses of vitamin C in an effort to prevent or to treat breast cancer in elderly dogs which might be very significant for human health.

The National Academy of Sciences (NAS) which sets standards for various nutritional matters has decided that guinea pigs in laboratories must have an amount of vitamin C that is 50 times higher than that recommended by the same bureau for human beings, in relation to weight. The RDA for human beings will, supposedly, keep a rested, healthy, well nourished young person free from symptoms of scurvy, which is apparently all that the NAS requires.

But in order to keep laboratory animals at their very best for growth, health, resistance to disease and trauma such as operations, these animals officially must have 50 times more vitamin C than the amount recommended for human beings! Why?

# Vitamin D Is . . .

*Fat-soluble*, meaning it is stored in the body, hence not essential in food or supplements every day.

*Responsible* for formation, growth and maintenance of bones and teeth, in combination with calcium and phosphorus, also maintains correct balances of these two minerals in blood.

*Present* in appreciable amounts in almost no foods. Fish liver oils contain large amounts. Among foods we eat at meals egg yolk, butter, herring, mackerel, sardines, shrimp, tuna contain very small amounts. Sunlight on bare skin produces vitamin D, so spending some time out of doors every day is helpful, especially for infants and children who need vitamin D for bone and tooth formation.

*Safe* in recommended amounts. Excessive vitamin D produces toxic symptoms: loss of appetite, nausea, thirst, diarrhea and so on. Following the recommendations on the label of any product is a good idea.

*Destroyed* in the body by mineral oil, as are all other fat-soluble vitamins.

*Required* officially: 400 International Units for adults and children alike. This is the reason most milk is fortified with 400 units of vitamin D per quart these days.

*Available* in capsules of not more than 400 International Units and in one-a-day brands.

# CHAPTER 47

# You Can Get Vitamin D from Sunlight or from Supplements

An ARTICLE IN the *Journal of the American Medical Association* in the year 1892 dealt with rickets, the bone-deforming disease that crippled so many children in those times. We know now that rickets is caused by deficiency in vitamin D and/or calcium. Since vitamin D is manufactured on the skin in the presence of sunlight, rickets attacked its victims usually in winter, when the sun's rays are feeble and children are bundled up in many layers of clothing.

In 1892 doctors had never heard of vitamins. They did not know that food contained anything but carbohydrate, protein and fat. So when they diagnosed rickets in 1892 they had to come up with some other reason for this painful deformity, which crippled many children for life because their bones did not grow normally.

Here are some of the suggestions the *JAMA* had for doctors treating rickets in 1892. They said, "Continuous bowel trouble often leads to rickets, but the earliest sign of the rickets is sweating, particularly at night and about the back of the head . . . The presence of rickets means that the child has been deprived of some important food element. Usually this is the fat, but not infrequently the protein constituents of the diet are deficient . . .

"By way of treatment," the 1892 article continued, "it is first necessary to get the child's stomach and bowels into a normal condition, so that the food administered can be

314

properly digested and absorbed. Then a diet rich in the element which has previously been deficient is to be prescribed. For the infant, protein food cannot be found outside of milk. But for its fats, not only is milk available, but also cod liver oil. This latter substance is usually taken readily by young children, and is well borne. . . ."

So, 100 years ago doctors did not know what was causing rickets but they did know that something in cod liver oil could prevent and even cure it. They thought it might be the fat in this oil. It was, of course, the vitamin D in the cod liver oil which worked the miracle cure.

A revolutionary scientific theory revealing the basic, elemental importance of vitamin D was described in the August 4, 1967 issue of *Science,* the publication of the American Association for the Advancement of Science. A biochemistry professor at Brandeis University, Dr. Farnsworth Lewis, explained how human beings happened to be able to migrate throughout the world, even into very cold regions like the Scandanavian countries, by developing, over millions of years, lighter skins through which the ultraviolet rays of the sun could penetrate.

This theory depends for its proof on the fact that vitamin D is manufactured in certain layers of the skin when the ultraviolet rays of the sun fall on the skin. Dr. Lewis said there is no essential function of ultraviolet rays so far as man is concerned except for the production of vitamin D. It is vitamin D which prevents rickets, allowing the bones of babies to develop straight and strong, helping to incorporate the minerals, calcium and phosphorus into the bone structure. Children who, for whatever reason, do not get enough vitamin D, develop rickets, which means twisted, deformed bones.

According to Dr. Lewis, the body has no mechanism for protecting itself against too much vitamin D. Human beings originally lived in the tropics. So how were they protected against getting too much of the intense ultraviolet light of the tropical sun? Originally, they had dark skins, says Dr. Lewis, for deeply pigmented skins do not allow much of the ultraviolet light to pass into inner layers of skin. So just enough vitamin D to prevent rickets is formed in a dark-skinned person, even though he or she may spend all day out in the hot sun. But what happened when those ancient people migrated farther north where the sun's rays contain much less ultraviolet light and where many cloudy days obscure the sun?

"These early people got rickets," says Dr. Lewis. For perhaps millions of years dark-skinned people trying to live in northern countries became so crippled with rickets that they could not hunt or find other food. So generation after generation, only the lighter-skinned people among them survived. Eventually, these lighter-skinned people became the people of Northern Europe and Scandanavia. It is noteworthy, says Lewis, that the coloring of skin among native peoples becomes lighter as one goes farther north. Vitamin D formation in the skin is the only explanation for this, he says.

There is only one exception to this general rule—the Eskimos. Here are people who live in the far North, where winters are very long and dark, where very little of the sun's rays penetrate for most of the year. For warmth, the Eskimos must wear thick, heavy clothing which also prevents ultraviolet light from reaching the skin. But rickets is unknown among these people. Why? They eat the livers of fish and animals which are the only dependable food source of vitamin D. Therefore they can keep their relatively dark skins and yet avoid rickets. Such is the magic of fish liver oil.

If this theory is correct, it becomes apparent that when light-skinned people come to live in northern countries they must pay strict attention to getting enough vitamin D in foods and supplements. If not, their children may develop rickets and adults may develop the adult form of rickets which is called osteomalacia or softening of the bones.

Today's commercial milk, our best source of calcium, is enriched with vitamin D almost everywhere in the Western world. We do this to prevent rickets in infants. Since most babies live largely on milk, the vitamin D enrichment program has prevented rickets on a nationwide scale even among children growing up in slums in the darkest winter months when air pollution prevents the ultraviolet light of the weak winter sun from reaching their skins.

By now physicians know well the cause of rickets, so children who cannot, for some reason, drink milk are given vitamin D supplements. What about older people? There is good evidence that they continue to need vitamin D in later life, although their bones are already formed. To be healthy we must be able to absorb calcium and phosphorus throughout our lives and these two minerals can be absorbed only when vitamin D is present.

In 1969 *Nutrition Reviews* reported the fact that a surprising number of children examined in Greece had rickets. Greece is a land of abundant sunshine even in winter. Among 137 babies examined by the physicians 15 percent already had rickets. One third of the babies had "clinical signs" of rickets, meaning that they had healed or inactive rickets. Of the 327 babies examined, only 116 had ever taken vitamin D in supplements.

All babies who had been taken outside on sunny days had a lower prevalence of the disease, even though their clothing covered all but their lower arms and face. Breast-fed babies had far less incidence, presumably because their mothers got plenty of vitamin D from exposure to sunlight. The physicians gave the children with symptoms of rickets vitamin D supplements for a number of weeks and all their symptoms disappeared.

Apparently Greek women at that time believed that infants should be fully clothed at all times, with only the head and upper arms exposed to sunlight. This is just not enough exposure, especially if the babies are not taken out every day when the sun is shining. The authors say that a similar condition was discovered in a southern part of Israel where the babies' clothing was to blame for the rickets, because it prevented exposure to the sun.

In 1969 the authors of the *Nutrition Reviews* article believed that a similar survey in our country might turn up some surprising facts about vitamin D and rickets. They say that no wide-scale tests to discover how many babies in any geographical area in our own country may be suffering from a degree of rickets which does not bend arm and leg bones out of shape, deform jaws and hands, but which is rickets nonetheless.

One specialist calls rickets the first air-pollution disease, since pollution in cities in winter can hide the sun for weeks on end and no one living in such a city can get much vitamin D from the sun no matter if he or she is outside much of the day. So rickets may not be an "historical curiosity" that we can write off casually as a "conquered disease."

"Nursing infants get more vitamin D from mothers taking doses of sunshine," says an article in *Medical Tribune,* June 11, 1984. A half hour of being out in the sun around noon on a clear summer day can significantly increase the vitamin D content of human breast milk for up to two weeks after exposure. Scientists at a Wisconsin Prenatal Center found that both mother's blood and breast milk increased dramatically in vitamin D within 24 to 48 hours of exposure to sunshine and remained elevated for seven to 14 days. Many nutrition experts think vitamin D should be called a hormone rather than a vitamin. It is, after all, manufactured in the body as are hormones. It is manufactured from compounds that appear on the skin after exposure to sunshine.

Drinking several glasses of milk a day and spending some time out of doors on sunny days the year round can probably give most of us enough vitamin D. Of course, for vitamin D to do its work, it must have calcium, as well. This is the main reason why milk is such a good source of vitamin D—the calcium that works with the vitamin to give us good health comes right in the milk along with the vitamin. Vegetarian children who eat no foods of animal origin have been reported to be very susceptible to rickets when they grow up in cold cloudy climates. Both Great Britain and Canada have reported some epidemics of rickets among vegetarian children who have emigrated to these northern localities from southern sunny countries.

At a Utah training school for retarded children in 1972 a visiting physician discovered that almost one fourth of the children were suffering from rickets. X-rays showed that, indeed, the children's bones were in very bad condition. Neither diet nor lack of sun appeared to be the cause of this condition. The visiting doctor eventually discovered that the serious deficiency in vitamin D was caused by the drugs being given to these children who had epilepsy. The drugs were phenylhydantoin and phenobarbital. Of the 70 children on drugs 63 had rickets. It seems that urinary excretion of vitamin D is excessive when these drugs are taken. Said Dr. John C. Leonidas in an article in *The Journal of the American Medical Association*, "It certainly cannot be denied that dietary vitamin D intake is very important in preventing the development of a deficiency state during anticonvulsant therapy."

Other drugs as well cause loss of vitamin D—oil-based laxatives such as mineral oil, also certain other drugs used in sedatives and sleeping pills as well as some antacids which contain aluminum hydroxide. Read labels.

No one knows for sure all the causes of the bone disease osteoporosis which bothers many older people, especially women. Most physicians today believe that lack of calcium may play a big part in this condition which results in pain, discomfort, shortening of the spine and, often, broken bones. Many doctors have found that broken hips, which many older people experience, are not the result of falls, but that the bones are so weak that they break first, causing the falls.

We have plenty of evidence that vitamin D is often effective in relieving this condition, along with plenty of calcium, of course. The British medical journal *The Lancet* in 1966 told of work with 60 elderly women living alone. All of them were over 70, but mentally alert, active and well. None was on any special diet.

The doctors studied the density of their bones. Obviously, thin bones tend to break more easily than very dense ones. Diet histories showed that those with the lowest levels of vitamin D intake had the bones most likely to be thin, hence most susceptible to fractures. Although these women were apparently getting enough calcium and phosphorus they lacked vitamin D which is the third factor—the third arm of the triangle of health.

Here are some histories of older folks with vitamin D deficiency as related in *The Journal of the American Geriatrics Society*. An 80-year old woman, living alone, was admitted to a British hospital unable to walk without great difficulty. Legs and feet were swollen. She seldom went out of the house since walking was so difficult. She was lonely and had lost interest in eating. She never ate liver, kidney, oily fish or eggs and for cooking she used only salad oil which contains no vitamin D. Tests showed gross deficiency in this vitamin. The doctors gave her calcium and vitamin D supplements. Within six months her bone pains disappeared and she could walk without aid.

An 82-year old woman who also lived alone was housebound and suffered from bone pain. Her appetite was poor. Doctors discovered she was living almost entirely on white bread and butter, getting only 10 units of vitamin D every day. Treated with massive vitamin and mineral therapy her bones healed rapidly, pain disappeared and she became fully mobile and independent. A 68-year old woman was breathless and had bone pain. Suspecting she had osteomalacia the doctors started her on calcium and vitamin D supplements. She improved rapidly and could walk unaided without pain when she left the hospital.

A 74-year old woman could not rise from a chair, had great difficulty getting around and had pain in her bones. Very apprehensive about her walking, she never went out. Her daily diet contained less than 80 units of vitamin D. Supplements of calcium and vitamin D brought her back to good health.

Dr. Masud Anwar, the British physician who made these reports added the following facts about people most likely to suffer from vitamin D deficiency: 1. Those with severe physical disability such as arthritis of hips and knees, strokes, severe heart and/or respiratory disease, all of which prevent them from spending much time out of doors. 2. Those with mental illnesses such as dementia, confused states, depression and psychoses. "Undernutrition and depression can combine to produce a self-sustaining downward spiral in an elderly person's clinical state," said Dr. Anwar. The elderly confused individual may avoid food because of illusions that he or she is allergic to it or that the food is poisoned.

3. People living in extreme isolation because their family and friends have died or live far away. Old women living alone tend to eat less than those living with their husbands, says the doctor. 4. People over 85 tend to eat less and to have less knowledge of what foods are essential. 5. People living in housing that is far from stores have difficulty shopping for food. 6. People who are ignorant of nutrition (and this includes most of us) tend to eat any food that is easy to prepare, especially if they never learned to cook. 7. Psychotics may neglect food just as they neglect proper clothing and washing. 8. Alcoholics are deficient in many nutrients because they substitute alcohol for food. 9. People with dental problems find it hard to chew, so they avoid many foods and eat mostly soft, mushy foods. They may also avoid milk which contains vitamin D. 10. People who have no physical disability but are nervous in traffic and may have lost their ability to do many things such as shop or cook are likely to eat whatever is easiest to obtain and prepare. This doctor also says that, whereas osteoporosis, the bone disorder afflicting many older folks, causes pain to be localized mostly in the spine, osteomalacia, caused by lack of vitamin D and/or calcium, is most likely to be diffuse, nagging, persistent and unremitting.

Lack of exercise also enters into the picture, Dr. Anwar continues. "Becoming sedentary as you age is an almost certain guarantee of bone troubles, since they must be moved to be healthy. This is especially true of the weight-bearing bones—pelvic, hip, thigh and shin bones as well as the spine."

It seems we need to move around every day and not ever lie motionless in bed for long periods of time. Adult rickets can also be found in women with closely spaced pregnancies where calcium is needed in large amounts for the growing unborn child and where vitamin D is deficient. In severe liver disease, also, the liver does not store vitamin D normally, so the patient is likely to suffer the consequences in weakened bones.

*Medical Tribune* in 1981 reported that, even though they got outside frequently in a sunny country, Israel, vitamin D was deficient in many older folks, apparently because of inadequate ways of absorbing the vitamin in the intestines.

Two to three glasses of milk every day may offer protection from colorectal cancer by raising levels of calcium and vitamin D, according to new research cited in *Medical World News*, April 22, 1985. Dr. Cedric Garland and colleagues at the University of California in San Diego had previously observed that rates of colon cancer were higher in areas of low sunlight. To extend this finding, they studied nutrition and outcome data from 1,954 telephone manufacturing workers at Chicago Western Electric.

These men were between 40 and 55 years old when enrolled in the study in 1957. Records were kept of the men's diets and health status throughout the 20 years of the study. The 49 workers who developed colorectal cancer by 1979 had lower vitamin D and calcium intakes than others in the group. Other elements of diet, including number of calories consumed, were similar.

According to Dr. Garland, those who drank *no* milk had nearly three times the risk of colorectal cancer as those who drank a couple of glasses of milk every day. Although previous researchers had begun to understand the role of calcium in protecting against cancer, the reasons for the benefit given by vitamin D have not been previously explored. Dr. Garland's findings do not provide final proof that drinking milk can prevent every incidence of this terrible cancer for which almost no therapy is known. Nevertheless, Dr. Garland suggests that we all drink two or three glasses of nonfat milk a day as a safe intervention against colorectal cancer.

In 1984 *The Journal of the American Medical Association* reported that preliminary studies by an English ear specialist point to a connection between vitamin D deficiency and certain types of progressive deafness. The doctor believes that vitamin D deficiency may lead to demineralization of a tiny bone in the ear called the cochlea, which is essential for normal hearing. Twenty-two patients studied by this doctor showed low or borderline vitamin D levels. The best idea, of course, is to *prevent* this loss of minerals due to vitamin D deficiency rather than trying to treat the deafness after it occurs.

Any disorder of the digestive tract that makes absorption of food difficult can result in deficiency in vitamin D, leading rapidly to disorders such as osteoporosis and osteomalacia. Here are some conditions that render assimilation and absorption difficult: disorders of the liver, pancreas, gallbladder, and intestines. When part of the digestive tract has been removed by surgery this is an added difficulty. Crohn's Disease results in such defective absorption of nutrients that it may bring on a deficiency in all the fat soluble vitamins.

Bone diseases brought on by lack of vitamin D may not show any symptoms of pain or other distress. The bones will be wasting away just the same. There is almost no vitamin D in food. We were apparently meant by nature to get our vitamin D from sunlight. Butter and egg yolk have a little vitamin D, also liver of all kinds, and certain fatty seafoods like sardines, salmon and shrimp. Fish liver oil is the most abundant source. Most dairy milk is enriched these days with 400 units of vitamin D to every quart. Other dairy products may or may not be enriched with vitamin D. Read the labels.

Can you get too much vitamin D? Yes. Symptoms may be lack of appetite, nausea, thirst, diarrhea, excessive urination, muscular weakness, joint pains and certain imbalances of minerals which will show up in blood tests from a laboratory. It's not likely to happen if you watch carefully the labels of your food supplements to see that no very large amounts of vitamin D are in the capsules.

*The Journal of the American Medical Association* reported in 1985 on an elderly woman who had been taking vitamin D and calcium to avoid osteoporosis. When she was brought to the hospital because of a broken bone she was given a prescription for vitamin D which was somehow misinterpreted by hospital personnel to be 50,000 units of vitamin D. She was to take this three times a day. Within three weeks she showed very disturbing symptoms as a result. The calcium level of her blood rose to disastrous heights and she went into a stupor. The doctors gave her vigorous therapy to counteract the vitamin and bring blood levels of calcium down and she recovered. The New York doctors who reported this case urged fellow physicians to administer this vitamin with close regard to possible risks of overdosage.

In general it's safest to stay close to 400 units daily either from milk or from supplements. Doses much higher than this can and have produced serious side effects. Of course, the best idea is to get as much of your vitamin D as possible from exposure to the sun. This does not mean baking yourself in the sunlight to "get a tan." The more tan you get, the less vitamin D you will absorb. And recently incidence of skin cancer has increased to what some specialists are calling an epidemic, mostly, they believe, from long exposure to brilliant sunlight which may be growing more dangerous because we are gradually losing the ozone layer in the atmosphere which protects us from the ultraviolet rays of the sun.

It isn't necessary to expose either old folks or children to long hours of "getting a tan." Just getting out of doors on any sunny day and walking, gardening, socializing, or engaging in any other pleasurable pursuit for half an hour or so, even if you stay mostly in the shade, will result in enough vitamin D being manufactured on your skin to keep you in good health where this nutrient is concerned.

# Vitamin E Is . . .

*Fat-soluble,* hence stored in the body.

*Responsible* for health and maintenance of circulatory system, and muscles in general, health of red blood cells, and healthful sex and reproductive life, detoxifying poisons, preventing oxidation of fats in the body.

*Present* in seeds, wholegrains, wheat germ, wheat bran, all salad oils, liver, eggs. Wheat germ oil is the best source in food. *Safe* in very large amounts. All reports show no disadvantages in extremely large amounts, even when taken over long periods of time.

*Destroyed* by mineral oil laxatives, iron medications, impaired fat absorption in certain disorders, heat in cooking and long storage in freezers. Iron medication should be taken at a different time from any vitamin E supplement.

*Required* officially in daily amounts of 8 to 10 International Units for adults, less for children.

*Available* in low or high potencies in one-a-day supplements or individual supplements.

# CHAPTER 48

# Your Need for
# Vitamin E

BECAUSE OF THEIR unpleasant smell, one would think that
rancid fats might not be good food. This is correct. Rancid
fats are very unhealthful. One reason is that they destroy
vitamin E. If you eat fats that are spoiled or rancid, they
will quickly destroy any vitamin E in your digestive tract
at the same time. Then, too, foods normally rich in Vitamin
E which have gone rancid will contain none of the vitamin.

On the other hand, one of the most important functions
of vitamin E is to prevent fats from becoming rancid. Fats
are spoiled by combining with oxygen. Vitamin E seems to
be an anti-oxidant, that is, it prevents this combination and
so prevents the fat from becoming rancid. In the same way,
this vitamin protects other vitamins, specifically vitamins A
and C, as well as certain other fats called the unsaturated
fats. This means that if you have plenty of vitamin E in
your diet you can get along successfully without suffering
so much from lack of these other vitamins, in case they are
short in your meals. This is one example of the way vitamins
work with and protect one another.

Throughout scientific literature vitamin E is linked over
and over again with the name of that substance without which
none of us can live for even a minute—oxygen. Vitamin E
and oxygen are important to one another. This alone indicates
that this vitamin, which has been identified and studied only
since 1936, must be essential for all of us.

326

Studying laboratory animals which have been made deficient in vitamin E, scientists have found that the muscles of these animals seem to need more oxygen than those of normal animals, so they have concluded that plenty of vitamin E in the diet enables us to get along on less oxygen than we would otherwise need. This discovery is very important, especially in modern times when so many things—environmental conditions and physical disorders—conspire to cheat us of much of the oxygen we need. Smoking, for instance, cuts off some of the supply of oxygen to the cells. The indoor, sedentary life most of us lead deprives us of the oxygen we might get in long country walks with fresh, unpolluted air filling our lungs.

Whether because of its relation to oxygen or because of something else as yet undiscovered, vitamin E seems to be involved in what goes on in an astonishing number of places in the body: reproductive system, muscles, brain, nerves, heart and circulatory organs, joints, skin and digestive tract, to name but a few. *An Annotated Bibliography of Vitamin E,* prepared by the Research Laboratories of the Distillation Products Industries, lists 195 pieces of important research reported just in the years 1958 through 1960, in which vitamin E was given to human beings in varying doses to see what the effect would be on whatever disorder they were suffering from.

Some of the researchers reported little or no success. Others were enthusiastic about the results they got. Here are some of the positive reports.

Premature infants with a disorder called scleroderma (a hardening and swelling of the skin) were given vitamin E. Mortality dropped from 75% to 27%. Children with cystic fibrosis of the pancreas were found to have some symptoms just like those of animals which are deficient in vitamin E. The children also had very low levels of the vitamin in their blood. The scientist who reported this discovery in *Pediatrics* in 1958 recommended that children with this disease be given vitamin E routinely.

A Russian scientific journal reported that the incidence

of miscarriage was reduced from 46% to 12% in women whose pregnancy was complicated by the Rh factor, when vitamin E was given along with vitamin C and vitamin K. A German scientist reported in 1959 that a certain kind of inherited muscular dystrophy responded well to doses of the B vitamins, vitamin A, C and E (300 milligrams a day). When started soon enough and continued for long enough, he said, this treatment relieved muscular distress and produced improvement. Note that these two physicians gave other vitamins along with vitamin E and have no way of knowing how much this combination of vitamins had to do with their success.

Evan Shute, M.D. of Canada, one of the earliest proponents of using vitamin E against disease, reported improved muscle strength in two patients with acute polio and three out of 14 patients with chronic polio. A South American physician at the National Institute of Public Health in Buenos Aires told of giving large doses of vitamin E to patients in a mental hospital, with resulting improvement in mental state and muscle coordination. Mentally handicapped children, given large doses of vitamin E, showed mental and physical improvement. He believes this vitamin plays some part in regulating glands and nervous system.

A Japanese scientist told of putting 40 surgical patients on vitamin E *before* an operation. Most of them were found safe from any possibility of blood clots after the operation. Of another group of 40 surgical patients who were not given the vitamin E, half showed evidence of risks of blood clots or strokes.

Dr. Shute offered convincing evidence of his belief that vitamin E is a natural anti-clotting agent. He also thought it is a vasodilator, meaning that it opens blood vessels so that plenty of blood can get through. He used it for heart trouble, varicose veins, phlebitis, hardening of the arteries, diabetic gangrene, burns, skin grafts and many other disorders. He believed that doctors who are not successful in using it as he did are just not giving the right dose or not continuing treatment long enough.

A Louisiana State University professor believed he found a key for preventing the aging process—vitamin E. Dr. William Pryor in *Scientific American,* August, 1979, said that effects of diets deficient in vitamin E are similar to effects of radiation damage and aging. In all these there is structural damage to membranes of cells.

"Free radicals" are unstable compounds which are very damaging to cells. When enough vitamin E is present free radicals are restrained. If it is not present, fatty substances collect into dark brown debris which is called "age pigment." Now it appears they may have nothing to do with just aging. They are, perhaps, just a sign of vitamin E deficiency.

Vitamin E, along with vitamin A, has been found to protect laboratory animals from damage from air pollutants in large cities. Those with plenty of vitamin E in their diets showed little damage when exposed to nitrogen dioxide and ozone, two ever-present pollutants. Animals deficient in the vitamin suffered extensive damage.

Dr. F. L. Money of Wellington, New Zealand, has found that baby pigs, kept in pens and fed artificially, are prone to sudden death just like the "crib deaths" of human infants. When the animals are examined, their hearts and lungs are affected and they bleed into the spinal cord. It is the same with human babies who die. These are almost always bottle-fed rather than breast-fed. Dr. Money's animals had low levels of vitamin E and selenium in their blood. Giving these nutrients to one group of animals and withholding them from another group, he found that those given the supplements did not die, while the second group continued to suffer many mortalities.

Vitamin E deficiency causes muscular dystrophy (MD) in monkeys. Lack of the vitamin causes accumulations of cholesterol in muscles with the crippling effects of dystrophy. Dr. Manford D. Morris of the University of Arkansas found that vitamin E deficiency alone could not be the *sole* cause of MD in human beings because almost total deficiency is extremely rare in them. *Medical World News* reported in May, 1960 that a pitcher on the Giants team credited vitamin

E with keeping his pitching arm in shape. He took the vitamin after a sore shoulder affected his pitching in 1967.

Premature babies of very low birth weight are often victims of an anemia which does not respond to iron supplements. Some researchers believe the anemia is caused by lack of vitamin E. Most babies are born with low levels of this vitamin, so unless enough is provided in breast milk they may suffer from a deficiency. Dr. M. A. Chadd and A. J. Fraser believe that "vitamin E deficiency be considered in any very small infant who had an anemia within a few weeks of birth."

It seems likely that low vitamin E levels in the infants' mothers may contribute to the reasons the babies were born prematurely. Veterinarians have known for years that horses and prize animals of many kinds are liable to abort their young or to deliver them prematurely when they are deficient in vitamin E. Many stock raisers use the vitamin routinely to prevent this.

In *Science,* March 1, 1968, two researchers at the University of California reported on the process of reproduction in rats deprived of vitamin E although the rest of their diets were complete. It is well known that sterility is the first indication of vitamin E deficiency in animals. Studying laboratory animals, the scientists discovered that their cells contained a given number of a particle in each cell that is not present in quantity when a cell is dividing normally. Animals getting plenty of vitamin E had fewer of these particles. They also found that animals breathing the air of the laboratory had a normal appearance, while the cells of those breathing pure oxygen looked more like those of the vitamin E deficient animals. The authors believe they may have shown that vitamin E has the basic function of giving direct protection to the apparatus responsible for the division of cells. All cells divide, so this finding is not applicable just to problems of reproduction. Cells of children growing from infancy must divide many times to produce that growth. As we grow older, cells wear out and must be replaced by new cells. Cancer is believed to be a disorder of cell division, where cells have lost their ability to limit their division and continue to divide wildly and profusely. If, indeed, vitamin E is essential to protect the apparatus which causes cells to divide, then it is tied in directly with life itself and almost every process that goes on in every living being.

# CHAPTER 49

# What Does Vitamin E Do in the Body?

THERE ARE MANY essential food elements whose full activity in the body is not known, not even guessed at by scientists who have made a life work of this study. This is no reason for not continuing to use them and to get them in every day's meals. In the case of vitamin E we know well what some of the activities of this vitamin are in the human body. Dr. Evan Shute of Canada answered some of these questions in his publication *The Summary,* volume 24.

Vitamin E is an antioxidant. It prevents the formation and deposition of certain harmful forms of fatty substances in the body. Vitamin E serves two purposes where oxygen is concerned. It is an antioxidant since it can prevent cells from being oxidized or rendered rancid by oxygen and it can also protect living cells from getting too little oxygen. "We tell patients it's like living in an oxygen tent to take vitamin E," says Dr. Shute.

Vitamin E serves a valuable function in preventing the formation of unwelcome blood clots. Although the clotting of blood is an essential body process, so we won't ever bleed to death, but when the clotting mechanism goes out of control, blood clots form where they are not wanted and serious or fatal circulatory complications result. Vitamin E helps to prevent such clots from forming. It also "eats away" at clots that have already formed, if they are fairly fresh.

332

So, you might say, vitamin E protects us from strokes in many ways.

Vitamin E also enlarges arteries permitting better circulation. One of the most dangerous complications of heart and artery disorders is the narrowing of arteries so that enough blood cannot get through. Vitamin E also promotes what Dr. Shute calls "collateral circulation" meaning that, when an artery or a smaller blood vessel is blocked, the vitamin helps the body to create a new artery around the damaged portion. Some patients have been given arterial grafts by surgeons to by-pass such useless arteries. Dr. Shute believes that a natural substance like vitamin E is much preferable to a surgical graft.

Vitamin E promotes formation of new skin in wounds and burns, doing away with the necessity for skin grafting. Vitamin E can be used in cases of gangrene which may help to avoid amputation, may decrease pain or save the other leg. Dr. Shute lists eight articles in medical journals supporting this use of the vitamin. Vitamin E eases the pain and swelling, prevents clots in thrombophlebitis. The problem seldom recurs and accompanying ulcers are almost unknown when vitamin E is given. He lists 57 papers in medical journals supporting this claim.

Indolent ulcers are common, neglected and painful. Vitamin E may cure them after years of failure with all other known therapy. He lists 61 papers on the subject in medical literature. Of burns, he says, "Pain, infection, long months of painful and expensive skin grafting with hideous cosmetic results" are the usual complications. Vitamin E relieves pain, promotes the growth of new skin, leaves flexible scars which seldom need grafting. "Such wound healing has never been seen before in the history of medicine," he says. "The effect of alphatocopherol on burns we regard as one of our most fortunate observations," he says.

Stroke victims are often left hopelessly crippled and helpless for many years. Giving the right amounts of vitamin E can sometimes help to rejuvenate old cases and can help to prevent the occurrence of strokes. Varicose veins and eczema are troublesome, common and usually neglected. Dr. Shute says they seldom disappear entirely when vitamin E is taken, but they do not become worse. There may be less itching and pain, less ulceration, less swelling and phlebitis. Buerger's Disease is a sinister and usually hopeless condition in which circulation in legs becomes so bad that recovery is impossible and amputation is needed. "Vitamin E saves many such legs," says Dr. Shute, and cites 13 papers in the medical literature attesting to this fact.

Intermittent claudication brings severe cramps in the legs, making it impossible for the victim to walk—a symptom of hardening of the arteries. Vitamin E is widely used for this condition, says Dr. Shute, and cites 32 medical papers on the subject. It is just as useful for night cramps, "little strokes," nephritis, some eye disorders, itchy keloid scars, thrombocytopanic purpura or hemorrhages and other conditions in the circulatory system.

Even scars that are years old may soften and relax under vitamin E therapy. It has been used for Depuytren's contracture, Peyronie's disease, stricture of the esophagus or anus or urethra. Vitamin E on fresh wounds prevents contracture, so that they heal smoothly, says Dr. Shute and cites 30 supportive papers.

In the field of obstetrics and gynecology, vitamin E can prevent miscarriage or abortion, threatened abortion, premature rupture of the membranes, prematurity and abruptio placentae. Female sterility is apparently not helped by vitamin E but 19 supportive papers indicate that vitamin E improves the quality of the sperm cells, so fathers may sire few or no congenitally damaged babies and their wives have fewer habitual abortions.

Vitamin E is no help in true eclampsia (convulsions or seizures associated with pregnancy) but in the non-convulsive or late type of this condition it is very helpful if used in time, he says. Nineteen doctors have apparently found it so helpful that they have written medical papers on the subject.

In lack of menstruation, vitamin E has occasionally been found helpful.

Kraurosis and other senile vulvur states associated with itching are often handled poorly by the usual medication which is estrogen, says Dr. Shute. Vitamin E is very valuable in shrinking tender vaginas due to aging, also for senile leucorrhea, vulvar itching, leukoplakia of the cervix and vulva, painful or difficult intercourse. Also in diabetic and anal pruritis (itching).

Chronic cystic mastitis is usually controlled brilliantly by vitamin E, says Dr. Shute, thus avoiding endless mastectomies and endless biopsies and alarm. He cites several supportive papers in the literature. He also says that birth trauma is less apt to be encountered if vitamin E is given to the mother before and during labor.

All these conditions were being treated with vitamin E by this physician and apparently many more physicians whom he quotes. None of them has any financial interest in the vitamin. All of them must have risked malpractice suits if their vitamin therapy had failed. So there seems to be no reason why they should have used vitamin E as therapy for all those years, if, indeed, it doesn't work.

In 1982 a professor of microbiology at Colorado State University, Dr. Robert Tengerdy, reported on his success in using vitamin E to improve the immunological state of the body—that is, it improves those blood cells and antibodies that protect the body from invaders of all kinds—bacteria, viruses, toxins and poisons.

His 12-year studies have shown the excellent effects of vitamin E on the immune systems of chickens, sheep, rabbits and mice. He has shown that animals given large doses of the vitamin are able to destroy bacteria faster and produce more antibodies to any body invaders. He says that vitamin E may also help out against disease by stimulating the production and activity of white blood cells. These are the protective cells that surround invaders and engulf them.

Dr. Tengerdy is an active sportsman, engaging in running,

cross-country skiing and sailing. He takes extra vitamin E himself every day. He uses a powdered form of the vitamin and sprinkles some of it on his food every day. He says, "My contention is that we really don't know if we get enough in our diet. Taking a little more may be helpful." He says that vitamin E, unlike vitamin A, is not toxic even in large quantities. "It breaks down and it isn't toxic," he says. "We have given chickens so much vitamin E they looked waxy, but there were no ill effects."

He agrees with the growing number of nutritionists who believe that the official RDA for vitamin E is inadequate. Minimum levels are set to keep people from getting vitamin deficiency disease, he says, but they cannot be used to obtain "optimal performance." The growing popularity of nutrition, exercise and good general health shows that society is interested in optimal performance. "There's a big gap between not being sick and performing optimally," he said in an August 27, 1982 press release from the University.

Confirming his comments on the safety of vitamin E is a letter to the editor of *The Journal of the American Medical Association*, September 3, 1982 from two physicians from Washington state. They are challenging an earlier *JAMA* article in which a physician found that many patients with circulatory disorders are taking vitamin E.

Say the two Washington physicians, "This is not surprising. Tens of millions of Americans take nutrients for various reasons. One could easily find a large group with just about any disease who have been taking vitamin E. If these observations imply that vitamin E may cause blood clots we had better also indict aspirin as a cause of strokes since many patients have strokes after starting a regimen of aspirin for transient ischemic attacks . . .

"We have given large doses of vitamin E to several thousand patients during the past decade. No case of thrombophlebitis or pulmonary embolus (stroke) has occurred even with longterm therapy . . . problems with this nutrient are negligible."

M. K. Horwitt, Ph.D., professor of biochemistry at St.

Louis University School of Medicine, had believed for many years that vitamin therapy for serious disorders is useless, since we all get enough of every vitamin in daily food to satisfy the official RDA. But at a symposium on vitamins he announced that he had changed his mind so completely that he was now recommending that all of us get as much as 800 milligrams of this vitamin daily as insurance against blood clots that complicate the lives of heart and circulatory patients.

And in the March, 1980 issue of *Nutrition Reviews* he published a lead article entitled "Therapeutic Uses of Vitamin E in Medicine." He discussed the nerve problems of those who cannot get enough vitamin E because of digestive difficulties. He spoke of muscle degeneration caused by lack of vitamin E. He told of adults who had symptoms of muscle degeneration as evidenced by a substance that appeared in their urine. Giving large doses of vitamin E to these people caused this urine constituent to disappear indicating that, at last, these people were getting enough vitamin E.

He described many cases of muscle problems which were treated successfully with large doses of vitamin E. He mentioned the importance of the vitamin for the health of the red blood cells, stating that the anemia of premature infants is related in part to vitamin E deficiency. He spoke of blood clotting abnormalities normalized with vitamin E, and hereditary deficiencies which make supplementation with this nutrient absolutely essential. These disorders include sickle-cell anemia and all the disorders of malabsorption which we have discussed in other chapters.

He listed many common toxic substances which vitamin E renders harmless. He suggested that vitamin E may be the answer to retrolental fibroplasia, an eye condition so serious that it may result in blindness and which appears to be increasing. He mentioned that a recent report showed that 600 milligrams of vitamin E could, in only 30 days, cause a redistribution of cholesterol so that the helpful HDL fraction of this fatty substance is increased and pointed out that smoking may bring about a decrease in this substance.

Dr. Horwitt's article has 86 references to medical and scientific literature in his bibliography. Our only comment is what a pity that all physicians have not done, as Dr. Horwitt has done—reverse their former skepticism about vitamin therapy and use it every day in treating their patients.

# CHAPTER 50

# Vitamin E in Circulatory Diseases

IN A LITTLE BOOK *Common Questions on Vitamin E and Their Answers* by the staff of the Shute Foundation for Medical Research, the physicians replied to questions about vitamin E in treatment of varicose veins. They said, in part, "We originally refused to treat such patients, thinking it was absurd to believe that vitamin E had anything to offer them. But so many patients with such leg conditions, whom we treated for other cardiovascular diseases, told us how much their varices (varicose veins) improved that we finally decided it was worthy of trial and now we have become thoroughly convinced of its value."

They go on to describe what happens when these unsightly veins occur and how vitamin E probably aids in mobilizing collateral or "detour" circulation around the obstructed veins, so some of the burden is taken from the disordered veins. Although the appearance of the legs may not be greatly improved, there is less swelling, less pain and ache in the lower legs and the natural tendency of the veins to get worse may be halted. "Certainly everyone with varicose veins should try vitamin E before he considers operation and should also remember how poor the results of operation usually are," say the Shute physicians.

How about Buerger's Disease? This is generally found in men, usually rather young men, and smoking apparently makes it much worse. It involves the "terminal twigs" of

339

the arteries in the legs. Say the physicians, "the gradual and very painful process of obliteration of circulation in the tips of the toes and fingers may go on to gangrene which eventually involves all the extremities and may lead to multiple amputations."

Vitamin E in proper dosage gives good and prompt relief, they say, including the cramps which may occur in walking and the clots or gangrene. "Certainly every Buerger's patient should use vitamin E because alternative treatments are very discouraging, and here is a simple, cheap and effective alternative. It is also absolutely essential to stop tobacco. No one who continues to smoke is apt to get relief. This means stop—not slow down."

A rather common complaint these days is "restless legs" and cramps in the legs. *Southern Medical Journal* in 1974 described treatment of nine long-standing cases of these complaints with vitamin E. The authors got complete remission of complaints in seven of their patients and some control in the other two. Of 125 patients they treated over the years, they say, many had cramps for long years every night or several times every night.

About half the patients responded to 300 units daily of vitamin E. When they stopped taking the vitamin their troubles began again. The response to vitamin E was usually prompt— within a week. It goes without saying that anyone who has successfully treated these painful conditions with vitamin E should continue to take it daily.

In a Hungarian medical journal Dr. F. Gerloczy told of the beneficial effects of vitamin E for various circulatory disorders. He gave the vitamin sometimes in enormous doses—up to 24,000 milligrams daily. He treated successfully thrombosis of arteries (blood clots), Buerger's Disease and other circulatory disorders. One patient with a leg ulcer for 20 years was healed after only six weeks on vitamin E internally, plus a vitamin E ointment on the skin.

Three Italian physicians used vitamin E to treat complications of hardening of the arteries in old folks. Symptoms were confusion, loss of memory, dizziness and generally decreased mental acuteness. Forty-eight patients were given six capsules (of 150 milligrams each) of vitamin E daily. Improvement followed measured by memory, general intellectual status and other evidence of improved circulation in the brain. All the patients became more talkative and lively.

An editorial by Dr. Walter Alvarez in *Geriatrics*, volume 29, 1974 talked about "little strokes"—a moment of confusion, loss of memory or dizziness. He said Dr. Evan Shute had found that these disorders are very common and are helped greatly by vitamin E. Intermittent claudication is a circulatory disorder of the legs and feet which makes it almost impossible to walk any distance because of the extreme pain which occurs. A Swedish physician wrote in a Swedish medical journal how he treated this condition with 300 milligrams of vitamin E daily and told the patients to exercise and walk daily. There was significant improvement within four to six months.

In the January 10, 1972 *Journal of the American Medical Association* two California physicians recounted their experience with vitamin E in cases of leg cramps and "restless legs." Said Dr. Robert Cathcart, III such symptoms are common among his patients. He prescribed vitamin E in doses of 300 milligrams daily and said, "the medication is almost universally effective on . . . nocturnal leg cramps . . . Certainly the dosage we have been prescribing and the dosages taken by the health food advocates are in excess of anything conceived of being a minimum daily requirement for the vitamin. The amount used is also far in excess of what could possibly be obtained through any reasonably normal diet."

Some of his patients who stop the vitamin E are bothered by leg cramps in excess of those they first complained of. But only for a few days. After that they disappear. It seems these cramps come and go so some people prefer to continue with the vitamin E. Some patients find that their troubles continue if they drop their dosage of vitamin E to 100 or 200 milligrams daily, but no one has needed more than 300 milligrams.

Another California physician Dr. Samuel Ayers, Jr. has

reported on 26 patients with leg cramps, restless legs and rectal cramps. All of them obtained relief with doses of vitamin E ranging from 300 to 400 milligrams daily. He has reported on 76 cases of his, including one young athlete training for the Olympics who had severe cramps after strenuous exercise including long distance running, swimming and weight lifting. "All these patients received prompt and gratifying relief from oral administration of vitamin E," he says.

*The British Medical Journal* in 1974 discussed the power of vitamin E to maintain the membrane of red blood cells. Low levels of the vitamin put circulating red blood cells "at risk" said the editorial. Children not getting enough protein or vitamin E may suffer from a kind of anemia which results from lack of this vitamin. Treating them with iron seems to worsen the condition.

This brings us to a consideration of medicinal iron in relation to vitamin E. The kind of iron given by the doctor to correct iron deficiency anemia tends to destroy vitamin E. So if you are taking an iron "tonic," take your vitamin E at another time, as far removed from the iron pill as possible. Take one at bedtime, the other in the morning, for example. Iron which is present in natural food supplements does not cause this destruction of vitamin E.

*The New England Journal of Medicine* reported on an experiment by a Canadian physician who gave vitamin E for angina pectoris. This is the severe chest pain which accompanies certain heart conditions. Dr. W. M. Toone treated 22 patients from 61 to 73 years of age. He gave eleven of them a capsule containing nothing and the other eleven a capsule of vitamin E (400 milligrams) to be taken four times daily. He had already instituted a program for good heart health in all 22 of the men. He studied their progress for two years. During this time three patients in each group reduced considerably the amount of nitroglycerin they had to take to relieve the angina pain. Four patients taking the vitamin E reduced their dosage of the drug to one or two tablets a month. No one in the group getting no vitamin E could do this.

# VITAMIN E IN CIRCULATORY DISEASES

In a letter to *Canadian Family Physician*, volume 19, 1973 Dr. M. Lattey reported on his personal experience taking vitamin E for paroxysmal auricular fibrillation. This is extremely rapid, irregular and dangerous heart contractions. He began with 400 milligrams of vitamin E which proved to be not enough. He doubled the dose, took 800 milligrams of vitamin E daily and his heart returned to normal. He reported that he could exercise with no difficulty and had never enjoyed such good health as he did now. He added that the medical profession should take another look at the use of vitamin E for heart disease.

In a Polish medical journal, volume 90, Supplement 913, 1972 a Polish physician reported on 29 patients with many of the heart and artery symptoms which are becoming common among people in Western industrialized countries. They ranged in age from 38 to 72 years. They were suffering from coronary and circulatory problems, plus angina pectoris, myocardial infarction (one kind of heart attack), claudication, fatty liver and high blood levels of fat.

All were given six daily capsules of vitamin E with 150 milligrams in each capsule. As their conditions gradually improved, the dosage was reduced by half. In all cases, levels of blood fats went down within a few weeks. In some cases cholesterol levels were lowered by 100 percent or more. Others had less decrease of these levels. Diastolic blood pressure (the lower one) fell by an average of 15 mm of mercury. There were no harmful side effects.

These days we hear many warnings about blood cholesterol levels. Cholesterol is a fatty substance that accumulates in arteries and eventually may close them off, creating hardening of the arteries and other circulatory troubles. Cholesterol is, however, an essential body compound. It is used in many body functions. It is manufactured in the human liver so that, when there is little cholesterol in the diet, the liver manufactures more. When we eat more cholesterol, the liver stops making it.

An article in *Physiology, Chemistry and Physics*, volume 5, 1973 states that the fat soluble vitamins A, D, E and K stop the liver from manufacturing too much cholesterol. In rabbits with muscular dystrophy there were high concentrations of cholesterol in blood and muscle. The animals were also deficient in vitamin E. In rabbits fed plenty of vitamin E cholesterol levels in both blood and muscle were much lower than in those animals fed diets lacking vitamin E.

One scientist has reported that, in human muscular dystrophy, muscles have a higher than normal accumulation of cholesterol. It seems possible, does it not, that lack of vitamin E, along with other factors, may play an important role in human muscular dystrophy. Studies of cholesterol manufactured in the livers of animals on diets deficient in vitamin E suggest strongly that vitamin E participates in controlling cholesterol.

The three authors of this article say it appears that vitamin E not only influences the production of cholesterol, but also the way it is used by the cells. This leads to the suggestion that lack of enough vitamin E may be one of the causes of high blood levels of cholesterol.

*Nutrition Reports International,* volume 10, no. 6, 1974 described experiments with mice which indicated that the older the animals are the more vitamin E they need to protect tissues from rancid fats caused by oxygen. This activity creates destructive compounds called "free radicals" and vitamin E is useful for destroying them.

# CHAPTER 51

# A Survey Reveals Vast Health Improvement from Vitamin E

In 1974 *Prevention* magazine asked their readers to answer a questionnaire on vitamin E and its effects on their health. They received 20,000 replies, a magnificent testimony to the loyalty of health seekers who take vitamin E regularly and are willing to take the time and trouble to tell the rest of us about their experiences.

The survey was conducted and studied by Richard A. Passwater, a biochemist, author of a fine book on vitamin therapy—*Super-Nutrition, The Megavitamin Revolution*. Reporting on the results in *Prevention*, Dr. Passwater stated that a critical level which appears to influence the possibility of developing heart disease is 300 I.U. of vitamin E daily. Occasionally, he says, "people taking 200 I.U. of vitamin E daily developed heart disease (generally in the late 80's) or showed little improvement. When they increased their dosage they experienced improvement. Only one case of heart trouble was reported to have developed at a higher dosage level." This was in the group of people responding to the survey who were 80 years old or older.

"The suggestion emerges," said Passwater, "that among persons over 80 taking 1,200 I.U. or more of vitamin E daily after a heart attack improves chances of complete recovery and that taking 300 I.U. or more of vitamin E daily for 10 years or more reduces the chances of ever developing heart disease. There is also a hint (in the replies that came in) that eating a balanced diet even in the absence of vitamin E supplements had a considerable protective effect against heart disease. The survey supports those observations but does not prove them.''

In following issues of *Prevention* Dr. Passwater reviewed comments from people of various age groups who replied to the survey. Testimony was almost unbelievable—of heart troubles overcome, circulatory symptoms overcome, much more vigor and freedom from pain, as well as many comments on conditions other than circulatory ones, comments which were volunteered by the respondents although they had not been asked to say anything on their ailments.

The 50 to 59-age group consisted of replies from 6,205 men and women. Of these, 818 had heart disease. Correlating the replies, Dr. Passwater found that:

1. Taking 400 I.U. or more of vitamin E is strongly associated with reducing the incidence of heart disease to one-tenth or less of the risk for this age group in a general population not taking the vitamin.

2. Taking 1,200 I.U. or more of vitamin E for four years or more is strongly associated with reducing the risk of heart disease to less than one-third of the risk for this age group in the general population.

3. More than 80 percent of the people who responded to the survey who already have had heart conditions (including tachycardia, angina and fibrillation) reported that their condition improved when they used vitamin E.

Here are some striking comments from people in this age group. A woman had had two heart attacks 15 years ago, had taken 400 units of vitamin E ever since. No more attacks. Another woman had fibrillation (rapid, disorganized heart beat) and high blood pressure. She had been taking 800 I.U. for 10 years, has had no more attacks and now has a normal heart rhythm. A husband with a heart attack is now taking 1,200 units of E, his wife, also victim of a heart attack, takes 800 units daily. The vitamin has lowered their blood pressure and their cholesterol count and "helped both hearts to heal." A woman whose heartbeat was 200 per minute put herself on 800 units of vitamin E when doctors could do nothing more for her. She has been well since then.

Of the group of people 60 to 69 years of age who responded to the survey, Dr. Passwater says, perhaps the single most important age group to study for heart disease is the 60 to 69 age group. This age group has the highest incidence of heart disease and still includes in its numbers those individuals who are destined not to survive beyond the average lifespan.

He had 6,459 replies to the questionnaire of whom 1,543 said they have heart disease. Their replies showed, in general, what the younger group had shown—that 400 units of vitamin E daily for 10 years or more reduces the incidence of heart disease to one-tenth or less of the risk of heart disease for people not taking the vitamin. Taking 1,200 units or more for four years or more seems to reduce the risk of heart disease to less than one-third of the risk for this age group. More than 80 percent of those with heart trouble reported that the vitamin improved their condition.

Says Dr. Passwater, "You can't take vitamin E as a preventive measure and do everything else wrong. If you smoke, drink, are inactive, overstrain, don't rest or eat properly, taking a pound of vitamin E daily won't completely protect you from heart disease, especially if you are genetically prone to it. However, you could be better off than if you didn't take any vitamin E at all."

Some comments from the respondents in their sixties are illuminating. A woman reported on curing her angina and a heart murmur with 400 units of vitamin E. When she stopped taking the vitamin for six months both of these conditions returned. She began again and her problems vanished. A woman with coronary thrombosis and phlebitis reported that both improved greatly while she took vitamin E. A man with three coronary attacks and hardening of the arteries reported that he gave up his nitroglycerin tablets one year after starting vitamin E—800 units daily. Another man testified that a number of friends *who are also MD's have had coronaries and all are taking from 800 to 1,200 units of vitamin E daily.* A man with severe pains from angina increased his intake of vitamin E from 100 to 400 units daily with slight improvement. When he increased it to 800 units "the improvement was fantastic," he said.

From the group of *Prevention* readers who are in their 70's, 4,060 replies were received. The same trend appears in this group: people who have taken 300 or more units of vitamin E daily for ten years or more are not likely to develop heart disease. And neither are people taking 1,200 units or more daily for more than three years.

Many of the people in their seventies wrote of pain treated with vitamin E. A 75-year old man said, "I would waken every morning early about four or five A.M. with my eyeballs hurting, severe pains in the temples and back of the neck. I was also nauseated. I felt like I was losing my mind. In just two weeks of 800 units of vitamin E the condition improved and has been relieved ever since."

A seventy-five-year old man with a coronary 30 years ago has been taking 1,200 units of vitamin E daily and has had no recurrence. A 75-year old woman had angina pectoris and weakness of heart valves. She has been taking vitamin E for 22 years. At the time of the survey she was taking 2,400 units daily. Her blood pressure had dropped to a healthy 120/80, her cholesterol level was down to 150.

A 71-year old woman has been taking vitamin E since 1958 after a Mayo Clinic diagnosis of such severe heart damage that she required surgery. She has been taking high doses of vitamin E since 1958 and was at the time taking 600 units daily. Her doctors said she had no heart damage and very little angina pain. A 71-year old woman had been taking two heart medications plus three kinds of diuretics and had been told by her doctors that she could not ever live without digitalis. She started to take 1,000 units of vitamin E daily. By gradually increasing all her vitamin and mineral intake, she was at the time able to do without the drugs. She was taking 800 units of vitamin E.

Dr. Passwater said, in part, ". . . these comments are

not accepted as scientific proof that vitamin E prevents or cures heart disease. Rigid controlled studies involving 'double-blind' tests are required for evidence of validity by most scientists. Yet the information is useful. I do not know of any large-scale well-controlled, double-blind test that proves aspirin cures headaches. But physicians and lay people 'know' it does through experience.

"Similarly many physicians know that vitamin E relieves angina pain and prescribe it, others have tried it and not seen the improvement described here, and still other physicians refuse even to try vitamin E. The main obstacle seems to be that many physicians have not considered the dose-time relationship required. They have tried too-little dosage for a too-little time. Now they should test the 300-plus units for 10-plus years or 1,200-plus units for three-plus years."

What about people in their eighties who replied to the questionnaire? Here are some comments from them. In this group the same general condition prevailed—the level of 300 units of vitamin E daily appeared to influence the risk to heart disease. Dr. Passwater believes the figures he collected show that in those over 80, taking 1,200 units of vitamin E daily after a heart attack improves chances of complete recovery and taking 300 units daily for ten years or more reduces the chances of having a heart attack.

One 84-year old woman had been taking vitamin E for 30 years. She had been experimenting with dosage and with other elements in diet and way of life. She was taking 500–600 units at the time of the survey and was in excellent health. An 86-year old man had two heart attacks years earlier, began taking 1,800 units of vitamin E daily and had been free from attacks for 25 years at the time of the survey. An 81-year old woman with phlebitis and a leg ulcer had been taking vitamin E for 25 years, mostly in doses of 1,000 units daily. All her circulatory problems cleared up. An 81-year old woman had a coronary thrombosis (heart attack caused by a blood clot) 20 years earlier. Fifteen years before the survey she began to take vitamin E and reported that she was in very good health. An 86-year old man had no more angina pains since he began to take 600 units of vitamin E daily for six years.

Many other fascinating bits of testimony turned up on the *Prevention* survey. Although no questions were asked about conditions other than circulatory ones, a great deal of evidence came in on improvement in other conditions as well. Most astonishing of all, 70 physicians replied to the questionnaire, 66 of whom had been taking vitamin E from one to 29 years. An 89-year old physician treated himself and his patients with vitamin E. He had had very serious heart trouble 26 years earlier. He has taken 800 units of vitamin E daily for 26 years. A man described as a "well-known" New York physician reported to *Prevention* that his last electrocardiogram and blood pressure were normal two years after taking 1,000 units of vitamin E daily after a coronary thrombosis. Another doctor claimed he cured his prostatitis with 800 units of vitamin E daily. That is the first such testimony we have ever seen on that condition.

It is cheering indeed to read such valuable and unsolicited remarks from people who had suffered for years from one or another disease. And not one word of any unpleasant side effects from really immense doses of vitamin E. One can only wonder why official medicine does not realize the significance of all this and take another look at the harm they may be doing with pills and surgery when the answer for most people may lie in a small capsule of a perfectly natural substance taken regularly every day for life.

# CHAPTER 52

# Vitamin E Is Powerful Against Ulcers and Open Sores

IN DECEMBER, 1974 a nurse in a small town hospital in Pennsylvania was using vitamin E against sores and ulcers. A 59-year-old diabetic woman with ulceration of the right foot was taking no drugs when she came to the hospital. The doctors immediately gave her insulin and 800 milligrams of vitamin E. Then they packed the ulcerated area with cotton saturated with vitamin E. Two months later all wounds were healed.

A second case is that of a 72-year-old woman with partial bowel obstruction and a huge bed sore (decubitus ulcer, doctors call it) which covered most of the upper part of her buttocks. The ulcer was treated with daily applications of vitamin E and the patient was given 800 units of vitamin E by mouth every day. Treatment was begun in February, 1974 and was completed in August, 1974. Said Dorothy Fisher, the nurse who wrote this article in Dr. Evan Shute's publication, *The Summary,* "In less than six months there was total healing and the area involved has remained well healed. The area now looks very healthy."

A 25-year-old man, a paraplegic, had been crippled in a car accident. Bedfast, he developed bed sores on the buttocks, in the right leg and left foot. He had been treated without success in five different hospitals and rehabilitation institutions. He was given 400 milligrams of vitamin E daily, plus 250 milligrams of vitamin C and his bedsores were treated

351

topically with vitamin E liniment. A month later the dose of vitamin E was increased to 600 milligrams daily, later to 800 milligrams daily. He was sent home completely healed and at the time the article was written he was still taking 400 milligrams of vitamin E daily along with applications to any body area where bed sores were developing.

The fourth case treated by this devoted nurse was a woman of 63 who had been operated on for cancer of the rectum. The surgeon performed a colostomy. The opening or *stoma* which he created for evacuation of the bowel became infected and ulcerated. It and the area around it were treated with vitamin E ointment daily and the patient was given 400 milligrams of vitamin E daily. Within six days all the area of badly ulcerated skin was completely healed.

In the same issue of *The Summary,* a Long Island (New York) doctor reported on 20 schizophrenia patients suffering from severe circulatory disorders in their legs. Three had gangrene, one had a perforating ulcer which had never completely healed in two years. Nine other patients had infected dermatitis on the insides of their legs.

All were diabetic, maintained on strict diets and an oral drug for diabetes. "The patients often committed breaches of diet," said their physician. They were given 20 to 40 capsules daily of vitamin E with 400 milligrams per capsule. Said the physician, "The gangrenous areas are healing. These dramatic results were described by visiting interns as incredible. The patients were maintained on a daily average of 20 capsules of 400 milligrams of vitamin E each and four months after healing of the ulcers the patients are well and without leg pain."

An Italian doctor reported in 1973 on experiments with rats in whom he had induced bed sores. They had suffered from these for five months when he gave them 65 milligrams daily of vitamin E—a very large amount for an animal as small as a mouse. Within two weeks of therapy the bed sores were healed.

In an editorial in *Geriatrics,* volume 29, page 159, 1974, Dr. W. C. Alvarez described what doctors call "little strokes"—common lapses of memory and speech with perhaps a moment of dizziness, which afflict many of us as we grow older. Dr. Alvarez said these are usually greatly improved by vitamin E taken regularly.

In a letter to the editor of *Archives of Dermatology* in 1973, two physicians reported using vitamin E for patients suffering from the neuralgia that afflicted them after a session of the nerve disorder, shingles. The doctors treated these patients with oral and topical vitamin E. Eleven of the patients had suffered for more than six months, seven for more than one year, one for 13 years and one for 19 years. These last two patients had almost complete relief from pain with the vitamin E treatment. Two were moderately improved and two were slightly improved. The doctors gave dosages of 400 to 1,600 milligrams of vitamin E per day.

One of the patients had angina, the agonizing pain that afflicts heart patients. Taking 1,200 milligrams of vitamin E daily she controlled the neuralgia. She also cured the leg cramps that had made her miserable and found that she no longer needed nitroglycerin, the drug she had been taking to control the angina.

A 53-year old diabetic man had a perforating ulcer of the foot so serious that he could not move the fourth and fifth toes. His ulcer was healed in two months with no treatment other than vitamin E. A 58-year old diabetic woman had an ulcer on the sole of one foot and advanced osteoporosis of the bones of her feet. The ulcer was healed in a few months and an ulcer on the same foot was healed later with no treatment other than vitamin E.

A five-year old boy, badly burned, with itchy keloid scars, had his discomfort ended when vitamin E ointment was applied locally. A 46-year old woman with second and third degree burns of the hand and forearm recovered within a week on vitamin E by mouth and applied locally.

These are only a few of the stunning case histories told in *The Summary* which was published by the Shute Foundation for Medical Research for many years. The Canadian physician, Dr. Evan Shute, was editor of *The Summary*. He worked with vitamin E for many years and used it routinely for treating a multitude of disorders and wounds. His success with complications of diabetes seems almost miraculous. The 53-year old man described above had been taking insulin for 15 years. He would not adhere to his diet. On 375 milligrams of vitamin E he healed completely in 71 days and could reduce his intake of insulin to about one-third of what it had been. He returned to work.

The diabetic woman who was obviously suffering from many kinds of malnutrition, including calcium, was given 600 milligrams of vitamin E daily. Within two months she was allowed to walk on her ulcerated foot. She was healed clinically and by x-ray observation within several months. Her second diabetic ulcer also healed quickly with vitamin E.

The burned child suffered from scars resulting from skin grafts. Vitamin E ointment was applied to the scars and, although he was given no vitamin E by mouth, just the ointment cleared all his problems within a few days. The woman who burned her hand was a long-time devotee of vitamin E. She began to take large doses of the vitamin immediately after she was burned. Then she wrapped her arm in a bandage and set off for the Shute Clinic. They treated her with saline bubble-baths and more vitamin E ointment applied three times daily. She was almost completely recovered within eight days, suffered no pain and had no contractures of the burned area and no scars.

Dr. Shute said he did not know why vitamin E relieves the pain of burn victims. He said he rarely had to send a burned patient for grafting and never had to repeat it. Since vitamin E is slightly anti-infective, wounds are usually clean, an important factor in the "take" of grafts. He said further that burned patients are rushed to the hospital and given the usual orthodox medical treatment so it is difficult to teach medical school patients the helpfulness of vitamin E, even if anyone at the hospital had any desire to learn. Scars left by the usual treatment, including grafts, can permanently cripple people and end their careers if the small joints involved are essential parts of their work—as with a surgeon, a musician or someone doing very fine, intricate work.

For burns of the conjunctiva of the eyes, Dr. Shute recommended opening a capsule of 400 to 800 milligrams of vitamin E and pouring the vitamin into the eye. Many readers of our books have reported similar incidents of curing many kinds of wounds, cuts, abrasions, as well as burns. Most of them took large doses of vitamin E as well as applying it locally.

"If vitamin E is useful for burns it should help frostbite or immersion foot," said Dr. Shute, "and be of great value to aviators and mountain climbers. I got in touch with Sir Edmund Hilary prior to his last climb in the Himalayas and suggested that vitamin E be included in their resources on that ascent. He courteously acknowledged my suggestion, but I heard nothing from his doctor. The sequel was tragic, as we all know."

"Vitamin E should be in every kitchen for convenient use. Every parent should have it handy for the children. As in coronary attacks the best results can be achieved only if treatment is prompt," said Dr. Shute. He says that, in treating skin ulcers, there are at least sixty reports in medical literature which mention the help that vitamin E has brought, mostly in cases of chronic ulcers.

"When everything else has failed," he says, "we suggest alphatocopherol (vitamin E) both orally and locally. The latter is what means most, we suspect. It must be remembered that many people are sensitive to local tocopherol. The latter may induce . . . a rash over part or all of the body. This means one should dilute the ointment or stop its use altogether, continuing with its oral exhibition only."

# CHAPTER 53

# Does Vitamin E Delay Aging?

THE STARTLING EVIDENCE came from human cells kept alive in a laboratory culture. Under normal laboratory conditions such cells might live for 50 generations of cell division. But when a small amount of vitamin E was added, the human cells in the test tube continued to reproduce beyond more than 120 divisions. Then the scientists conducting the research discontinued the experiment.

Drs. Lester Packer and James R. Smith of the University of California stated that the cells appeared to show no signs of old age. They were still completely normal and going on about the healthy business of dividing, just as they had when the experiment began. Scientists generally accept the theory that cells have a built-in life-span depending on the inheritance of the individual. You inherit a set of cells which will see you through to a healthy old age, other things being equal. Or, because of a long line of short-lived, unhealthy ancestors, you may have inherited a tendency to succumb to many diseases and die at an early age.

But now it seems that the magic of vitamin E may have proved this theory to be false. Perhaps just getting enough and more than enough vitamin E may enable the individual with a poor heritage to live much longer than expected.

The California scientists deny that their research demonstrates anything like this, of course. According to *The New York Times* for September 2, 1974, they stated that the most immediate benefits of this world-shaking discovery will be to benefit scientists. Now they can keep human cells alive long enough in a laboratory to investigate human genetics and develop ways to tinker with the genetics of human cells. Then, too, researchers can use such long-living cells to evaluate the effects of environmental stress, like pollutants, on cell life.

So, said they, this doesn't mean at all that taking vitamin E will prolong life or will turn the clock back for a 40-year old and make him or her feel like 18. And why not? Well, said another California researcher who has done much work with vitamin E, everybody gets so much vitamin E in their food that the body has large stored reserves to draw upon, hence getting any more would be useless.

This is the kind of argument some scientists use when they are confronted with laboratory experiments which prove beyond a shadow of a doubt that some extraordinary vital substance exists in a given vitamin which performs almost magically on individual cells. Now consider for a moment that the human cell under the microscope which went right on behaving like a young, vital cell way past the time when it should have stopped dividing, apparently contained enough vitamin E to be a healthy cell. There was no indication that these cells were deficient in vitamin E. But when more vitamin E was added, the effects were entirely different from what happened to other cells being studied, which had not been given extra vitamin E. Is it not possible that whole human beings might expect this same effect, since the vitamin affects individual cells that way and since human bodies are nothing but collections of human cells?

Drs. Packer and Smith went on to make two of the most highly contradictory remarks we have ever heard from scientists. "Vitamin E won't extend life in humans," they said, "except in the possible case where humans are subjected to severe environmental pollution." (Aren't we all?) And then they went on to say, according to the *Times*, "Even if vitamin E can't turn a 40-year old into a 14-year old, it might prevent an early death, or brain disease, heart attacks or senility. Of course, we don't know these things at all, yet."

And the two scientists, who have presumably been told for years that we all get plenty of vitamin E in our food, are now taking 200 milligrams of vitamin E daily in capsules!

In the tenth volume of *Executive Health*, Dr. Linus Pauling speaks his mind on vitamin E. As one would expect, it is very much worth listening to.

He begins by outlining the course of vitamin E in present-day medicine. More than 40 years ago three Canadian physicians began to use it in their treatment of disease. These were Drs. Evan and Wilfrid Shute and their father, Dr. R. James Shute. They reported excellent results. But official medicine on this continent refused to accept these results and steadfastly averred that vitamin E has no place in human health in amounts larger than the officially recommended amount of 12 milligrams per day, as it was at that time. Says Dr. Pauling, "It is my opinion that the authorities are wrong about vitamin E as they were about vitamin C."

In 1956, Dr. Pauling tells us, a researcher experimented with a diet which contained only three milligrams of vitamin E. Nine volunteers ate a diet containing only this small amount of vitamin E while a comparable group of volunteers had diets containing 18 milligrams of vitamin E. Within six months the people getting the small amount of vitamin E began to develop fragile red blood cells resulting in anemia and the concentration of the vitamin in their blood began slowly to decline. The volunteers on larger amounts of vitamin E had no such problems.

Dr. Pauling explains that the main function of vitamin E is its ability to prevent the rancidity or oxidation of fats in the tissues of the body. "Vitamin E is the principal fat-soluble antioxidant," says he, "and vitamin C (ascorbic acid) is the principal water-soluble antioxidant. They probably co-operate in providing protection for our bodies and slowing the aging process."

The late Dr. Roger J. Williams is quoted as saying in his book *Nutrition Against Disease:* "Vitamin E is thought to be the leading agent for the prevention of peroxidation and the free radical production which is associated both with it and with radiation. Vitamin E—along with . . . other antioxidants—do their jobs in a complicated manner. They protect the body against the damaging products formed when oxygen reacts directly with the highly unsaturated fatty substances which are essential parts of our metabolic machinery.

"We do not know all the details of how these antioxidants do their work in practical situations, and the information probably would not be of interest to laymen anyway. As a practical matter, providing plenty of vitamin E and ascorbic acid (vitamin C)—both harmless antioxidants—is indicated as a possible means of preventing premature aging, especially if one's diet is rich in polyunsaturated acids."

Dr. Williams goes on to describe the brown pigments (like freckles) which are often found on the skin of older people. Such deposits are not just on skin. They are also found in the brain, the heart, the adrenal gland and many other parts of the body. They seem to represent lack of vitamin E, since they are symptoms of rancidity which has not been prevented and which vitamin E and vitamin C can and do prevent.

The stubborn refusal of the medical hierarchy to accept thousands of pieces of evidence of the healthfulness of vitamin E could be settled easily, says Dr. Pauling, by setting up a series of tests in which one large group of heart and circulatory patients are given vitamin E dosages recommended by specialists like the Shutes and other physicians who use the vitamin, while another matched group of volunteers with circulatory problems get the usual medical treatment with no vitamin E. The Shutes themselves can not conduct such trials, he says, since their duty is to treat all their patients with the very best treatment they know, which is of course, vitamin E.

Dr. Pauling quotes Dr. Alton Ochsner, the distinguished surgeon, as saying that for many years he has used vitamin E (100 I.U. three times a day) for surgical patients to prevent blood clots in veins. The vitamin is a "potent inhibitor" of the blood clots which are such a fearful aftermath of surgery in many instances. Drugs which prevent blood clots are likely to bring about hemorrhages unless they are regulated with extreme care. Vitamin E presents no such problems.

A "free radical" is defined as a highly reactive compound in which the central element is linked to an abnormal number of atoms or groups of atoms, along with the presence of at least one unpaired electron. This doesn't mean much to the layman, but free radicals are apparently very destructive of health. One scientist, J. M. Washburn, speculates in *The Gerontologist,* volume 13, page 436, 1973, that free radical reactions in the arteries which carry blood may be the cause of hardening of the arteries. A layer of fat collects on the inner lining of the artery, more fat collects on top of that and the damage that ensues appears to be caused by "free radicals."

Studying animals, this researcher discovered that the liver of an animal on a diet deficient in vitamin E contains a large amount of free radicals—50 times more than would be produced by a damaging amount of radiation. Thus, vitamin E may be very important, says he. Along with other antioxidants it may increase the life span of animals. And, we would add, presumably also human beings.

In line with these findings, it is not surprising to find, in *Chemical and Engineering News* for September 30, 1974, that one scientist treated human cells enriched with vitamin E in a test tube and found that he could prolong their lives for as much as 120 generations of cell division, compared to a span of 50 generations, for untreated cells. The vitamin was apparently acting as an antioxidant in this experiment.

While we cannot, from this, decide finally that getting plenty of vitamin E will enable us all to live longer lives in good health, it does seem wise, does it not, to make certain we get lots of the vitamin at meals and in food supplements, since it seems to have a protective action in so many areas of health, and since it seems to be totally harmless in any amounts?

And finally, here's an account of an experiment reported in the May 1973 *Proceedings of the National Academy of Sciences*. Damage to chromosomes, the genetic material in cells, has been linked to cancer and the aging process. If we could prevent the damage to chromosomes perhaps we could prevent cancer and retard aging.

Vitamin E, vitamin C and two other antioxidants have now been shown to reduce damage to chromosomes in blood cells exposed to chemicals known to be cancer-causing. Vitamin E gave 63.8 percent protection against chromosome breakage and vitamin C gave 31.7 percent protection.

The Cleveland Clinic Foundation scientists who conducted the experiment believe, they say, that "The protection against chromosomal breakage provided by antioxidants may have important relationships to aging and carcinogenesis (cancer)."

Certain nutrients that help to protect us against aging were reported in the March, 1980 issue of *Executive Health*. Dr. Al Tappel, Ph.D., of the University of California mentioned oxidation as one of the causes of aging. The "free radicals" caused by this process can be controlled by vitamin E among other nutrients, he said. When tissues suffer from attacks by free radicals a dark pigment is formed—called "age pigment." We are most familiar with them when they occur on face, arms and hands.

"It has been long known," says Dr. Tappel, "that if dietary levels of vitamin E are below the RDA, the body will be subjected to much free radical damage through life." Dr. Tappel has fed mice with doses of vitamin E equivalent to 2,000 milligrams a day for a human being, also giving them some vitamin C and trace minerals. At the end of a year the mice given these supplements showed far less of the "age pigment" in their tissues than a similar group of mice not given the supplements.

Dr. Tappel has also shown definite protection from certain elements of air pollution when these nutrients are given, especially vitamin E. So it seems that our present epidemics of bronchitis, emphysema and lung cancer might prove less overwhelming if all of us were getting enough vitamin E. Dr. Tappel has found that vitamin E protects us to some extent from heavy metal pollutants that we may encounter frequently in our environment: cadmium, lead and mercury which harm many of us who work in industries where these metals are used or because they live in areas where the metals pollute soil, air and water. The PCB's and chloroform found in some areas as water pollutants are also rendered less harmful by vitamin E.

Dr. Tappel reminds us that no human being who lived previous to the past 50 years or so was ever assaulted by the variety and persistence of pollutants that surround us every day of our lives, so it seems possible that our need for supplementation with vitamin E increases with the amount of exposure we have to these poisons. Vitamins are among the least expensive protective items you can buy. Can you suggest any surer guarantee against harm from environmental pollutants, short of moving to a desert island?

*Medical Tribune* reported January 8, 1986 that Dr. Jeffrey Blumberg of the U.S.D.A. Human Nutrition Center on Aging at Tufts University had found evidence that vitamin E given in high doses to aging animals causes several characteristics of immune function in those animals to be equal to those functions in younger animals. "This may mean," he said, "that old animals have higher requirements for vitamin E than young animals in terms of immune system responsiveness." Studies with elderly human beings were in progress at this Center, where volunteers are being given 800 milligrams of vitamin E daily. Dr. Blumberg also reminded us that some over-the-counter drugs popular with older folks can cause depletion of some nutrients.

In a discussion of Alzheimer's Disease and Parkinson's Disease, four researchers from British Columbia and New York theorize in *The Lancet,* November 8, 1986 on the usefulness of vitamin E because of its ability to detoxify "free radicals," those destructive substances formed in cells by oxidation of fats. Alzheimer's Disease and Parkinson's Disease are both more common in older folks.

# CHAPTER 54

# Using Vitamin E in Medicine

So MANY USES of vitamin E are reported in medical literature that one does not know where to begin to describe them. And one cannot help but wonder why, with all this information available to physicians, vitamin E is not being used in every doctor's office to treat a wide variety of disorders.

A report from Japan states that giving vitamin E helps to cure liver damage by protecting certain fatty tissues in the liver from oxidation. Japanese physicians also use vitamin E to boost that very helpful kind of cholesterol—high density lipoprotein (HDL). They used the vitamin in groups of the elderly and in post-stroke victims.

Since vitamin E is fat soluble, it is to be expected that this vitamin might be deficient in people whose digestive tracts do not handle fats normally. Vitamin E would disappear along with the fats that are excreted undigested. Those individuals who suffer from these conditions are generally well aware of their problems with retaining all the fat soluble vitamins. Celiac-sprue disease, Crohn's Disease, cystic fibrosis, chronic diarrhea—all these are conditions in which fat soluble vitamins are lost and must be replaced by supplements.

Said John G. Bieri, Ph.D. in *The New England Journal of Medicine* May 5, 1983, "Among the conditions for which vitamin E has been prescribed are angina, muscular dystrophy, infertility, purpura (easy bruising), scleroderma and diabetes. Conditions still being investigated include cystic mastitis, certain types of ulcers and wounds, intermittent claudication and habitual abortion."

Very significant statements on vitamin E appeared in an editorial in *The New England Journal of Medicine*. Frank A. Oski, M.D., wrote of this vitamin's power as an antioxidant. Free radicals, he says, can damage membrane lipids (fats) and even denature DNA. DNA is the substance in every body cell that carries hereditary information for the production of all future cells in that individual and all of that individual's offspring. To produce perfect offspring born to perfect parents the DNA must be undamaged. Vitamin E can provide just such protection.

In individuals who cannot normally digest and absorb vitamin E, fat soluble vitamins cannot maintain normal amounts of red blood cells. These are the blood cells that carry oxygen to all body cells. Red blood cells are susceptible to destruction by oxygen (oxidation) if all the body mechanisms—enzymes for example—which protect them from this are not functioning normally. In some cases people are born with deficiency in these enzymes so they will probably have difficulty maintaining blood levels of red cells throughout life.

Some such patients have been found to respond to vitamin E in very large doses. Others, with a different kind of enzyme deficiency, were treated with 800 milligrams of vitamin E daily and the life of their red blood cells was extended up to normal. The authors of this study stated, "This study demonstrates that supplementation with vitamin E at a dose without known toxicity, was associated with a reduction in the mild chronic hemolysis (destruction of red blood cells) in patients with inherited deficiency in the essential enzymes."

High density lipoprotein (HDL) is a waxy, fatty substance found in the blood which appears to be very helpful in preventing heart attacks and other circulatory problems. Another fatty substance, called LDL (low density lipoprotein) is apparently harmful. A group of Japanese scientists measured the red blood cells in a number of patients—elderly people who had had strokes and healthy people. They found that vitamin E levels were low in the red cells of the elderly and in patients who had had strokes. Then they measured the amount of vitamin E in various kinds of body fat. In the healthy people they found that vitamin E was most abundant in HDL. By comparison, the elderly had lower levels of vitamin E in their HDL and higher levels of LDL, the kind of fat known to be harmful.

A research scientist at the Ludwig Institute for Cancer Research in Toronto, Canada has described studies indicating that deficiencies in both vitamin C and vitamin E may be related to cancer. Dr. Elizabeth Bright-See said, "Some research indicates that populations with a high incidence of esophageal or stomach cancer do not eat enough foods containing vitamin C. And the effects of vitamin C and E are already being studied in people at high risk for colon cancer."

She continued, "Both vitamins block the conversion of nitrates and nitrites to nitrosamines, which have produced tumors in experimental animals. Although we lack conclusive proof that nitrosamines cause cancer in humans, it is only prudent to reduce our exposure to them as much as possible." Nitrates and nitrites are in many processed meats such as delicatessen lunch meats. They also occur naturally in drinking water in some localities and in many foods, especially vegetables, probably due to nitrogen fertilizers.

"Although the food industry has reduced the amounts of nitrates and nitrites used to cure meats and is already adding vitamin C to some nitrate-cured products, even the most stringent control won't protect us from the nitrates in water and foods," says the Canadian scientist, "Thus the practical approach may be to use nitrosamine-blocking agents such as vitamin C and E."

An article in *Science* described a laboratory experiment using liver cells incubated with three different toxic chemicals. Adding vitamin E to the medium in which the cells were growing completely protected the cells from injury from the poisons. The authors of the article from the Department of Biochemistry and Biophysics at Oregon State University state that vitamin E is an antioxidant and a scavenger of free radicals. Antioxidants protect cells against being oxidized or made rancid. Free radicals are segments of cells that react with the fats in cell walls generating a chain reaction that produces more and more free radicals. These can be held in check, say the scientists, by ample amounts of vitamins A, C and E. In this experiment it was the vitamin E that kept the cells healthy in spite of their exposure to toxic chemicals.

In modern industrialized nations we are exposed every day to an unknown number of toxic pollutants in air and water, as well as in food and in the household products we use. Many of us are also exposed to toxic chemicals at work. There is abundant evidence that just one vitamin E capsule a day can give lots of protection. It also helps to get plenty of vitamin C and vitamin A.

The prestigious *New England Journal of Medicine* published a lengthy article titled "Medical Uses of Vitamin E" in its May 5, 1983 issue. The three authors were from the National Institutes of Health, that branch of the federal government which deals with various diseases and their possible cure or prevention.

The article says, "It should be recognized at the outset that nutritional inadequacy or frank deficiency of vitamin E is found only in patients with various genetic or acquired diseases with the exception of premature children in whom the deficiency may be iatrogenous (caused by medical treatment)."

They continue to say that "the average American diet contains from eight to 11 milligrams of vitamin E." One of the references they give for this statement is an article which appeared in 1964 in the *American Journal of Clinical Nutrition*. The NIH spokesmen did not mention that the researchers who wrote this 1965 article planned highly nutritious diets which were purposely rich in vitamin E with plenty of wholegrain cereals and breads, lots of eggs, meat and green leafy vegetables as well as salad oils and margarine. They then analyzed these diets and discovered that they contained only seven milligrams of vitamin E, whereas the RDA for vitamin E at that time was 15 milligrams. So the article proved without a shadow of a doubt that even people who eat every day the most perfectly planned diets with vitamin E-rich foods emphasized cannot get more than seven milligrams of vitamin E per day.

At this point the official body which sets the RDA's, the National Academy of Sciences, decided that since nobody seems to show any deficiency disease from not getting enough vitamin E, they would reduce the official RDA. And they did—reduced it to 10 milligrams for adult males, eight milligrams for adult females. Since nobody was assigned officially to study what various diseases in our society might be related to vitamin E deficiency, the official opinion now is that there is no such disease!

*The New England Journal of Medicine* article states that vitamin E, being fat-soluble, is not absorbed by people who have no ability to digest and absorb fats. Since there must be a very large number of such people among us, there must be a large number of Americans who get not nearly enough vitamin E at meals, no matter how well planned their diets are. However, try as they might, officials from NIH could not come up with any evidence that large doses of vitamin E could be harmful in any way. They said, "The bulk of evidence to date indicates that a daily intake in the range of 200 to 600 milligrams is innocuous in most people."

The February, 1980 issue of *Runner's World* published an article on the use of vitamin E by long-distance runners. Dr. Michael Weiner, the author, pointed out that in long-distance running the chief requirement is endurance. Vitamin E is known to improve the utilization of oxygen by the heart, hence improve endurance.

"Fatigue is a result of oxygen starvation in the blood," said Weiner, "Numerous studies have proven that vitamin E levels decline as oxygen requirements increase, and are related to fatigue. Vitamin E combined with aerobic exercise, increases the oxygen-carrying capacity of hemoglobin in the blood, leading to greater dynamic capabilities of the lungs.

Since stores of this vitamin are depleted during stress, a case can be made for the need of vitamin E supplements to ensure physical stamina in the long-distance runner.''

Vitamin E also protects against the stresses of any vigorous exercise, says Dr. Weiner. ''For many long-distance runners in our clinic,'' he says, ''megadoses of vitamin E (up to 1,000 milligrams a day) are valuable in reducing night leg cramps.'' He stresses again the usefulness of vitamin E in protecting us against environmental poisons, such as the nitrates and nitrites in food, also the toxic metals lead, cadmium and mercury. He reminds his readers, too, that many people are taking relatively large amounts of unsaturated fats to improve their health. Taking these fats increases our need for vitamin E since it is needed to prevent oxidation of these fats, to make them harmless.

It's becoming popular these days to schedule marathon runs in cities where air pollution is ever present. Any individual just walking outside in some cities under certain weather conditions is threatened with serious harm from air pollutants. So a runner, trying to conserve as much energy as possible, is faced, under these conditions, with having to contend with urban air pollution as well.

It is well known that vitamin E can help to protect lungs from air pollution and, in the process, provide more oxygen to reach those organs whose oxygen demand is enormous. Vitamin E was beneficial for runners in the 1968 Olympics which were held in Mexico City where the high altitude has a deleterious effect on lung efficiency. Runners had less trouble breathing when they had enough vitamin E.

As reported in *The Journal of the American Medical Association*, March 14, 1980, Dr. John Trevthick, Ph.D. at the University of Western Ontario, London, placed lenses from the eyes of diabetic rats in test tubes with a high sugar solution which could be expected to produce cataracts on the lenses. Placing vitamin E in the same test tubes seemed to prevent the formation of the cataracts.

Later studies were with live rats made diabetic. If such animals are not treated, they *always* develop cataracts. It seems obvious that the subject of sugar comes up often when we speak of eye health. Consumption of sugar is closely related to the formation of cataracts, also to troubles with the retina of the eyes. In the Canadian experiments the diabetic rats were given vitamin E in amounts 35 times greater than their normal, highly nutritious diets provided. No cataracts had appeared in the eyes of these animals when the report in the *Journal* was made. The vitamin was given intravenously, presumably so that none of it might be lost due to inability to absorb it. The Canadian researchers planned to do further experiments along these lines using members of the primate family. They are also anticipating experiments to determine if cataract damage can be reversed by large amounts of vitamin E. Their studies are financed by the National Institutes of Health and several other government bureaus in Canada.

*Science News* for April 19, 1980 carried word of research at Columbia University College of Physicians and Surgeons which seems to show that cataract formation may be caused by extensive oxidation of the proteins in the lens of the eye. Cataract is a clouding of the lens which produces failing vision. It is usually treated surgically by removing the lens and substituting appropriate glasses or lenses placed surgically in the eyes.

Dr. Margaret H. Garner and Dr. Abraham Spector reported they had found no oxidation of proteins in the eye lenses in young people, some oxidation in lenses from healthy older people and "dramatic oxidation" in the lenses of people with cataracts. Oxidation is the process whereby oxygen combines with susceptible tissues to create unhealthy conditions. Fats that combine with oxygen become rancid. The brown cut surface of an apple or banana shows oxidation when it becomes brown. Vitamin C can prevent this browning in fruit. The Columbia researchers remind us that vitamin C protects the lens of the eye from certain types of oxidation damage which comes from light. Vitamin E has the same function.

"Therapeutic Uses of Vitamin C in Medicine," is the

369

title of an article in *Nutrition Reviews* for March, 1980. M. K. Horwitt, Ph.D., a specialist in this field, reviewed a number of articles on the subject. A disease of chicks called encephalomalacia causes gross destruction of brain cells. It is caused by deficiency in vitamin E. The same thing has happened, said Dr. Horwitt, in premature babies fed intravenously with no vitamin E in the intravenous fluid.

"Most cases of muscular dystrophy do not respond to vitamin E," said Dr. Horwitt, "But there have been cases in which vitamin E deficiency associated with inability to absorb nutrients from food have resulted in muscular diseases . . . indicating destruction of muscles." One adult man with muscle atrophy due to vitamin E deficiency, secondary to a disorder of the pancreas which caused diarrhea, responded to vitamin E supplements with improvement in muscle health.

A seven-year-old boy who suffered from severe malabsorption problems from birth had severe muscle weakness and low levels of vitamin E in his blood. Over 16 months he was given 400 to 800 units of water soluble vitamin E by mouth daily and produced a remarkable increase in muscular health.

Dr. Horwitt also tells of patients who had suffered from alcoholism and a disorder in absorbing the nutrients in their food. They were given vitamin E and there was a marked increase in both health and life expectancy of important red blood cells. In a number of inherited diseases, vitamin E can alleviate the distress such conditions impose. Patients with Cooley's Anemia (also called thalassemia major) appear to suffer from vitamin E deficiency. In one case the fragility of the red blood cells returned to normal when 750 milligrams of vitamin E were given daily for up to six months.

Another inherited disorder called glutathione synthetase deficiency benefits from vitamin E. A two-year old boy with this condition improved after three months of vitamin E therapy. Another victim of this disorder suffered from frequent ear infections and a drastically reduced level of white blood cells. After three months of treatment with 400 units of vitamin E daily the blood cells returned to normal and the infections disappeared. The child's brother, similarly afflicted, had the same experience.

Victims of sickle-cell anemia may also benefit from vitamin E. Eye and nerve conditions from this disorder improved when large doses of vitamin E were given. In another hereditary disorder vitamin E levels in the blood are low because the condition causes failure of the blood to transport the vitamin through the body. Eye and nerve disorders related to this disease improved when large doses of vitamin A and vitamin E were given. An eleven-year old girl, treated for two and a half years, showed improvement in both eyes and nerves when treated with the vitamins.

Children who must be given oxygen therapy for lung problems may suffer further lung complications because the oxygen may form free radicals which injure lung tissues. Giving vitamin E at the same time can prevent this injury.

Vitamin E can also protect against a number of extremely toxic compounds, said Dr. Horwitt. Adriamycin, a drug used in cancer treatment, is potentially lethal to hearts. It increases the oxidation of the fatty tissues in hearts. Vitamin E is an antioxidant and could be used to protect hearts from this damage. A large dose of acetaminophen (the pain killer used in Tylenol) can cause liver damage much like that caused by the toxic carbon tetrachloride. Giving vitamin E to animals before exposing them to this drug protects them from liver damage.

Sickle cell anemia (referred to by Dr. Horwitt) is a congenital disorder in which red blood cells take on a peculiar shape (like a sickle) and are unable to perform their function of supplying oxygen to cells. According to an article in *American Journal of Clinical Nutrition,* May, 1980, researchers have known for some time that vitamin E is deficient in the blood of victims of this disorder. The authors of the article from the Department of Medicine and Pathology of Columbia University gave 450 milligrams of vitamin E daily to patients with sickle-cell anemia and found that there were "profound" decreases in the number of defective cells after this daily treatment. The vitamin was given for 35 weeks and for all that time this great improvement in the condition of these blood cells continued.

*Medical Tribune,* February 15, 1984 reported that a team of researchers at Hiroshima University in Japan has found that giving vitamin E in large doses alleviates liver damage. It does so, said these experts, by stopping the production of "free radicals" which are believed to be the cause of this condition.

Methylmercury is a potent toxin which attacks nerves. Vitamin E can protect against its effects. Increasing the vitamin E doses from 50 to 100 parts per million in rats increased growth and survival in these animals when they were exposed to this poison. Lead poisoning becomes more serious in rats when they are made deficient in vitamin E.

*Science News,* March 31, 1984 reported on an experiment spraying vitamin E into the lungs of animals. Scientists have known for some time that this vitamin can destroy those destructive body chemicals known as free radicals. But researchers at the University of California believed that you cannot get enough and absorb enough vitamin E through the digestive tract to destroy all the free radicals present in the oxone-laden smog that hangs over most large urban centers.

Why not spray the vitamin into the lungs, asked one of the UCLA researchers. Working with rats, Judy Berliner made up an aerosol preparation of vitamin E in a mineral oil base and sprayed it into the lungs of the animals. They were then exposed for 30 minutes to the harmful constituents in smog.

According to *Science News,* "Viewed under an electron microscope, tissue taken from the animals that had not received the vitamin treatment looked about as bad as tissue from the lungs of chronic smokers . . . By contrast, tissue from the vitamin E-treated animals 'looked almost normal'." The scientists had found that the vitamin's protection against pollution lasts for about five days. Are our lung problems from air pollution solved? Not quite. The scientists believe they must put in a lot more work with laboratory animals before they can recommend a vitamin E spray for human beings.

In the June 1984 *Journal of Pediatric Gastroenterology and Nutrition,* F. Alvarez and colleagues report that children with malfunction of the bile tract may develop severe deficiency in vitamin E. Preliminary results of a study conducted in France seem to show that giving vitamin E by mouth or injection may be necessary to maintain blood levels of the vitamin.

*The New England Journal of Medicine,* December 19, 1985 reported on work being done by professors at the University of Colorado School of Medicine in which they treated 14 children with a chronic disease called cholestasis, meaning a malfunction of the bile ducts which are involved with normal digestion. The researchers gave the children up to 120 milligrams of vitamin E per kilogram of weight every day either orally or by intramuscular injection.

All the children improved greatly, although it took some four years of therapy in some cases. Say the authors, "We conclude that vitamin E repletion therapy should be initiated at an early age in children with chronic cholestasis complicated by vitamin E deficiency to prevent irreversible neurological (nerve) injury."

Vitamin E may be deficient in any condition that makes absorption of food difficult. All the fat soluble vitamins are not absorbed under such conditions. Celiac disease is one such condition. Also cystic fibrosis and other enzyme deficiencies, Whipple's Disease, Hirschprung's Disease, Giardiasis, tuberculous and lymphomatous infiltration of mesenteric nodes are all conditions which are called "malabsorption" diseases.

Two Swedish physicians writing in *Anticancer Research,* volume 1, 1981 reported that giving laboratory animals vitamin E before exposing them to radiation for cancer treatment enhanced the effect of the radiation so that less radiation was needed when vitamin E was given. Since no one has been harmed by massive doses of vitamin E one cannot help but wonder why it is not given regularly to all hospital patients and all seriously ill patients just to see if the vitamin may produce some improvement. Why not, as Dr. Roger Williams always said, "try nutritional therapy *first!*"

Vitamin therapy is not like drug therapy. You can't stop it as soon as it appears to have brought some improvement. If it's caused by longterm deficiency in the nutrient it won't clear up if you stop giving the nutrient.

In the 1970's a researcher at the University of California School of Dentistry found that diseased gum tissues contain ten times the normal level of a harmful substance called prostaglandin. It increases inflammation and causes bone to resorb or dissolve. Dr. J. Max Goodson found that this harmful compound was greatly increased in the diseased gums. He knew that vitamin E has the reputation of inhibiting the body's manufacture of this harmful compound.

He worked with 14 patients suffering from periodontal disease—the condition that causes loss of more teeth than any other disorder in middle and old age. Dr. Goodson gave each of his volunteers 800 milligrams of vitamin E and told them to bite the capsule open and swish the contents around in their mouths before swallowing it. He hoped to get a local effect on the gum tissues as well as an effect from the increased amount of vitamin E in the body. After only 21 days of treatment he found that the vitamin reduced inflammation, while a similar group of patients who had not been told to use the vitamin E treatment showed no improvement.

Dr. Goodson believes that from two to 12 percent of all Americans have blood levels of vitamin E that are less than 0.5 milligrams percent. At this level, he says, red blood cells are destroyed. One-third of us have blood levels of vitamin E below one milligram—the level required to completely eliminate this destruction of red blood cells.

Studies have shown that there is considerably less trouble with bleeding gums in people with high blood levels of vitamin E. Others have shown that just getting more vitamin E, with higher blood levels as a result, is associated with better gum health. In patients with muscle-wasting diseases, says Dr. Goodson, 30 milligram doses of vitamin E, given in intramuscular injections once or twice weekly, have improved the condition of the gums usually by the fourth week. Teeth which had been very loose generally became tighter in their sockets. He says that certain air pollutants such as ozone and nitrogen oxide are destructive of vitamin E, so perhaps some of our gum troubles may result from exposure to urban air pollutants.

In the 1970's two Israeli physicians, testing a drug for arthritis, gave a similar shaped capsule to a group of arthritics not getting the drug. This capsule contained vitamin E. The doctors were sure they would get no reports of improvement from the patients taking the placebo (the vitamin E). But at the end of the test 22 percent of the people getting the vitamin E reported improvement. Drs. I. Machtey and L. Ouknine decided to do a real test of vitamin E. Twenty-nine patients volunteered. Some suffered from a kind of osteoarthritis called spondylosis (completely stiff or fixed joint), some from arthrosis (inflammation of a knee joint), Heberden's Nodes (deformity of fingers) or osteoarthritis of other joints. All the diseases had been confirmed by x-ray. Some of the patients had suffered for nine years.

One group was given 600 milligrams of vitamin E a day while the other group was given a look-alike pill containing nothing. The patients kept daily records of how they felt. Almost 52 percent of the patients taking vitamin E had marked relief of pain as compared to only one patient who thought he felt better on the placebo. Minor relief was also reported by 24 percent of the vitamin E group. It seems quite possible that any of us suffering from any of these arthritis disorders might find the same improvement. In any case, vitamin E costs pennies and is totally harmless, so there is certainly no harm in trying it, in addition to whatever treatment the doctor is giving, if necessary.

# CHAPTER 55

# Vitamin E for Breast Disorders

"LUMPY BREAST TISSUE" affects up to 20 percent of all American women, according to a lead article in *The Journal of the American Medical Association* for September 5, 1980. It is also called fibrocystic breast disease, mammary dysplasia or fibrous mastopathy. Women with such a condition are, presumably, two to eight times more likely to develop breast cancer. Even those whose "lumps" remain non-cancerous often experience "extreme discomfort," according to the *Journal*. Breasts may ache before the menstrual period.

Robert S. London, M.D. at Mt. Sinai Hospital in Baltimore and assistant professor of obstetrics and gynecology at Johns Hopkins University Medical School told the *Journal* that many of his patients seeking treatment for this painful disorder come from all parts of the country, since their own doctors can give them no relief.

Several years earlier Dr. London and his colleagues gave vitamin E to women with this condition and brought relief in a majority of the women. They were proceeding on a theory developed in 1965 when a Boston physician relieved premenstrual tension in patients with fibrocystic breast disease. Dr. London gave 26 women so afflicted 600 milligrams of vitamin E daily for four weeks. Ten of the women found, after the test was over, that pain and tenderness had disappeared and the lumps were gone. Twelve of the women had results not quite so dramatic but meaningful nonetheless. Four reported no improvement.

Asked how he explained these results, Dr. London said, "I can give you five pages of theory, but I'm really not sure. I think the important thing is that vitamin E has profound effects on the homeostatic mechanism both in normal women and in women with mammary (breast) dysplasia." Homeostasis means the ability of the body to maintain a "steady state" or normalcy of all physiological mechanisms.

Dr. London does not know, he says, why some of the women responded differently in the experiment. He thinks perhaps some women just need more of the vitamin for good health. Perhaps there are differences in the way people metabolize this vitamin. Dr. London said he could not perform further experiments along this line because he cannot get any money to finance them.

Money for experimenting with drugs is easy to come by, but not vitamins. Dr. London mentioned one drug that has been used to treat menstrual disorders and other sex-related problems. In *The Physician's Drug Manual* this drug is accompanied by a list of frightful side effects that take up half a page—effects on skin, glands, central nervous system, muscles and bones, digestive and intestinal tract and blood pressure, plus allergic reactions. Dr. London reports no unpleasant side effects in the women who took the vitamin E.

The fine book *Women and the Crisis in Sex Hormones* by Barbara Seaman and Gideon Seaman, M.D. recommended the use of vitamin E in 600 milligram doses daily for fibrocystic breast disease; the authors quoted Dr. London as their source.

In the *Journal* article Dr. London recommends that all physicians try prescribing vitamin E "for their patients with cystic breast." He says, "We found absolutely no side effects in terms of clinical derangements, and it worked in a high percentage of patients. If the clinicians can get symptomatic relief in patients with something as benign as vitamin E, I think it's reasonable therapy. The other therapies are all more dangerous or have more side effects."

Other research has shown that overuse of coffee and other

foods like chocolate and tea, which contain certain harmful compounds may also be involved with cystic breast disease, so it is recommended that these be avoided or used in very small amounts by women. Smoking and alcohol have also been indicted as possible causes of this widespread breast disease.

An article in *New Scientist,* a British publication (March 10, 1983), described the work of Dr. D. F. Horrobin of Canada who studied incidence of breast cancer in 20 countries and found that these figures were related directly to the consumption of sugar in those same countries. Five of the countries are England, Netherlands, Ireland, Denmark and Canada. Countries with the highest incidence of breast cancer in descending order are England, Netherlands, Ireland, Denmark and Canada. The lowest figures are for Italy, Spain, Portugal, Yugoslavia and Japan.

England has the highest consumption of sugar, next Netherlands, then Ireland, Canada and Denmark. Countries with the lowest sugar consumption are Italy, Yugoslavia, Spain, Portugal and Japan. In Japan the average consumption of sugar is only 15 teaspoons a day. In Canada it is 30 teaspoons a day. In the United States it is about 36 teaspoons of sugar a day. Isn't it possible that these figures partly explain the high incidence of breast problems in our country?

Dr. London reported in the *Journal of the American College of Nutrition,* 1983 that painful premenstrual symptoms can also be treated with vitamin E. In a double-blind test, 75 women between the ages of 18 and 45 years were given a "nothing" pill or 150, 200 or 600 milligrams of vitamin E daily. Patients rated some 20 common premenstrual symptoms on a scale of zero to three. Treatment with vitamin E helped to decrease or diminish these unpleasant symptoms in three out of four categories. No adverse side effects were reported.

Vitamin E appears to be important for other aspects of sexual life, especially in women. The U.S. Department of Agriculture announced in 1978 that a progressively fatal disease affecting the central nervous system of guinea pigs can be prevented by supplementing pregnant females with vitamin E. A disorder called Spontaneous Hemorrhagic Necrosis (SHN) has interfered seriously with commercial hamster production. Entire litters have been born with the disease and have died before reaching maturity. A Colorado scientist has found that giving "high level doses" of the vitamin prevents the occurrence of the disease and reduces its severity.

Veterinarians have known for many years that prize animals must be given supplements of vitamin E to insure successful pregnancies. These valuable animals need supplements of vitamin E even though they are eating perfectly balanced diets (unlike human beings), they are not smoking or drinking alcohol or eating sugar. Since they are so valuable to their owners, no expense is spared in giving them nutritional supplements. We cannot say the same for human beings.

# CHAPTER 56

# Vitamin E Is Deficient in Those Who Cannot Absorb Fats

THE DECEMBER 12, 1981 *Lancet* reported on four children who suffered from inability to absorb fat normally. "Chronic steatorrhea" is the name given to this condition. It may result in extremely serious nerve symptoms. It occurs in a number of disorders including cystic fibrosis. One patient, 19 years old, had no detectable vitamin E in his blood. He was given vitamin E by mouth and did not improve. After three years he was given vitamin E by intramuscular injection—100 milligrams a week. Blood levels of the vitamin increased to normal and the young man's nerve symptoms greatly improved.

A second patient suffered from liver cirrhosis from birth. He was given one gram of vitamin E which kept levels of this nutrient in his blood fairly normal. He suffered from severe nerve disorders. When he was 29 years old he complained of great difficulty in walking. He had stopped taking the vitamin and no vitamin E at all could be detected in his blood.

A third patient was born with severe problems of many kinds. As he grew older he was unable to walk normally or use hands and arms normally. His reflexes were abnormal. No vitamin E at all was detectable in his blood when he was 15. Given 200 milligrams of vitamin E three times a day he showed "marked improvement." A fourth patient had cystic fibrosis. At 15, she came to a hospital in England with extreme deficiency in vitamin A and calcium. This latter was undoubtedly caused by lack of vitamin D which is essential for absorbing calcium. She had progressive unsteadiness in walking, with tremor in hands, and eye disorders. Two years later she developed diabetes. At the age of 31 no vitamin E could be detected in her blood.

The three physicians who made this report recommended that blood concentrations of vitamin E be regularly determined in anyone who has difficulty in absorbing fats and, when levels are low, supplements should be given by injection, if they are useless when given by mouth.

*The New England Journal of Medicine* printed an article by four physicians from St. Louis area hospitals who described a progressive nerve disorder in children who were unable to absorb fat. Blood levels of vitamin E were very low. Studies of nerve function in two of three fatal cases showed nerve degeneration similar to that found in animals with induced vitamin E deficiency.

There is an hereditary disease called abetalipoproteinemia in which there is almost complete absence in the blood of certain substances containing both protein and fats. Children born with this disorder develop conditions like celiac disease early in life. This is a disorder which brings many unpleasant and dangerous consequences. The intestine is abnormal. The child cannot eat any food that contains gluten, a protein found in many cereal foods. Eating any such food produces severe diarrhea in the celiac-sprue patient, also bloating, gas and great abdominal discomfort. There is no cure for this disease except a diet which eliminates all sources of gluten.

Since the diarrhea causes lack of absorption of many essential nutrients, the child with celiac disease is likely to be deficient in many such nutrients including vitamins, minerals and trace minerals. A child born with the disease mentioned above has other complications as well. These are nerve problems such as ataxia (incoordination of muscles), especially those used in walking or reaching for things. In addition, we are told in an article in *The Lancet*, January 29, 1983 that trouble with the retina of the eye usually follows. A child born with this trait may show severe nerve disorders and eye disorders by the time he or she is ten years old.

D. P. R. Muller, June K. Lloyd and O. H. Wolff of the Institute of Child Health at St. George's Hospital in London, England, told in *The Lancet* that tests of such children for vitamin E show that it is *entirely* absent in the blood. Experiments with chicks and several animals have shown that, in the absence of vitamin E, severe nerve disorders develop, difficulty in walking and many of the same characteristics of children with the congenital disease.

The London doctors treated some such young people with very large doses of vitamin E—as much as 7,500 milligrams daily, depending on the weight of the individual. They followed the progress of these patients for periods from nine to 15 years. At that time vitamin E levels could be detected in their blood and their red blood cells indicated that the normal activity of these cells had responded to the vitamin E.

At the time the article was written, the five youngest patients were attending school and "show no clinical abnormalities." All tests showed that both nerve function and eye function were normal. The three oldest patients had some deterioration of nerve activity before the vitamin therapy was started. Patient number 6 had received vitamin E from the age of three years. At eleven years of age all that remained of his nerve troubles was a slight reduction in his ability to feel vibrations. By the age of 17 almost all nerve symptoms had disappeared. This young man was at the time working in a car-body repair shop and attending college.

Patient number 7 was diagnosed in 1960 at the age of 17 months. She had no normal reflexes, due to nerve damage, and had some retinal problems. Treatment with vitamin E was started when she was eight. She was 24 when this article was written. She had no nerve or eye problems at that age except for very slight difficulties with reflexes. She teaches school and has a university degree.

The oldest patient, number 8, was 25 at the time the

article was written. He was diagnosed at seven and got his first vitamin E when he was ten. By this time he was walking very abnormally, had no tendon reflexes and great trouble with eyesight. Within two years after vitamin E therapy was started, his gait, motor nerve conduction and measurement of eye movements had greatly improved, although some reflexes remained unchanged. Over the next 13 years there was further improvement in his gait. Nerve conduction and retinal function tests returned to normal. He was employed making furniture in a sheltered workshop and was able to drive a car.

The doctors of the *Lancet* article describe other cases where vitamin E brought similar improvement. They theorize on the possibility of giving large doses of the vitamin in all conditions where there is chronic inability to absorb fats. This condition is called "steatorrhea." It occurs in chronic liver disease and in chronic gall bladder conditions where there is stoppage or slowing of the flow of those digestive juices which digest fats.

The London doctors said that large doses of vitamin E have been given to such patients in the past with great success. In some cases the vitamin must be given intravenously since these patients could not absorb much of the vitamin internally. These individuals, too, had suffered from serious nerve disorders which were corrected by the vitamin. In six adults (two with chronic liver disease, two with cystic fibrosis and two who had sections of their intestines removed) no vitamin E could be detected in their blood. In two of these, large doses of vitamin E resulted in clinical improvement. Some of the others required injections of the vitamin to bring about improvement.

Autopsies of patients with cystic fibrosis who died between 1970 and 1980 had less degeneration of nerve tissues than those dying between 1952 and 1969. This change coincides with the introduction of vitamin E therapy in cystic fibrosis patients in the mid-1960's. The doctors conclude that "The evidence linking vitamin E deficiency with nerve abnormalities is now sufficiently strong to make vitamin E supplementation advisable, not only in patients with abetalipo-proteinemia but also in those with chronic fat malabsorption who have low blood vitamin E concentrations. The object . . . is to restore and maintain normal blood concentrations of the vitamin.''

Here is a list of the normal functions of vitamin E according to *Handbook of Vitamins, Minerals and Hormones* by Roman J. Kutsky. It is an antioxidant. It is essential for normal growth and health, fertility and pregnancy. It protects the essential unsaturated fatty acids in body tissues. It is necessary for intercellular respiration. It maintains normal muscle metabolism. (Remember that the heart is a muscle). It maintains the integrity of the circulatory system and the central nervous system. It is a detoxifying agent. It maintains kidney tubules, the lungs, the genital structures, the liver and red blood cell membranes. If it is missing or at low levels in the blood all these functions are likely to suffer.

# CHAPTER 57

# How Can You Tell Synthetic Vitamin E from Natural Vitamin E?

THERE IS A way to tell natural from synthetic vitamin E. It is outlined here by a spokesman from Eastman Chemical Company which manufactures much of the natural vitamin E we see in food supplements. Although some of this discussion is a bit difficult for a non-chemist to follow, the basic way to determine at a glance the difference between natural and synthetic vitamin E is clearly indicated.

Vitamin E was discovered in 1922 in the course of biochemical research with laboratory animals. Over the years, thousands of scientific papers have been published on the subject. Much research on it is still going on in well-respected laboratories around the world.

Despite this half century of research, much less is known about the extent of the biological role of vitamin E than of a number of other vitamins.

In research, the effects of a lack of a vitamin can be studied by controlling the diet fed to animals. However, vitamin E is unusual in the large variation of effects among animal species from insufficient vitamin E.

For example, in male rats the lack of vitamin E results in sterility; in calves, heart failure; in lambs paralysis of the hind quarters; in chicks, leakage from the capillaries and brain deterioration, and in milk cows, bad flavored milk.

385

Even deciding on the recommended daily allowance of vitamin E is complicated. It depends very much on what else the animal is getting. For example, in cat food switching from one kind of fish product to another resulted in greatly increased need for vitamin E. When these increased needs were not met, pets died . . .

To serve the human need to make one's own choices, the marketplace offers such things as dietary supplements in such forms as capsules, tablets and liquids. Some of these are represented as "natural" in origin in contrast with "synthetic."

As one of the companies that supplies manufacturers of these products with the naturally derived form of vitamin E, we want to explain what we mean by "naturally derived" and how to make sure you get it.

The particular kind of molecule that gives vitamin E effects is a structure of carbon, hydrogen and oxygen atoms. Molecules composed of these atoms are called "organic" because of a belief among early chemists that a certain category of substances could come only from living organisms. Today, scientists know how to make millions of kinds of "organic" molecules that never occur in nature, in addition to other thousands that do occur in nature. A "synthetic" molecule may be absolutely identical in every known property with one made by the body of a plant or a creature other than a human chemist.

It may be. It may also be slightly different. The difference, if any, may not matter for some purposes. For others it may matter.

Look at a glove for the right hand and its mate for the left hand. Same design, same material, but different. Molecules made by nature can differ from otherwise identical ones made by the chemist in just this property of "handedness." Only certain molecular structures have handedness, just as some familiar objects like dishes, for example, have no inbuilt handedness, while gloves and screw threads do have it. Vitamin E molecules have it, too.

When factories make molecules, the processes have to

be efficient. Efficient methods of quantity production leave it to chance whether the parts of each individual molecule will be assembled left-handed or right-handed where either twist is possible. Nature, using subtle methods, tends to put them together with all the same twist.

In the case of vitamin E, a difference in twist makes a difference in biological potency. This is officially recognized in National Formulary's definition of the International Unit of vitamin E, the unit required by regulatory authorities for stating vitamin E potency on labels. It recognizes that handedness affects potency, just as one of a person's hands is stronger than the other.

One milligram of the synthetic vitamin E, dl-Alpha tocopheryl acetate, is equal to one International Unit of vitamin E. The two letters "d" and "l" in combination is a chemist's way of indicating that the molecules are built on both the left-handed and right-handed pattern.

The same National Formulary goes on to specify that one milligram of d-Alpha tocopheryl acetate equals 1.36 International Units (36% more).

It takes careful reading to note the difference in those chemical names:

dl-Alpha tocopheryl acetate

d-Alpha tocopheryl acetate

That small "l" results in a lower potency. When it is NOT there you are being informed that the molecules have indeed all been assembled nature's way.

This doesn't mean that it is necessarily a better nutrient. It just means that less of it is required to do whatever essential biochemical job is to be done in your body by the vitamin E. It doesn't say that the chemist hasn't tinkered with the molecule nature made. The absence of that little "l" doesn't even prove that nature actually built those particular molecules, although actually building them in a laboratory from their constituent atoms would have been exorbitantly expensive. If the consumer wants "d" rather than "dl" it is far more practical to let nature do the molecule building out in the field where she makes vegetable oil.

387

If, for reasons of your own, you prefer the naturally derived form of vitamin E, just look at the label carefully. Find that little "d" that goes with tocopheryl (sometimes it's tocopherol). Be sure that it applies to all the vitamin E in the product. If there is a little "l" after the little "d," there is vitamin E in it that did not start out from natural vegetable oils, whatever else may be stated about natural oils contained.

Not that synthetic vitamin E would harm you.

It's just that you have a right to know.

# CHAPTER 58

# How Much Vitamin E Do You Need?

OFFICIALLY WE WERE TOLD, a number of years ago, that a minimum of 10 to 30 milligrams of vitamin E daily should be sufficient for most adults. And we were told that "the estimated average daily adult consumption of vitamin E has been calculated to be about 14 milligrams."

Some time ago a survey was conducted by four researchers who chose food from a supermarket which, they thought, might be typical of the food we Americans eat every day for breakfast, lunch and dinner. They made a special effort, however, to include as many foods as possible that are rich in vitamin E—salad oils, for example, and margarine, butter and mayonnaise.

They planned menus for eight days, and, by careful investigation in a laboratory, found out just how much vitamin E each day's menus contained. They were very well-planned, highly nutritious menus—far bigger meals than most of us eat, probably.

A typical breakfast, for instance was tomato juice, cooked cereal, two slices of ham, one egg, two slices of whole grain bread with margarine, coffee with cream and sugar. How many people you know eat that big a breakfast? Lunches and dinners were equally well planned, with an eye to including as many foods as possible in which vitamin E is abundant.

They found that the daily average intake of vitamin E was only 7.4 milligrams, or just about half the amount that has been officially announced as the average daily intake of the average American. The authors of the survey say in their article in the *American Journal of Clinical Nutrition*, July, 1965, that it indicates the possibility of relatively low vitamin E intake in a portion of the population. We'd say it certainly indicates that even if you eat well planned meals with nothing much but their vitamin E content in mind you will still be getting only half the amount officially recommended for you.

How does this happen? Have human beings always been short on vitamin E? No, of course not. The richest source of vitamin E is the germ of cereals—that little nubbin which is removed when we process grains to make white flour or commercial cereals. At present it is estimated that about half of our meals consist of foods made of sugar and these highly processed grains, from which all the vitamin E has been removed. It's no wonder that large numbers of us are probably not getting even the 7.4 milligrams of vitamin E which turned up in the survey described above.

Another reason for a possible shortage in vitamin E is that many of the foods we eat today have been frozen. If we eat commercially processed foods which have been fried in deep fat, these foods contain almost no vitamin E at all, for it is destroyed in the fat when they are frozen.

In a letter to *Chemical and Engineering News* for October 9, 1972, a reader protested a previous article in which it was stated that the only demonstrated function of vitamin E in man is as an antioxidant. Richard A. Passwater lists a number of other functions performed by this vitamin in the human body. Then he objected to another statement made in the earlier article—that vitamin E deficiency is practically unknown in man.

"It may be unknown," he said, "but borderline deficiencies may exist in more than half our population, if the arbitrary 20–30 milligrams per day RDA established by the Food and Nutrition Board of the National Research Council is used as a guideline. Surveys . . . indicate typical diets may contain less than 7 milligrams a day of vitamin E. These surveys do not consider the vitamin losses due to preparation or storage, nor analytical problems. Blood level measurements are inconclusive . . . An antioxidant deficiency state existed in 90 percent of those studied.

"As vitamin E deficiency in animals leads to tissue degradation and gross changes in biochemistry, we should err on the high intake side, rather than the low.

"Today's typical vitamin E consumption is only a fraction of that of 50 years ago, even when adjusted for lipid intake. Degermination, bleaching, processing and longer storage periods have depleted foods. The long-term effects of this, along with decreased (physical) activity and other factors may explain our worsening morbidity/mortality rates of cardiovascular disease and other diseases.

"In conclusion it is difficult to assess, but borderline vitamin E deficiencies are widespread, based on both the RDA and the diene test (for antioxidants). It is difficult to assume that the long-term consequences are not a major problem."

*The Journal of the American Geriatrics Society* for August, 1974 published an article by E. Cheraskin, MD, DMD, W. M. Ringsdorf, Jr., DMD, and B. S. Hicks on "Eating Habits of the Dentist and His Wife: Daily Consumption of Vitamin E." They tell us that they collected information from a group of 369 dentists and 288 wives on what they ate every day for one week. They kept very careful records, with special attention to the frequency with which they ate certain foods—in this case, foods in which there is lots of vitamin E.

The information was analyzed by a computer. The results were discussed with the people involved. They were told of the relationship between good nutrition and good health, especially, in this case, getting enough vitamin E. They were told how they could increase their intake of vitamin E and why they should.

About one year later, the survey was made again. Every participant kept account of every food eaten during one week. Similar surveys were taken every year for four years for the same group of people, so that the researchers now have a good idea of just what foods are eaten daily by each member of this group and how much vitamin E is contained in each day's diet.

At the same time, the same group of volunteers were being given certain tests to determine just what their condition was in regard to heart and circulatory health. Some of them showed improved health in this area. Others showed no improvement or little improvement. These facts were then correlated with the amounts of vitamin E which each individual got in his daily diet. It's hard to imagine a more comprehensive and convincing way to arrive at the facts.

One object was to see if those who had not been getting enough vitamin E would increase their intake after a period of nutritional education. Another object was to see if an increase in the amount of vitamin E in the daily diet would improve heart and circulatory health and if a decrease in the amount of vitamin E in the daily diet would cause lack of improvement or even a turn for the worse in heart and circulatory health.

The results are enlightening. First of all the Alabama scientists found that there was a wide range of vitamin E intake among the volunteer dentists and their wives. Among the dentists, some got as little as 6 units of vitamin E daily, some as much as 212 units. Forty-six percent of all the dentists got, at meals, less than 30 units daily, which was the recommended daily allowance until recently. Their wives also got widely varying amounts of vitamin E. Some got as little as 4 units, others as much as 213. Forty-five percent of the wives were getting less than the 25 units daily which were until recently recommended by federal experts.

How did they do after the nutritional education course? The average amount of daily intake of vitamin E at the beginning of the test was 21 units in a selected group of 84 paired subjects. At the second visit, after the nutritional instruction, these same people were getting an average of 51 units. And at the third visit they were getting 127 units of vitamin E. So there is no doubt that a simple course of instruction in nutrition can improve the intake of nutrients among those who wish to show improvement. In other words, it's perfectly possible to learn how to get more of a given vitamin at meals, if you want to.

And what happened to the health of the people who arranged their eating patterns so that they got more vitamin E? You have perhaps guessed what happened. As the intake of vitamin E went up, so did the heart and circulatory health improve. When the intake went up only slightly there was little or no noticeable improvement. But when daily intake went up considerably, there was considerable improvement in circulatory conditions.

This was determined, incidentally, by use of the Cornell Medical Index Questionnaire on which various facts in regard to heart and circulation are recorded.

The Alabama researchers report that the dose of vitamin E seems to be very important in regard to benefits received. Dosages twice as high as those officially recommended appeared to be the most beneficial.

As we have pointed out, in other chapters of this book, the National Academy of Sciences-National Research Council, which sets these standards, lowered their estimate of daily needs of vitamin E in the 1974 edition of *Recommended Dietary Allowances*. They lowered it from 30 and 35 milligrams down to 15 milligrams for a man, and 12 milligrams for a woman. Their reason was, generally speaking, that there does not appear to be any national deficiency in vitamin E and it appears that all of us get at least this much in our food. The 1980 edition of the RDA booklet lowered the recommendation even farther—down to 10 milligrams for men and eight for women.

It is noteworthy that, when a new edition of the RDA book was proposed in 1985 the controversy over what changes should be made in the 1980 booklet was so prolonged and so vociferous that the committee finally decided not to go ahead with it. They stated in a press release that "the Research Council Committee on Dietary Allowances on the one hand and a panel of independent reviewers and the Food and Nutrition board of the Research Council on the other, were unable to agree—despite exhaustive deliberations over the last six months—on interpretation of scientific data on several of the nutrients and consequently on RDA's for those nutrients." So both the 1980 and 1989 RDA's remain at the low level of 10 mg for men and 8 mg for women.

The Alabama test referred to above showed that almost half of us may not be getting the basic recommended requirement of vitamin E. It also showed that the more vitamin E you get, apparently, the more improvement there will be in your circulatory health. And remember that the subjects of this test were dentists and their wives—people who would, one imagines, have a fairly good basic education in nutrition, unlike most of the rest of us.

In a previous article these Alabama doctors showed much the same thing in regard to refined carbohydrates, using the same group of professional men as volunteers. The less of the refined carbohydrates eaten, the better the health of the subjects. The more refined carbohydrates eaten, the worse the general condition of health, as determined by the Cornell test.

Now we find the same general condition in regard to vitamin E. The better the diet eaten—that is, the more vitamin E it contains—the better the cardiovascular health. And as the diet grows worse, just in regard to vitamin E, the circulatory health declines.

How can you improve your intake of vitamin E? The best sources of this fat-soluble vitamin are seeds, cereals and their oils. But they must, of course be wholegrain, for refining and bleaching of cereals destroys vitamin E wholesale. And nothing is done to replace what has been lost from white flour and commercially refined cereals.

Here are some of the best food sources of vitamin E. Think of them in relation to the amount of each that you might eat in the course of a day. You eat liver and oatmeal in average servings. You eat a serving of peas or baked beans, brown rice, turnip or other greens at a meal. All these contain ample vitamin E. Although soybean oil along with other salad oils, is very rich in vitamin E, you cannot get down "a serving" of soybean oil at one meal, and you shouldn't. Salad oils are highly concentrated foods. But you can and should use them in smaller quantities wherever appropriate—in salads, for instance, and recipes where you might otherwise use butter or hydrogenated shortening.

As might be expected, wholegrains contain more vitamin E than white flour or processed cereals, since most of the vitamin E in grains is concentrated in the germ and bran which are removed during processing. Adding insult to injury, bleaching of flour to make it chalky white destroys the last of whatever vitamin E was in the white flour or processed cereal to begin with. The two parts of the grain which are removed, the germ and the bran, are rich sources of vitamin E.

A serving of wheat germ (3½ ounces) contains 27 units of vitamin E. All whole, unrefined seeds contain it, as well as green leafy vegetables and eggs. There are, of course, many food supplements containing vitamin E. It is possible to take it in very large amounts if you feel that you need it. And there is much research in medical journals showing the health advantages to large doses of vitamin E.

In *The American Journal of Clinical Nutrition* for September, 1972 Karen C. Davis of the Agricultural Experiment Station, University of Idaho, tells us about the amount of vitamin E in baby's diets in this country.

As might be expected she found that the situation in regard to vitamin E in commercial baby food is chaotic, completely chaotic. Since American parents spent $344,700,000 for baby foods every year, it is apparent that most babies are fed out of drug store bottles and supermarket cartons. Breast feeding being generally considered too inconvenient most babies live on formulas which are bought at the store. It's also too inconvenient to prepare baby's formula at home apparently.

Because of the nationwide scare over cholesterol, commercial baby's formulas these days are loaded with unsaturated fats, rather than good, old saturated fats that come in human milk and cow's milk. But unsaturated fats must be accompanied by very sizable amounts of vitamin E or they create a deficiency in this vitamin. And most of the commercial formulas Dr. Davis studied contained little or no vitamin E.

So, in consultation with a local pediatrician, she designed complete all-day feeding schedules for babies of different ages using 23 different commercial formulas, plus fruit, cereal and vegetables. And she carefully calculated the amount of vitamin E the infants might get from such diets. She found that the minimum amount of vitamin E was 1.38 milligrams, the maximum was 14.92 milligrams, depending on which formulas were used!

She came to the conclusion that the range of vitamin E varies so greatly that "it becomes a matter of real concern

## Vitamin E Content of Some Common Foods

| Food | Vitamin E in one serving |
|------|-------------------------|
| | mg. |
| Beef | 0.63 |
| Liver | 1.62 |
| Haddock | 1.20 |
| Baked potato | 0.05 |
| Baked beans | 1.16 |
| Fresh peas | 1.73 |
| Whole wheat bread, 4 slices | 2.2 |
| Oatmeal | 3.23 |
| Corn oil margarine, 1 tablespoon | 2.60 |
| Mayonnaise, 1 tablespoon | 3.16 |
| Wheat germ, ½ cup | 11.0 |

to choose formulas and foods that are adequate with respect to both vitamin E and the ratio of vitamin E to the unsaturated fats. . . . Baby foods generally do not supply much vitamin," she says, mostly because the cereals are all refined cereals, and fruits and vegetables are not very good sources of the vitamin. So, she says, we should fortify the commercial formulas with vitamin E. Some of them are already fortified but probably have too little of the vitamin.

Interestingly enough, whenever cereal appears on her list of foods, the infant always gets one teaspoon of sugar, plain white sugar, along with the cereal—just to make sure, we guess, that the child will be addicted to sugar by the time he can toddle. Or maybe pediatricians and nutritionists simply do not know that children have no need of added sugar, don't especially like it but very soon become addicted to the taste. Adults apparently go right on assuming that babies are born with the same perverted sense of taste their parents have developed, over the years, in regard to sugar and salt.

What to do? We suggest if there's a new baby at your home, that breast-feeding is infinitely superior to any formula and that all babies should be breast-fed as long as possible. We also suggest that homemade formulas are infinitely superior to commercial ones, that they should be made of cow's milk or goat milk diluted to make them as nearly identical to human breast milk as possible and that early foods should include cooked cereals with as much vitamin E as possible, as well as egg yolk and pureed meat along with fruits and vegetables.

And finally, *Nutrition Reviews* for March, 1972 reported on the great difficulty found in trying to calculate the amount of vitamin E actually in food. The article tells of testing the diets of 40 ambulant patients in a hospital. Twenty-nine of the forty diets contained less than five milligrams of vitamin E per day. (Remember, this is a hospital where, supposedly, highly trained nutrition experts plan the meals!)

Part of the reason for all the confusion, said the article, is simply that the same food may contain widely varying amounts of vitamin E depending on where and when it is bought.

The other day in an animal feed store, we saw gallon cans of wheat germ oil, enriched with considerable amounts of vitamin E, vitamin A and vitamin D. These preparations are available for use in the diets of cows, horses and other valuable stock animals. The stock raiser cannot take any chances on poor health in his animals. It's too costly.

So even though they are eating the best possible diet, even though they suffer from almost none of the daily stresses to health which we human beings suffer from, stock animals are regularly plied with massive doses of the fat soluble vitamins. Nobody—least of all the FDA—says a reproachful word.

But the minute anybody suggests in print that perhaps human beings, too, might benefit from the addition of vitamin supplements to their diets, a hue and a cry goes up from every regulatory bureau in Washington.

"What are you saying!" they shout. "Don't you know that every American eating 'the average American diet' is already getting enough vitamins and minerals? Why waste your money buying vitamins?"

Gentlemen, the hard-headed raisers of prize horses and cows don't consider vitamin supplements a waste of money. Why do you?

For a list of some common foods which contain vitamin E, refer to the chart on page 396.

# Vitamin K Is . . .

*Fat-soluble,* hence stored in the body.

*Responsible for* maintenance of the blood's clotting system.

Without vitamin K we would bleed to death with the slightest scratch. So a deficiency in vitamin K results in a tendency to bleed or hemorrhage.

*Present* in cabbage, cauliflower, soybeans, spinach, liver, kidney, wholegrains, wheat germ, wheat bran, egg yolk, potatoes, tomatoes.

*Usually safe* in large amounts. Given by doctors to prevent bleeding, it may eventually cause clotting, though it is safer than drugs given for this purpose.

*Destroyed* by mineral oil laxatives, impaired absorption of fat in the intestine, antibiotics given by mouth, certain liver disorders.

*RDA* of 1 milligram per kilogram of body weight for adults and children established for first time in 1989.

# CHAPTER 59

# Vitamin K Stands
# for Well-Ordered
# "Koagulation"

TWO WORRISOME CIRCUMSTANCES of modern life are the reasons why we are especially concerned about vitamin K. First, the fact that coronary thrombosis is a leading cause of death, and "strokes" take an additional toll of life, as well as crippling and disabling many thousands each year. The second reason for our concern is that the FDA has recently granted permission for the irradiation of various foods and we are promised that eventually almost everything we eat will be irradiated.

Why do these two circumstances worry us so and what do they have to do with vitamin K? Vitamin K is so-called because it is involved chiefly with the process of blood coagulation. The letter K stands for Koagulation—the spelling of this word in Danish. The vitamin was discovered by a Danish scientist. Vitamin K is necessary for manufacturing, in the liver, the substance which causes blood to coagulate normally. Without vitamin K we would bleed to death.

In fact, many newly-born children do not survive precisely because their small bodies are lacking in this important substance during the early days of life. Many obstetricians now give vitamin K to pregnant women to prevent any hemorrhaging accident in their newly-born children. The reasons why any prospective mother might be deficient in vitamin K are abundant. If her liver does not function well this may interfere with the manufacture of the coagulation substance by vitamin K in this organ.

If she suffers from some disease affecting the digestive tract, she may not absorb the vitamin from her food. Sprue, diarrhea, dysentery, colitis, and other disorders of this kind prevent the absorption of many vitamins. If she has been taking mineral oil, the fat-soluble vitamin K in her digestive tract would be destroyed, along with the other fat-soluble vitamins A, D and E. Bile is essential for the absorption of vitamin K, so if some disorder prevents the presence of bile in the intestine, vitamin K will not be absorbed.

Strokes are, of course, hemorrhages of blood vessels. We do not know what causes them. But it seems quite possible that one cause may be lack of vitamin K. That is, lack of the substance in the blood which helps it to clot in the way it is supposed to when some small blood vessel is broken. Coronary thrombosis may be caused by a blood clot in the main artery of the heart. After such an attack, the patient is usually given some anticoagulant drug—that is, a drug which interferes with the process of coagulation so that further clots will not form. These drugs must be administered with great care, for serious accidents can occur when the blood loses some of its ability to clot.

Vitamin K can be given to help regulate this delicate balance, since it will provide materials to help the natural and healthful clotting process.

So we see that this vitamin is absolutely essential to health. The older we are the more important becomes an ample supply of vitamin K because it is in these later years that problems with the circulatory system become most troublesome. Also, as we become older, we tend to have more problems with the proper absorption of food elements. Up until quite recently we were told that vitamin K is manufactured by helpful bacteria in the intestine, so it isn't necessary to have a certain supply in the diet.

Such conclusions were arrived at by studying laboratory animals. We do not know, however, how much of this information can be applied directly to all human beings. There is, we must not forget, the problem of decreased numbers of helpful bacteria in the human intestine as a result of the antibiotic drugs which are given so widely these days. Antibiotics and sulfa drugs destroy bacteria, both harmful and helpful. So anyone who has been taking these drugs is quite likely to be unable to synthesize any vitamin in his digestive tract. The helpful bacteria must first be re-established there, preferably by daily intake of considerable quantities of yogurt or other products which contain the same helpful bacteria yogurt contains.

The October 11, 1965 issue of *The Journal of the American Medical Association* printed an article by an Arizona physician which seems to show that we cannot depend on intestinal bacteria for manufacturing our own vitamin K, but must get it in our food. Dr. John A. Udall gave human volunteers diets completely lacking in vitamin K and found that the normal clotting ability of the blood decreased almost at once.

By giving vitamin K he could raise the level of this substance. As soon as he took vitamin K out of the diet, it decreased once more. He concluded, "Foods, rather than intestinal bacterial synthesis, probably provide most vitamin K for humans."

In a long-awaited move, the National Research Council established an RDA for vitamin K for the first time in 1989. The 10th edition states: "The RDA for adults and children is set at approximately 1 mg/kg of body weight. There is no recommended increment during pregnancy and lactation, because the effects of pregnancy on vitamin K requirements are unknown and lactation imposes little additional need for this nutrient."

The RDA book continues, "Because human milk contains low levels of vitamin K and the intestinal flora are limited, exclusively breastfed infants who do not receive vitamin K . . . at birth are at very real risk of developing fatal intracranial hemorrhage secondary to vitamin K deficiency. Home-delivered, breastfed infants require particular attention in this regard . . . Newborn infants are routinely given a supplement of vitamin K by intramuscular injection to prevent hemorrhage."

It seems that such help for newborns is not always given. Medical journals in the 1980's were describing what happens as a result. *The Lancet,* June 25, 1983 told of four cases in which hemorrhage of brain tissues resulted in death of the infant or recovery only after vitamin K had been administered. The authors, from the Royal Hospital for Sick Children in Bristol, England, stated that "Some of these units have not decided to give prophylactic vitamin K and we feel that their example should be followed. Our cases suggest that more than one milligrams of vitamin K be given."

*The Lancet* (August 3, 1985) carried an article from Japan comparing a group of infants who were given vitamin K to another group which did not get the vitamin shortly after birth. Said the authors, from Kumamoto University Medical School, "The findings support the view that vitamin K given prophylactically at birth will help to prevent neonatal bleeding." Considering the seriousness of such bleeding and the low cost of vitamin K treatment one can only wonder why any physician would hesitate to give the newborn infant this completely safe treatment just as insurance against any circulatory accident.

In addition to infants, those at most risk of deficiency in vitamin K are individuals with some digestive complaint which makes absorption of fat soluble vitamins difficult or impossible. Vitamin K is fat soluble. An article in *Nutrition Reviews,* January, 1986 stated that "Biochemical evidence of vitamin K deficiency was found in about one-third of patients with gastrointestinal disorders. The incidence was higher in patients with inflammatory bowel diseases afflicting the ileum." The ileum is the lower part of the small intestine which leads into the large intestine.

In Crohn's Disease, almost half of all the patients studied had mild vitamin K deficiency. Five of 17 patients with ulcerative colitis had vitamin K deficiency. The authors say that it was not clear if the deficiency was related to not enough vitamin K in the diets eaten or if it was caused by lack of enough healthy intestinal bacteria to manufacture enough vitamin K. They conclude, "Further studies will provide the evidence to identify other persons at risk for vitamin K deficiency.''

An October, 1980 *Nutrition Reviews* article pointed out the serious effects of various antibiotics given by mouth on the body's ability to manufacture enough vitamin K. The article described a woman seriously injured in an accident whose wounds became infected and who was fed a liquid diet which did not include any vitamin K. She was given large doses of antibiotics to fight the infections. She developed bruise marks, bleeding gums and other symptoms of lack of vitamin K which persisted until she was finally given injections of the vitamin, and later given the vitamin by mouth.

Still another article in *Nutrition Reviews* (April, 1984) described three cases of patients given antibiotics for various infectious conditions all of whom developed the bleeding characteristic of vitamin K deficiency. The authors recommend, ''Since parenteral (intravenous) vitamin K is safe and inexpensive, it behooves all physicians to administer vitamin K prophylactically when these antibiotics are used.''

Now for our second worry in regard to this vitamin. The Army and the Atomic Energy Commission have been experimenting with irradiated foods—that is, perishable foods sterilized by subjecting them to massive doses of radiation. It seems that such foods will keep, without refrigeration, for several months. This is economical. Many of the earlier experiments showed damage to animals who ate these foods. A professor at the St. Louis University School of Medicine reported in *Federation Proceedings,* December, 1961, that laboratory animals which were fed a diet, 35 percent of which consisted of irradiated foods, died of hemorrhage. Animals given a supplement of vitamin K did not succumb to hemorrhaging.

It is known that radiating food destroys its vitamin K. Now we know that, unless enough vitamin K is obtained in foods and supplements other than the irradiated ones, hemorrhaging and possible death will result. The St. Louis physician adds that there are many mysteries surrounding vitamin K which he hopes will be speedily resolved.

One of the mysteries, we would add, is the fact that anybody authorized the radiation of foods, declaring that no harm could come to anyone from eating them. So far as vitamin K is concerned, it seems that this may be true, provided you are getting plenty of vitamin K in other foods to make up for the vitamin K destroyed in the radiation process. How do you know that you are? Since there is no official estimate of the amount of vitamin K needed by the average person, how could anyone safely work out this problem for himself?

The Army has been experimenting with irradiated foods since 1945 and those involved in the federally funded experiments state that such food is entirely acceptable and tasty. Congressional opponents and many nutrition experts contend that the Army experiments were a complete failure and the final products were inedible. Champions of irradiation point out that any processing of food—cooking, freezing, canning—changes the texture and taste of food, so why object only to those changes brought about by radiation?

Many nutrients other than vitamin K are sensitive to radiation and are destroyed in the process of irradiation. During the past years seventeen important irradiation studies conducted by an industrial laboratory were rejected by the Food and Drug Administration as not valid. This laboratory had performed several hundred such studies purporting to show that irradiation of food is perfectly safe and healthful. FDA scientists have judged that 99 percent of these studies were inadequate.

John W. Gofman, M.D. who has worked in the field of radiation for many years, has said, about irradiated foods, that "to be really able to say that this technique has serious effects on humans would require epidemiological studies of 20 to 30 years on 100,000 or more subjects. That study has not been done . . . We don't know what the longterm safety is."

Nevertheless, the government is now allowing radiation of certain foods and it is not clear at this time just how any consumer will be able to identify the foods thus treated in order to avoid them.

Vitamin K is abundant in "the average diet," we are told by experts. Is it? Check over the list of foods below and see for yourself. As you read the list, think of all the surveys that have been done showing that a great many older folks are trying to nourish themselves on tea and toast with a little processed cereal and cookies.

How much vitamin K would such a diet provide for these older people, those who are most susceptible to circulatory disorders? How many times have you read of the appalling diets of many of our young people, who eat no breakfast, have sketchy hamburger, soft drink and potato chip lunches and badly planned dinners? How much vitamin K would such a diet contain?

It is true, apparently, that only a very small amount of vitamin K is necessary to maintain the normal clotting ability of the blood. But you must get this vitamin K in your diet—nothing else can take its place. And your digestive tract must be in such good shape that you will absorb it all.

Keep well in mind in planning everyday meals just which foods contain most vitamin K. Green leafy vegetables are excellent sources. Since they contain many other essential vitamins and minerals as well, make them part of every day's menus. For someone who can't eat them either cooked or raw, because of plain dislike or because of some condition of ill health, use a juicer. But get plenty of these green leafy vegetables. Wheat bran and wheat germ are other fine sources.

Foods that contain most vitamin K are: pork liver, soybean oil, spinach, kale, carrot tops, cabbage, alfalfa and other green leafy vegetables, cauliflower, tomatoes, eggyolk, corn, mushrooms, oats, peas, potatoes, soybeans, strawberries, wheat bran and wheat germ.

# Vitamins in the Nineties: Where We Are Now

So WHAT HAS HAPPENED in the field of vitamins since 1988 when the latest edition of this book was published? *A LOT*. The single most important thing was a conference on *Antioxidant Vitamins: Good News for Healthy Hearts* held in New York City in May 1991.

Antioxidants are those nutrients which protect fatty tissues of the body from going "bad" or become rancid with very serious consequences. The three most important antioxidant vitamins are beta carotene (which is the plant form of vitamin A), vitamin C and vitamin E.

Specialists in this field came from many areas of our country and abroad to this conference. Michael Oliver, M.D. of the Wynn Institute in London, England studied 110 angina patients and found low blood levels of beta carotene and vitamin C and E. He said "The relative risk of developing angina was 2.7 times higher at the lowest plasma concentration of vitamin E, as compared to the highest . . . Vitamin E is an excellent scavenger of free radicals and thus mitigates some of their damage."

David Kritchevsky, Ph.D of the Wistar Institute of Anatomy and Biology in Philadelphia, Pa. explained that these vitamins appear to play several beneficial roles. They may help to protect against high blood pressure and smoking. They may increase the level of the protective type of cholesterol known as HDL.

Data showing an association between high blood levels

409

of vitamin C and reduced blood pressure was presented by Paul Jacques, Sc.D of the U.S. Department of Agriculture Human Nutrition Research Center on Aging at Tufts University. "Limited experimental data suggest that vitamin C supplementation may reduce blood pressure in borderline hypertensive patients," said Dr. Jacques.

Judith Hallfrisch, Ph.D., an investigator with the National Institute of Aging, found a correlation between higher blood levels of HDL cholesterol and vitamin C in a large sample of people enrolled in the Baltimore Longitudinal Study on Aging.

"After adjusting for age, gender, smoking status and other variables, plasma vitamin C was directly and significantly associated with HDL," said Dr. Hallfrisch. "These findings suggest that high plasma levels of vitamin C may reduce the risk of developing atherosclerosis by increasing the amount of protective HDL."

Cigarette smoking is a known risk factor for the development of coronary heart disease. Although it is not clear exactly how cigarette smoking affects heart health, the association is so strong that smoking is considered a major independent risk factor for the disease. One theory suggests that cigarette smoking causes an increase in the presence of destructive oxygen radicals, which are generated by smoke itself, and also by the inflammation of body tissues induced by smoking.

Vitamin C is an excellent neutralizer of these harmful oxygen radicals, particularly in blood plasma. However, according to research presented by Raymond B. Bridges, Ph.D. of the University of Kentucky, cigarette smokers have significantly depressed levels of vitamin C. Dr. Bridges hypothesized, "The increased risk of cardiovascular disease in smokers could be mediated by the synergistic effects of an increase in destructive oxygen radicals, along with a decrease in blood levels of antioxidants such as vitamin C. Both of these have been associated with smoking."

Joseph Witztum, M.D. of the University of California, San Diego explained that when major cholesterol-carrying blood fat—LDL or low density lipoprotein—becomes oxidized, it assumes properties that can promote hardening of the arteries.

## Preventing atherosclerosis

Oxidation is a chemical alteration of the fat similar to the way in which butter turns rancid. It can be triggered in the body by a variety of factors including compounds in cigarette smoke or polluted air; inflammation and by essential metals such as iron and copper. Dr. Witztum's group has demonstrated that once oxidized, LDL is preferentially taken up by cells of the immune system called macrophages. This is a crucial step in the process of atherosclerosis, because the macrophages die and eventually make their way into the lesions in artery walls.

Ishwarlal Jialal, M.D. and his colleagues at the University of Texas Southwestern Medical Center showed that antioxidant vitamin C and vitamin E can stop LDL from becoming oxidized and taken up by macrophages. They found that vitamin C inhibited uptake for LDL by 93% and vitamin E by 45%.

"These findings appear to support a role for vitamin C supplementation in the prevention of atherosclerosis, if the oxidized-LDL hypothesis is correct," said Dr. Jialal.

Another series of studies was reported by Balz Frei, Ph.D. a researcher and professor of nutrition at the Harvard School of Public Health. "We compared the effectiveness of different antioxidants that are present naturally within LDL, as well as those present in plasma, the fluid component of blood in which LDL is transported," said Dr. Frei. "We found that under all different types of oxidizing conditions, vitamin C completely protected the lipoproteins against detectable oxidative damage, and the other antioxidants provided partial protection. Our data suggest that dietary antioxidants, especially vitamin C, are capable of preventing atherosclerosis in humans or slowing down its progression by inhibiting the oxidation of LDL," he said.

411

Direct evidence of the ability of antioxidants to counter oxidative damage to heart tissue was cited by Donald Mickle, M.D. of Toronto General Hospital. Dr. Mickle presented evidence that vitamin E, the only membrane-soluble antioxidant, helps minimize the damage that occurs in heart tissues during medical procedures such as bypass surgery.

"When the heart is deprived of oxygen, then resupplied with oxygen-rich blood, a high concentraition of free radicals is released. This overwhelms the tissues' defense systems and causes severe damage. Vitamin E mitigates some of this damage because it is an excellent scavenger of free radicals," he said. He also said that preliminary results have been so encouraging that a water-soluble analogue of vitamin E is currently being developed for emergency treatment of heart attack patients.

A summary of the conference states that vitamin C appears to minimize certain heart and artery risks associated with high blood pressure, high cholesterol levels and even smoking.

All these findings assume great importance when, as was pointed out at the conference, approximately 68,090,000 Americans have one or more forms of cardiovascular disease. It takes a human life every 32 seconds in the U.S.A. An estimated 61,870,000 Americans older than six years have high blood pressure resulting in more than 30,000 deaths in 1988. An estimated more than three million Americans have angina. Some forty-six million Americans are smokers, placing them at increased risk of heart attack.

To summarize, vitamins C and E and beta carotene appear to be among the body's arsenal of weapons against the development of coronary heart disease which is, at present, our greatest killer.

## Vitamins against cancer

In her *New York Times* column, September 25, 1991, Jane Brody wrote at length of cancer and these three vitamins. She quoted a Swiss study of nearly 3,000 men which found that cancer deaths were significantly higher in those with low blood levels of carotene. In women with precancerous changes in the cervix, abnormal tissues were far more common in those with low blood levels of carotene and vitamin C. Other studies have shown that precancerous lesions in the mouth can be checked by a diet enriched with beta carotene. Animal studies have suggested that vitamin C can protect against sunlight-induced skin cancer. A recent Cornell University study showed that beta carotene can prevent impairment of the human immune system by ultraviolet light. The immune system is that coalition of body parts that helps to protect us against almost any harmful invaders. Ms. Brody suggests that you make every effort to include in every day's diet plenty of dark green, leafy vegetables plus bright orange vegetables and fruits since these are loaded with beta carotene.

Scientists and physicians have known for many years that beta carotene or vitamin A is essential for the health of the eyes. *Medical Tribune,* August 22, 1991, reported that lack of just this one vitamin leads to blindness in India and says that vitamin A deficiency affects 10 to 40 million children worldwide, about half of whom live in India. In addition to blindness such children are more likely to have respiratory or gastrointestinal problems.

*Medical World News,* August, 1991 reported on beta carotene as a shield against colon cancer according to Australian doctors. An Italian team slowed cell proliferation among 20 polyp patients by treating them with 30,000 units of vitamin A, 70 milligrams of vitamin E and one gram of vitamin C daily. We would point out that such high doses of vitamin A itself must be carefully watched. Beta carotene has no such risks.

*The Washington Post,* September 25, 1990 reported that a chemical cousin to vitamin A—an anti-acne drug marketed as Accutane—can help to prevent development of additional tumors in cancer patients. In our country one individual in every four will develop cancer at some time in their lives.

The *Post* quotes an article in *The New England Journal of Medicine* which showed that high doses of Accutane could help to prevent tumors from recurring in patients who had one bout of cancer of the larynx, pharynx or the mouth, and were thus at great risk of developing cancer of the lung, throat or mouth. However, Accutane "is not a vitamin and there are side effects from taking it," the expert warned. It is a synthetic form of vitamin A. As usual, the *Post* article suggests that we eat diets rich in fresh fruits and dark green vegetables rather than depending solely on vitamin pills.

*Medical Tribune* reported in October, 1991 that children with low levels of vitamin A display more serious symptoms than those who have plenty of vitamin A. In fact, vitamin A-deficient children must usually be treated for measles in a hospital! Both the severity of the disease and the morality figures show clearly that children deficient in vitamin A are at higher risk from just this difference and who knows, perhaps other contagious diseases as well.

**Update on B vitamins**

What has been discovered about the B vitamins during the early days of the 1990's? *The Lancet* October, 26, 1991 reported on findings that thiamine deficiency has been found in some AIDS patients. The Canadian authors suggest that AIDS patients be given supplements of thiamine. *The Lancet,* August 3, 1991 describes the risk of sudden death among Southeast Asian men. They died suddenly in their sleep. The authors, Ronald Munger and his colleagues state that this sudden death in sleep may be related to lack of thiamine. They state that among refugees in Thailand lack of thiamine was related to sleep disorders. So it appears that deficiency in thiamine may be a cause of sudden death in this region. The authors suggest that they be given thiamine supplements if they have a tendency to this disorder.

*Archives of Internal Medicine,* Volume 151, 1991 reported on an experiment giving a slow-release form of niacin (vitamin B3) to 200 volunteers and getting a decided decrease in low density fat (LDL) the harmful kind. The author was Joseph M. Keenan, et.al. Department of Family Practice, Minneapolis, Minnesota.

*Better Nutrition for Today's Living* reported in the March, 1991 issue on an experiment giving niacin (B3) in a study lasting nine years. At the end of the test researchers from the Coronary Drug Project, funded by the National Heart, Lung and Blood Institute found that there were 79 fewer fatalities among those taking the vitamin than in those who took other drugs.

*Diabetologia* reported in May, 1991 that 14 children at risk of diabetes were given one form of niacin (nicotinamide) and only one child of those did get the disease.

## Vitamin B12

Much new research was done on vitamin B12. Dr. E. H. Reynold et al. from the Department of Neurology, King's College Hospital, London worked with 10 patients with multiple sclerosis and vitamin B12 deficiency. Eight cases occurred before the age of 40, which is a rare age for B12 deficiency. He says, "The nature of the association of multiple sclerosis and vitamin B12 deficiency was explained. A vitamin B12 binding and/or transport defect is suspected . . . Further studies of vitamin B12 metabolism binding and transport in multiple sclerosis are indicated, as these cases may offer a clue to the understanding of a still mysterious neurological disorder."

*The New England Journal of Medicine* reported in its July 14, 1988 issue that lack of vitamin B12 affects bone growth. Giving B12 to one group of patients and not to the second group, the five researchers discovered that those who got the vitamin showed improvement indicating that osteoblastic activity depends on vitamin B12 and bone metabolism is affected by deficiency of the vitamin.

The same journal, June 30, 1988, published an article showing that an inherited tendency to disorders of dealing with vitamin B12 may lead to nerve problems in later life which may be diagnosed as multiple sclerosis.

## Niacin and biotin

Dr. Carl C. Pfeiffer in his book *Mental and Elemental Nutrients* stated that the Research Directory of the Miami Heart Institute used the B vitamin niacin for heart patients in more than 1000 cases. In one group 600 patients' insurance companies had predicted probably 62 deaths over a 10-year period. Only six deaths occurred among those who were taking niacin.

*Science News* reported, April 27, 1991, on a form of niacin which releases the vitamin very slowly into the blood. A Minnesota physician, using this form of the vitamin in a 16-week trial reduced the harmful form of cholesterol in his patients who were given massive doses of niacin with almost no unpleasant side effects. However, medical journals do report side effects from massive doses of niacin. Some of them are quite serious, so if you plan to take niacin to reduce your cholesterol level, it's a good idea to make the experiment under a physician's care.

Biotin, another B vitamin, has been shown to be essential for normal bone growth. *Nutrition Reviews,* May, 1989 told of chicks raised on diets deficient in biotin whose bones grew abnormally. The same publication in April, 1989 told of biotin deficiency altering the fatty acid composition of infants placed on total feeding through tubes. Just the lack of this one vitamin resulted in this condition.

*The American Journal of Clinical Nutrition,* January, 1989, reported findings that individuals being treated with anti-convulsant drugs are likely to become deficient in biotin. In 1991 a physician at Columbia Center in New York City became interested in stories of Swiss researchers who used biotin to correct brittle fingernails. *Prevention* for July

1991 told of Swiss researchers in a controlled experiment who gave one group of 32 volunteers with brittle fingernails six to nine months of daily treatment of only 25 milligrams of biotin. The subjects' nail thickness was boosted by 25%. This experiment was reported in the *Journal of the American Academy of Dermatology* in 1990.

## Vitamin B6

"Doses of B6 [pyridoxine] Cited as Too Low for Elderly" was a headline in *Medical Tribune* September 19, 1991. Andrea Kott told of a Tufts University study of elderly people showing that even those who were eating nutritionally balanced meals providing the recommended amount of B6 were deficienct in the vitamin, according to Stanley Gershoff, Ph.D. head of the School of Nutrition. "We believe," said he, "that the B6 recommended dietary allowance isn't likely to meet the real requirements of the elderly. Prolonged absence of vitamin B6 could compromise the health of older Americans . . . The RDA's which were introduced at that time do not meet the needs of elderly people."

People in a three-month study had vitamin B6 measured before the study and during a three-week period when they were fed a vitamin B6 deficient diet. Blood and urine samples collected during this time revealed deficiencies, according to D. Ribaya-Mercado, D. Sc. of the Tufts University School of Nutrition.

A 1991 press release from the U.S. Department of Agriculture stated that older people, especially older women appear to need more of this vitamin than currently recommended. Since the vitamin plays an important role in control of nervous system function, a low intake of this vitamin could result in depression, lethargy, confusion or nervousness. At that time 1.6 milligrams of B6 were recommended. But the women tested needed almost 2 milligrams daily before their tests returned to normal. These tests

417

showed that such levels provide a small safety margin for women and a little larger margin for older men.

*Prevention,* August, 1991, told of a report in *Quarterly Report,* October-December, 1990, recounting an experiment in which four men and four women, all in their sixties, were given a short-term diet virtually devoid of vitamin B6. In less than three weeks the men's insulin levels climbed 131% over normal, even though their blood sugar levels went up only slightly. Oddly, the women were relatively unaffected. B6 was added to their diets and the men's insulin levels returned to normal.

*The Journal of the American Medical Association,* November 20, 1990, reported that vitamin B6 is effective in treating nausea and vomiting of pregnancy. The amount of the vitamin needed was only 25 milligrams every eight hours. Infant rats from mothers on diets deficient in B6 were found to be likely to have convulsive disorders. *FDA Consumer,* September, 1991, stated that deficiency in B6 can cause anemia, dermatitis and convulsions. In infants it can lead to "a variety of neurological disorders and abdominal distress."

*Better Nutrition for Today's Living* (October, 1990) reported on vitamin B6 as successful in treating the wrist disorder called carpal tunnel syndrome, found most commonly in people who do daily work using their hands in repetitive motions. Dr. John Ellis of Texas has used B6 in treating other manifestations of arthritis. He says that numbness, tingling and pain and stiffness in fingers and hands are an early symptom of vitamin B6 deficiency. A dose of 50 milligrams of vitamin B6 daily and indefinitely can be helpful, he says.

**Folic acid**

Folic acid has been in the news in recent years because of the finding that lack of this vitamin in the pregnant woman's diet may result in a child with "neural tube defects"—

that is, some defects in the baby's spine leading perhaps to spina bifida. *The Journal of the American Medical Association* in December, 1991 reviewed a *Lancet* article on this subject that showed in these words, "Folic acid supplementation starting before pregnancy can now be firmly recommended for all women who have had an affected pregnancy and public health measures should be taken to insure that the diets of all women who may bear children contain an adequate amount of folic acid."

Deficiency in folic acid may also be responsible for cancer of the cervix and cervical dysplasia (abnormal cell development or growth in women). A lead article in the *Journal of the American Medical Association,* January, 1992 reported on a study of 726 young women among whom were found 294 cases of dysplasia. Low blood levels of folic acid "enhanced the effect of other risk factors for cervical dysplasia," say the authors, all physicians from various medical centers. They add that lack of folic acid may also be a cause of cervical cancer. *Nutrition Reviews,* October, 1989 discussed these risks, adding that folic acid deficiency may also be a cause of cervical cancer.

*American Journal of Clinical Nutrition* (September, 1989) presented a survey of some 11,000 Americans to determine their intake of folic acid. The researchers found that it was uniformly low. The authors concluded that, "Folate intake along with vitamin C, vitamin A and dietary fiber would show a substantial increase if Americans consumed more vegetables and legumes." The authors were Amy F. Subar, Gladys Block and L. Denise James.

## Vitamin C

So many things have happened with vitamin C research these recent years that there is hardly room to list them. In 1991, Dr. Linus Pauling, the world's greatest champion of vitamin C, had his 90th birthday and stated, "Some people say I'm the best evidence that my regimen works." His regimen contains large amounts of vitamin C along with all the other essential nutrients.

In September 1990 The National Cancer Institute held a conference on *Vitamin C, Biological Functions and Relation to Cancer*. The conference contained a great deal of evidence that vitamin C is powerful against cancer, both in test tubes and in living animals. Vitamin C was found to be powerful against breast cancer. It protected skin from becoming cancerous when it was exposed to ultraviolet light.

Vitamin C protected against cancer in animals exposed to various cancer-causing hormones. Other topics at the meeting covered the antioxidant and free-radical scavenging activities of vitamin C, its relation to iron metabolism, immune functions and data on how best to prevent cancers from occurring by giving vitamin C. Complete copies of abstracts of the conference are available from Gladys Block, Ph.D. National Cancer Institute, EPN 313, 9000 Rockville Pike, Bethesda, MD, 20892.

*Medical Tribune*, January 16, 1992, reported that daily vitamin C protects sperm from genetic damage. A study of men who cut back on their dietary intake of vitamin C going from 250 milligrams a day to five milligrams of vitamin C, found that a form of DNA damage in their sperm nearly doubled, according to Bruce N. Ames, Ph.D., a researcher at the University of California at Berkeley. When the men increased their intake of vitamin C, taking either 60 milligrams or 250 milligrams a day, DNA damage dropped. Dr. Ames commented, "This is the first study to link low levels of vitamin C to DNA damage." His study did not examine whether vitamin C doses greater than 250 milligrams a day provide even more protection.

Vitamin C is found normally in semen where it is believed to protect the DNA of sperm cells from toxic oxygen radicals. Studies have shown that children of male smokers are at greater risk of leukemia and immune-system cancer than children of male non-smokers. Dr. Ames said this is due to the significant drop in vitamin C that occurs in semen when a man smokes.

In 1991 *Medical Science Research,* volume 19, printed a full-page editorial by Linus Pauling titled "Vitamin C and Cardiological Disease." Pauling said, among other things, that almost 11 animal species synthesize vitamin C and the amounts synthesized per day, corrected for body weight, are in the 3,000 to 18,000 milligram range. Moreover, ascorbate is involved in many biochemical reactions and "there is considerable evidence that a high intake of supplementary ascorbate improves the health and helps to control various diseases." He said further that Linus Pauling Institute researchers studied the guinea pig and showed that guinea pigs' blood contains lipoproteins. Laboratory guinea pigs are fed a diet very high in ascorbate (vitamin C). "We accordingly verified that when guinea pigs are placed on a low ascorbate diet, corresponding to the usual human intake of this vitamin, they rapidly develop atherosclerotic plaques similar in nature to human plaques. Accordingly, there is now available a satisfactory animal model for the study of atherosclerosis."

The *Washington Post* in 1991 quoted a National Institute for Mental Health spokesman as saying that Pauling's recommendation of treatment for schizophrenia—massive doses of vitamin C—remains "on the fringe." Pauling himself opposes the RDA for vitamin C (60 milligrams for most adults) and states that this is not nearly enough to assure good health. He himself takes 18,000 milligrams of vitamin C daily in divided doses.

For those troubled with what doctors call "atropic dermatitis," a slow-release ascorbic acid preparation might be the answer as University of California researchers found. The report in *Medical World News* (April, 1989) stated that the vitamin might be given along with antibiotic drugs which are frequently given. Eczema and psoriasis are two such skin disorders.

In 1990 Dr. Pauling criticized *Consumer Reports* for its

denial that vitamin C has any value in controlling the common cold. He also reminded them that large doses of vitamin C are not dangerous and do not have serious side effects. The only possible side effect, he said, is a laxative effect. No cases of formation of kidney stones or other harmful effects of vitamin C have been reliably reported.

*Medical World News,* August, 1991, reported on two studies on vitamin C in hardening of the arteries and heart health. The National Institute of Aging found that, in a large group of volunteers, vitamin C was associated with lower LDL levels of cholesterol (the harmful kind) and higher levels of HDL (the helpful kind).

**Vitamin D**

Vitamin D is manufactured on the skin in sunlight. So people who are not outside very much in summer are apt to be short on this vitamin. On October 2, 1991 the U.S. Department of Agriculture reported that older women can increase spine bone by getting more of the "sunshine vitamin"—vitamin D—along with extra calcium during the short and gloomy days of winter. Leader of the U.S.D.A. study, Bess Dawson-Hughes, stated that "We find that postmenopausal women living in the temperate zone benefit from increasing their vitamin D intake to about 500 international Units (I.U.) daily."

Dr. Dawson-Hughes and her colleagues at USDA's Human Nutrition Research Center of Aging at Tufts University in Boston measured bone density in 247 women past menopause three times during a year-long study. They reported their findings in the October, 1991 *Annals of Internal Medicine.* Both groups studied had an increase in spine bone during the first measurement period from June or July to December or January. Both had loss during the second measurement from December or January to June or July. But the group getting the vitamin D supplement had less than half as much loss as the group getting the placebo, she said.

*The Washington Post,* July 31, 1990, reported on another study at the Boston University School of Medicine which showed that of 50 aged residents of the Hebrew Rehabilitation Center, nearly 80% were deficient in vitamin D by the end of winter.

## Vitamin E

Research on vitamin E is proceeding in many countries. One 1991 finding showed that a low blood level of vitamin E is the most important risk factor in death from ischemic heart disease, significantly more important than high cholesterol levels, elevated blood pressure or smoking. These were results of a World Health Organization sponsored study published in the January, 1991 issue of the *American Journal of Clinical Nutrition.* The study is the first large-scale study in humans that correlates dietary factors other than cholesterol. It is particularly significant because the results show that factors in addition to cholesterol levels should be considered when assessing risk of ischemic heart disease.

In this international study, blood plasma levels of antioxidants (nutrients including vitamins C, E and A and beta carotene), cholesterol levels and blood pressure were measured in middle-aged men selected at random in 16 European cities. Smokers and nonsmokers were included in the study. It was found that cholesterol and diastolic blood pressure had only moderate association with death caused by blockage of coronary arteries. But low plasma levels of vitamin E were *of major importance* in predicting death from this type of heart disease. A finding of low vitamin E predicted IHD mortality in 62% of the cases. A total of four factors combined—low vitamin E, elevated total cholesterol, low vitamin A and elevated blood pressure predicted death from ischemic heart disease by 87%. In this study vitamin C showed only moderate relation and vitamin A a weak relation to death from ischemic heart disease.

Current scientific hypotheses link initial development of

atherosclerosis with oxidation of fats circulating in the blood, especially LDL's (low density lipoproteins). It is believed that vitamin E, which is an antioxidant, protects LDL's from oxidation in the blood stream, thereby slowing or preventing deposits that build up on the walls of arteries and eventually restrict blood flow to the heart. This study made headlines in many American newspapers.

*Science News,* October 12, 1991, presented a short article showing that vitamin E may be a shield against lung cancer. The article describes three reports from the September, 1991 *American Journal of Epidemiology.* One research group followed 4,538 Finnish men for 20 years. Among the 117 men who developed lung cancer smoking proved to be the biggest risk factor. But the data also suggest that non-smokers eating diets high in antioxidants—mainly carotenoids, vitamin C and vitamin E—lowered their lung cancer risk by at least 60%. And these agents appear to act independently since non-smokers with diets low in all three faced nearly four times the cancer risk of those whose diets contained the most. Among plant-derived foods fruits conveyed the biggest benefits, although the study also linked red and yellow vegetables and cereals to lower lung cancer risks.

In 1989 at a symposium on Vitamin E, John D. Trevichick, Ph.D., Professor of Biochemistry at the University of Western Ontario, Canada, stated that in a study that compared the self-reported intake of supplementary vitamin E in 175 cataract patients and 175 matched cataract-free patients, it was found that those who were cataract-free took significantly more vitamin E and C.

At the same symposium Lester Packer, Ph.D., Professor of Molecular and Cell Biology at the University of California in Berkeley, showed that vitamin E may exert benefits to slow the aging process. He said in part, ''Research has shown that free radical damage accumulates during the aging process. Such damage is also implicated in the process of cancer initiation and promotion. Free radical mediated damage processes have also been implicated in other degenerative diseases such as arthritis and arteriosclerosis. In these instances, vitamin E has been shown to exert various benefits which appear to slow and reduce the severity of these diseases.''

"Vitamin E May Help Us Breathe a Little Easier" is the headline on a news release from the Henkel corporation. It states that the threat of ozone pollution is high in the summer, ozone being one of the most noxious of all air pollutants. Scientific studies conducted over the last decade show that vitamin E may offer one remedy. In a study at the University of California in Los Angeles Nabil M. Elsayed, Ph.D. published a report in the December, 1988 issue of *Drug-Nutrient Interaction* showing that "The results suggest that an absence of vitamin E exacerbates lung injury from ozone inhalation while its presence protects from injury. When we are exposed to polluted air, the need for vitamin E protection is increased."

## Cataracts

Older people who consume plenty of vitamins run far lower risk of cataracts, the leading cause of blindness, researchers say. Both vitamin A and E, being antioxidants, decrease the risk, according to Leo T. Chylack, co-author of a study at Brigham and Women's Hospital in Boston. The study was directed by M. Christina Leske of the State University at Stony Brook and was based on 1,380 people aged 40 to 79 who were treated at the Boston hospitals. The study was published in *The Archives of Ophthalmology*, February 1991.

A similar study by James M. Robinson of the University of Western Ontario, Canada, demonstrated the same thing. Commenting on the research in volume 135 of *Science News*, Allen Taylor of the USDA Human Nutrition Research Center on Aging in Medford, MA said, "If you could delay cataract formation by just 10 years you would eliminate the need for half of the cataract extractions." Such surgery mounts up to half a million operations each year. Studying 175 cataract patients over 55 with another 175 cataract-free adults, the scientists found that the only significant difference betweeen the two groups, other than the presence of cataracts, was that the cataract-free individuals had taken at least 400 International Units (one regular capsule) of vitamin E and/or a minimum of 500 milligrams of vitamin C per day over the last five years. Researchers assumed the volunteers ate similar diets because they came from similar backgrounds. This article appeared in *Science News*, Volume 135. These researchers have also shown that diabetic rats given high levels of vitamin E develop fewer cataracts than those animals who did not get the vitamin.

Tardive dyskinesia is a disease usually of elderly people. It is caused usually by drugs prescribed for various ailments. It consists of abnormal involuntary movements of the facial structure and limbs. A recent double-blind crossover study showed that vitamin E is effective in treatment of this very disturbing illness. Eight individuals with the disease took 400 I.U. of vitamin E a day for the first week, then 400 I.U. twice a day for the second week and 400 I.U. of vitamin E three times a day for the final two weeks.

The authors of the study, A. M. Elkashef, P. E. Ruskin, N. Bacher and D. Barrett said in their report in the *American Journal of Psychiatry,* Vol. 147: 505–506, 1990 that, although conclusions based on a small group of people must be made with caution, they parallel the results obtained in another experiment and the researchers ask for additional research on this matter.

At a 1991 vitamin E symposium, Alfredo Lopez-s, M.D., Ph.D., Professor of Medicine and Nutrition at Louisiana State University, spoke on vitamins A, E and C and lung cancer.

In his laboratory he compared the blood levels of vitamin A, carotene, vitamin C and vitamin E and smoking habits in a group of hospitalized persons who were newly diagnosed with primary lung cancer with a control group of hospitalized patients matched for race, sex and age but without cancer. He found that persons with lung cancer had lower blood levels of the carotene group and vitamin E compared with the controls. He says that his results suggest there is a relationship between low levels of vitamin E and lung cancer, regardless of levels of blood cholesterol. This association, he found, is greater for vitamin E than for beta carotene or vitamin A.

## Antioxidants and exercise

New studies show that a vigorous workout can cause damage to the body's cells if vitamin E levels are not adequate. During vigorous exercise the body takes in and uses oxygen at a high rate—up to 10 to 20 times as much as in normal day-to-day activity. The greater the use of oxygen, the more free radicals are created and the higher the potential for cell damage. If we exercise in an environment where the air is polluted, the free radical threat is exacerbated.

The body has an antioxidant defense system consisting of enzymes and nutrients that protect the body from oxidative cell damage. When there is an ample supply of these antioxidants, free radical damage is not a problem. But Dr. Lester Packer of the University of California at Berkeley has demonstrated in his studies of runners and cyclists that the body's antioxidant supply gets used up more quickly under conditions of increased oxygen consumption during exercise. Packer found that increasing the intake of certain nutrients—especially vitamin E—helps to bolster antioxidant defense and protects against cell damage.

*The International Journal of Biochemistry,* Vol. 21 (1989) published a study of male college students engaging in exhaustive exercise. The exercise was followed by an increase in blood fat peroxide levels. When the exercisers were given 300 milligrams of vitamin E per day for four weeks, the blood levels of peroxide returned to normal. The conclusion to this and other research along the same lines is that "While research is continuing on the protective role of vitamin E in exercise, results to date demonstrate an increased requirement for vitamin E to prevent free radical-related tissue damage associated with strenuous exercise."

My file on vitamin E research during the early 1990's is so large that there is no way even to list the titles of the research articles, all of which have shown vitamin E to be extremely valuable in almost every aspect of health. It is also totally without any deterimental side effects in doses up to eight International Units taken throughout the day. From all the above interest in vitamin E it seems obvious that it will continue far into the future and we and our descendants will benefit greatly from using these wholly natural compounds for good health.

# Suggested Further Reading

Atkins, Robert C., M.D., *Dr. Atkins' Nutrition Breakthrough,* William Morrow and Co., New York, 1981.

Berkley, George, Ph.D., *Arthritis Without Aspirin,* Prentice-Hall, Inc., Englewood Cliffs, N.J., 1982.

Bland, Jeffrey, Ph.D., *Bioflavonoids,* Keats Publishing, Inc., New Canaan, CT, 1984.

Brighthope, Ian M. D. with Peter Fitzgerald, *The AIDS Fighters,* Keats Publishing, Inc. New Canaan, CT, 1988.

Burkitt, D. P. and H. C. Trowell, *Refined Carbohydrate Foods and Disease,* Academic Press, New York, 1975.

Burkitt, Denis, M.D., *Eat Right to Stay Healthy and Enjoy Life More,* ARCO Publishing, Inc., New York, 1979.

Cameron, Ewan, M.D. and Linus Pauling, Ph.D., *Cancer and Vitamin C,* Linus Pauling Institute of Science and Medicine, Palo Alto, CA, 1979.

Cheraskin, Emanuel, M.D., D.M.D., W. Marshall Ringsdorf, Jr., M.S., D.M.D., Emily Sisley, Ph.D., *The Vitamin C Connection,* Harper and Row, New York, 1983.

Cheraskin, E., M.D., D.M.D., W. M. Ringsdorf, Jr., D.M.D., M.S. and J. W. Clark, D.D.S., *Diet and Disease,* Keats Publishing, Inc., New Canaan, CT, 1987.

Cheraskin, Emanuel, M.D., D.M.D., *The Vitamin C Controversy: Questions and Answers,* Keats Publishing, Inc., New Canaan, CT, 1988.

Cleave, T. L., M.D., *The Saccharine Disease,* Keats Publishing, New Canaan, CT, 1975

Cousins, Norman, *Anatomy of an Illness,* W. W. Norton and Co., Inc., New York, 1979.

Ellis, John, M.D. and James Presley, *Vitamin B6, The Doctor's Report,* Harper and Row, New York, 1973.

Fredericks, Carlton, Ph.D., *Breast Cancer, a Nutritional Approach,* Grosset and Dunlap, New York, 1977.

Fredericks, Carlton, Ph.D., *Arthritis, Don't Learn to Live With It,* Grosset and Dunlap, New York, 1981.

Fredericks, Carlton, Ph.D., *Eat Well, Get Well, Stay Well,* Grosset and Dunlap, New York, 1980.

Garrison, Robert H., Jr., M.A., R.Ph. and Somer, Elizabeth, M.A., R.D., *The Nutrition Desk Reference,* Keats Publishing, Inc., New Canaan, CT, 1990.

Goodman, Sandra, *Vitamin C, The Master Nutrient,* Keats Publishing, Inc., New Canaan, CT, 1991.

Gruberg, Edward R., Ph.D. and Stephen A. Raymond, Ph.D., *Beyond Choelsterol: Vitamin B6, Arteriosclerosis and Your Heart,* St. Martin's Press, New York, 1981.

Hawkins, David and Linus Pauling, *Orthomolecular Psychiatry,* W. H. Freeman, San Francisco, CA, 1973.

Hendler, Sheldon Saul, M.D., Ph.D., *The Doctors' Vitamin and Mineral Encyclopedia,* Simon & Schuster, 1990.

Hoffer, Abram,. M.D., Ph.D., and Morton Walker, D.P.M., *Orthomolecular Nutrition,* Keats Publishing, Inc., New Canaan, CT, 1978

Kalokerinos, Archie, M.D., *Every Second Child,* Keats Publishing, Inc., New Canaan, CT, 1981.

Kirschmann, John D., Director, *Nutrition Almanac,* 2nd edition, McGraw-Hill Book Co., New York, 1984.

Kowalski, Robert E., *The 8-Week Cholesterol Cure,* Harper and Row, New York, 1987.

Kugler, Hans, Ph.D., *The Disease of Aging,* Keats Publishing, Inc., New Canaan, CT, 1984.

# SUGGESTED FURTHER READING

Kutsky, Roman J., Ph.D., *Handbook of Vitamins, Minerals and Hormones*, Van Nostrand-Reinhold Co., New York, 1981.

Lesser, Michael, M.D., *Nutrition and Vitamin Therapy*, Grove Press, Inc., New York, 1980.

Lewin, Sherry, Ph.D., *Vitamin C, Its Molecular Biology and Medical Potential*, Academic Press, New York, 1976.

Lieberman, Shari and Nancy Bruning, *The Real Vitamin and Mineral Book*, Avery Publishing Group, Inc., Garden City Park, N.Y., 1990.

Mindell, Earl, R. Ph., Ph.D. and William H. Lee, R. Ph., Ph.D., *The Vitamin Robbers*, Keats Publishing, Inc., New Canaan, CT, 1983.

Modell, Walter, M.D., *Drugs in Current Use, and New Drugs*, Springer Publishing Co., New York, 1978.

Newbold, H. L., M.D., *Vitamin C Against Cancer*, Stein and Day, Briarcliff Manor, N.Y., 1979.

Newbold, H. L., M.D., *Meganutrients for Your Nerves*, Keats Publishing, Inc., New Canaan, CT, 1993.

Passwater, Richard A., Ph.D., *Cancer and Its Nutritional Therapies*, Keats Publishing, Inc., New Canaan, CT, 1983.

Passwater, Richard A., Ph.D., *Beta-Carotene*, Keats Publishing Inc., New Canaan, CT, 1984.

Passwater, Richard A., Ph.D., *A Beginner's Introduction to Vitamins*, Keats Publishing, New Canaan, CT, 1983.

Pauling, Linus, Ph.D., *Vitamin C and the Common Cold*, Bantam Books, New York, 1971.

Pauling, Linus, Ph.D., *Vitamin C, the Common Cold and the Flu*, W. H. Freeman and Co., San Francisco, CA, 1970.

Pauling, Linus, Ph.D., *How to Live Longer and Feel Better*, W. H. Freeman and Co., New York, 1986.

Pfeiffer, Carl C., M.D., *Zinc and Other Micro-Nutrients,* Keats Publishing, Inc., New Canaan, CT, 1978.

Pfeiffer, Carl C., Ph.D., M.D., *Mental and Elemental Nutrients,* Keats Publishing Inc., New Canaan, CT, 1975.

Price, Weston A., D.D.S., *Nutrition and Physical Degeneration,* Keats Publishing, Inc., New Canaan, CT, 1990.

*Recommended Dietary Allowances, 10th Ed.* 1989, National Academy of Sciences, Washington, D.C.

Reed, Barbara, Ph.D., *Food, Teens and Behavior,* Natural Press, Manitowoc, WI, 1983.

Roe, Daphne, M.D., *Drug-Induced Nutritional Deficiencies,* The AVI Publishing Co., Inc., Westport, CT, 1976.

Rosenberg, Harold, M.D. and A. N. Feldzamen, Ph.D., *The Doctor's Book of Vitamin Therapy,* G. P. Putnam, New York, 1974.

Ross, Harvey, M.D., *Fighting Depression,* Keats Publishing, Inc., New Canaan, CT, 1992.

Seaman, Barbara and Gideon Seaman, M.D., *Women and the Crisis in Sex Hormones,* Rawson Associates, Publishers, New York, 1977.

Shute, Evan, M.D., *The Heart and Vitamin E,* Keats Publishing, Inc., New Canaan, CT, 1977.

Shute, Wilfred E., M.D., *The Complete Updated Vitamin E Book,* Keats Publishing Co., New Canaan, CT, 1975.

Smith, Lendon, M.D., *Feed Yourself Right,* McGraw-Hill Book Co., New York, 1983.

Smith, Lendon H., M.D., *Happiness is a Healthy Life,* Keats Publishing, Inc., New Canaan, CT, 1992.

Stone, Irwin, *The Healing Factor, Vitamin C Against Disease,* Grosset and Dunlap, New York, 1972.

Weiner, Michael, Ph.D., *Reducing Risk of Alzheimer's Disease,* Stein and Day, Publishers, Briarcliff Manor, N.Y., 1987.

Werbach, Melvyn R., M.D., *Nutritional Influences on Illness*, Keats Publishing, Inc., New Canaan, CT, 1990.

Williams, Roger J., Ph.D., D.Sc., and Dwight K. Kalita, Ph.D., *A Physician's Handbook on Orthomolecular Medicine*, Keats Publishing, Inc., New Canaan, CT, 1989.

Williams, Roger J., Ph.D., *Nutrition Against Disease*, Pitman Publishing Corp, New York, 1971.

Williams, Roger J., Ph.D., D.Sc., *Physician's Handbook of Nutritional Science*, Charles C. Thomas, Publisher, Springfield, Ill, 1975.

Williams, Roger, J., Ph.D., *The Wonderful World Within You*, Keats Publishing, Inc., New Canaan,. CT, 1977.

Wright, Jonathan V., M.D., *Dr. Wright's Guide to Healing Nutrition*, Keats Publishing, Inc., New Canaan, CT, 1990.

Yudkin, John, M.D., *Sweet and Dangerous*, Peter H. Wyden, New York, 1972.

# Index

# INDEX

Cameron, Ewan, M.D., 210, 222, 251, 275, 281ff, 287
*Canadian Family Physician,* 343
*Canadian Medical Journal,* 113, 214
Canadian Schizophrenia Foundation, 170, 233
Cancer, 22, 26, 34, 53, 63ff, 117, 174, 205ff, 260
*Cancer and Vitamin C, a Discussion of the Nature, Causes, Prevention and Treatment of Cancer With Special Reference to Vitamin C,* 281
Cancer of the colon, 322
Cancer of the lung, 165, 286, 361
Cancer, statistics on, 294
*Cancer Therapy by Nutritional Means,* 286ff
Cancer, vitamin C and vitamin E, 365
Candida infections, 264
Canker sores, 262
Canner, Paul L., Ph.D., 124
Canthaxanthin, 89
Carbon Monoxide, 34, 218
Carbuncles, 80
Carotene, 67, 68, 69, 70, 303
"The Carotene Bunch," 70
Carpal Tunnel Syndrome, 146
Cataract, 22, 47ff, 116, 241, 243, 293, 299, 368, 369
Cathcart, Robert F., M.D., 222, 259ff, 267, 275, 305, 341
Celiac disease, 106, 177, 363, 381
Cereals, processed, 13
Cervical dysplasia, 303
Chadd, M. A., M.D., 330
*Chemical and Engineering News,* 147, 226, 299, 360, 390
Chemical poisons, 293
Chemicals and vitamin B6, 154

*Chemtech,* 259
Cheraskin, Emanuel, M.D., D.M.D., 90, 113, 186, 191, 234, 235, 290, 302, 391
Chickenpox, 219, 270
Children, need for vitamin C, 302
Chinese Restaurant Syndrome, 154, 155
Chlorine, 30, 291
Chloroform, 362
Cholecalciferol (Vitamin D3), 37
Cholestasis, 373
Cholesterol, 17, 44, 55, 107, 125, 126, 133, 136, 191, 195, 196, 202, 219, 223, 227, 260, 329, 337, 343, 346, 348, 363
Choline, 15, 190, 193ff, 235
Chromium, 126, 244
Circulation, 230, 283, 293, 327, 333, 340, 343, 384
Clark, J. W., D.D.S., 408
Cleary, John P., M.D., 129, 131
*Clinical Nutrition,* 11
*Clinics in Endocrinology and Metabolism,* 107
Cobalt, 15
Cod liver oil, 30
Coffee and breast disease, 378
Cohen, Benjamin, M.D., 75
Cohen, Louis, M.D., 136
Colds, 259, 270, 283, 293, 301, 302
Cold sores, 221, 261, 267
Colitis, 22, 106, 401, 403
Collagen, 293ff
Colon cancer, 65
*The Common Form of Joint Dysfunction: Its Incidence and Treatment,* 138
*Common Questions and Their Answers,* 339
Confusion, 99
Constipation, 22, 276
*Contemporary Nutrition,* 174

437

# INDEX

## H

Haddow, Sir Alexander, 71
HBLV Infections, 270
Hair, falling, 22, 161, 162, 183, 191
Hair, white, 200
Haldol, 274
Hallucinations, 166
*Handbook of Vitamins, Minerals and Hormones*, 158, 384
Hardening of the arteries, 99
Harrell, Ruth, Ph.D., 112
Hartnup's Disease, 130
Hartz, Stuart C., Sc.D., 238
Hay fever, 259, 264, 293
Headaches, 22
*The Healing Factor, Vitamin C Against Disease*, 34, 215, 221, 242, 244, 293ff
Hearing loss, 162, 283, 323
Heart attack, 14, 22, 26, 124, 224, 346, 349
Heart disease, 53, 69, 96, 100, 104, 320, 345, 346
Heart rhythm changes, 96
Heberden's Nodes, 375
Helen Keller Foundation, 82
Hemorrhages, 334, 399
Hepatitis, 221, 257, 264, 267, 270
Herbert, Victor, M.D., 175
Heredity, 20
Hernia, 69
Herpes, 257, 261, 270
Hicks, B. S., 391
High density lipoprotein, 264
Hirschprung's Disease, 373
Hodgkins Disease, 68, 282
Hoffer, Abram, M.D., Ph.D., 43, 98, 101, 110, 127, 131, 144, 185, 233, 234, 300
Homocysteine, 150
Horrobin, D. F., M.D., 378

Horwitt, M. K., Ph.D., 336, 370
*How to Live Longer and Feel Better*, 285
*How to Live With Schizophrenia*, 128
Huxley Institute for Biosocial Research, 42, 113, 133, 233
*Huxley Institute-CSF Newsletter*, 144
Hyperactive children, 128, 154
Hypertension, 20, 22, 34, 59, 306, 346

## I

Ichthyosis, 73, 79
Immune system, 76, 272, 335
Immunizations, 298
Impetigo, 80
Impotency, 167
Indigestion, 22
Infertility, 180, 300, 363
Infiltration of mesenteric nodes, 373
Ingelfinger, F. J., M.D., 248
Inositol, 15, 145, 188, 189ff
Interferon, 271
Intermittent claudication, 334, 341, 363
*International Journal for Vitamin and Nutrition Research*, 151, 161, 302
*International Journal of Biosocial Research*, 112
International Units, 37
Intestinal disorders, 323
Intestinal polyps, 300
Iodine, 15, 17, 18
Iron, 15, 19, 32, 33, 46, 75, 168, 170, 206ff, 278ff, 342
Irradiation of food, 400, 404
Irritability, 57
Isoniazid, 154

# Index to "Vitamins in the Nineties"